Praise for *Population-Based Public Health Clinical Manual, Second Edition*

"*The second edition of* Population-Based Public Health Clinical Manual: The Henry Street Model for Nurses *is an excellent primer on public health nursing (PHN) practice and serves as a valuable resource book for undergraduate students as well as PHN staff. This comprehensive and inspiring text invokes the timeless perspectives of public health nursing's founder, Lillian Wald; builds on Minnesota's rich tradition of PHN practice; and guides readers' understanding of PHN cornerstone beliefs, values, and principles. The authors skillfully thread contemporary competencies, essentials, and standards into local and global practice scenarios with individuals and families, communities, and populations. They create a mind-set that challenges, questions, and encourages actions to promote the public's health.*"

–Pamela A. Kulbok, DNSc, RN, PHCNS-BC, FAAN
Theresa A. Thomas Professor of Nursing and Professor of Public Health Sciences
University of Virginia School of Nursing

"*Relevant, current, timely, inspiring, rigorous, and compelling—this volume is an exceptional resource for those teaching, learning, and practicing public health or community health nursing. Thanks to the Henry Street Consortium and the authors who have brought this remarkable collaboration and uniquely powerful resource that will serve the needs of academicians and practitioners alike. Lillian Wald would have loved this book.*"

–Marla E. Salmon, ScD, RN, FAAN
Senior Visiting Fellow, Evans School of Public Affairs
Professor, Nursing, Global Health, and Public Health
University of Washington

"*The Henry Street Consortium continues in this second edition to use the innovative and historically important Henry Street model to inspire and guide beginning students and novice nurses in learning and applying the arts and sciences of nursing care in home and community. Competency-based resources, case applications, and reflective learning exercises are now enhanced by attention to technological applications, national and international goals, and global public health issues. Partnerships of students, practicing nurses, and clinical preceptors will find this manual a practical and inspiring resource.*"

–Mary W. Byrne, PhD, DNP, MPH, FAAN
Stone Foundation and Elise D. Fish Professor of Clinical Health Care for the Underserved
Columbia University School of Nursing and College of Physicians and Surgeons

"*The Henry Street Consortium brings the second edition of its textbook based on public health nursing competencies written from the student's perspective. New features in this volume include a discussion of social marketing; a comparison of evidence-based practice, research, and quality improvement; and motivational interviewing. Woven throughout the chapters are activities related to the Healthy People website, with practical examples on how to use the information from this site as well as updated resources related to the Affordable Care Act.*"

–Linda Spencer, PhD, RN
Associate Professor of Nursing
Nell Hodgson Woodruff School of Nursing

Population-Based Public Health Clinical Manual, Second Edition

The Henry Street Model for Nurses

Carolyn M. Garcia, PhD, MPH, RN, PHN
Marjorie A. Schaffer, PhD, MS, RN, PHN
Patricia M. Schoon, MPH, RN, PHN

Sigma Theta Tau International
Honor Society of Nursing®

The Honor Society of Nursing, Sigma Theta Tau International (STTI), is a nonprofit organization whose mission is to support the learning, knowledge, and professional development of nurses committed to making a difference in health worldwide. Founded in 1922, STTI has 130,000 members in 86 countries. Members include practicing nurses, instructors, researchers, policymakers, entrepreneurs, and others. STTI's 488 chapters are located at 628 institutions of higher education throughout Australia, Botswana, Brazil, Canada, Colombia, Ghana, Hong Kong, Japan, Kenya, Malawi, Mexico, the Netherlands, Pakistan, Portugal, Singapore, South Africa, South Korea, Swaziland, Sweden, Taiwan, Tanzania, the United Kingdom, the United States, and Wales. More information about STTI can be found online at www.nursingsociety.org.

Sigma Theta Tau International
550 West North Street
Indianapolis, IN, 46202 USA

To order additional books, buy in bulk, or order for corporate use, contact Nursing Knowledge International at 888. NKI.4YOU (888.654.4968/U.S. and Canada) or ׀1.317.634.8171 (outside U.S. and Canada).

To request a review copy for course adoption, email solutions@nursingknowledge.org or call 888.NKI.4YOU (888.654.4968/U.S. and Canada) or +1.317.634.8171 (outside U.S. and Canada).

To request author information, or for speaker or other media requests, contact Marketing at the Honor Society of Nursing, Sigma Theta Tau International, at 888.634.7575 (U.S. and Canada) or +1.317.634.8171 (outside U.S. and Canada).

ISBN: 9781938835346
EPUB ISBN: 9781938835353
PDF ISBN: 9781938835360
MOBI ISBN: 9781938835377

Library of Congress Cataloging-in-Publication Data

Garcia, Carolyn, author.
  Population based public health clinical manual : the Henry Street model for nurses / Carolyn M. Garcia, Marjorie A. Schaffer, Patricia M. Schoon. -- Second edition.
    p. ; cm.
  Includes bibliographical references and index.
  ISBN 978-1-938835-34-6 (book : alk. paper) -- ISBN 978-1-938835-35-3 (EPUB) -- ISBN 978-1-938835-36-0 (PDF) -- ISBN   978-1-938835-37-7 (MOBI)
  I. Garcia, Carolyn M., author. II. Schoon, Patricia M., author. III. Sigma Theta Tau International, issuing body. IV. Title.
  [DNLM: 1. Henry Street Consortium. 2. Public Health Nursing--education. 3. Competency-Based Education. 4. Education, Nursing--standards. 5. Models, Educational. WY 108]
  RT97
  610.73'4--dc23
                    2013050299

First Printing, 2014

Publisher: Renee Wilmeth	**Principal Editor:** Carla Hall
Acquisitions and Development Editor: Emily Hatch	**Project Editor:** Heather Wilcox
Editorial Coordinator: Paula Jeffers	**Copy Editor:** Heather Wilcox
Cover Designer: Katy Bodenmiller	**Proofreader:** Erin Geile
Interior Design and Page Composition: Rebecca Batchelor	**Indexer:** Joy Dean Lee

Dedication

We dedicate this book to the public health nurses and educators who work together to create effective and meaningful learning experiences for nursing students. Your commitment and passion will live on in the public health nursing workforce of the future.

Acknowledgments

We wish to thank our colleagues in the Henry Street Consortium who generously shared their knowledge, experiences, and examples of the essence of public health nursing. Linda Olson Keller and Sue Strohschein's vision for developing the public health nursing workforce of the future led to a federal Division of Nursing grant obtained by the Minnesota Department of Health. The "Linking Public Health Nursing Practice and Education to Promote Population Health" grant provided support for the development of the Henry Street Consortium. As a result of this support, public health nurses and nursing educators collaborated to develop the Henry Street Consortium competencies.

We wish to thank Liz Fine Weinfurter, health sciences librarian, who conducted literature searches for each of the competencies. The colleges, universities, health departments, and agencies represented by Henry Street Consortium members are listed below.

Public Health Agencies
Anoka County Community Health & Environmental Services Department
Carver County Public Health Department
Chisago County Public Health Division of Health and Human Services
City of Bloomington Division of Public Health
Dakota County Public Health Department
Hennepin County Human Services & Public Health Department
Isanti County Public Health
Kanabec County Public Health
Metropolitan Area School Nurses
Minnesota Department of Health
Minnesota Visiting Nurse Agency
Saint Paul-Ramsey County Public Health
Scott County Public Health
Sherburne County Public Health Department
Washington County Department of Public Health & Environment
Wright County Human Services Agency

Colleges and Universities
Augsburg College
Bethel University
St. Catherine University
Crown College
Globe University & Minnesota School of Business
Herzing University
Metropolitan State University
Minnesota State University, Mankato
Saint Mary's University of Minnesota
University of Minnesota

About the Authors

Carolyn M. Garcia, PhD, MPH, RN, PHN, is an associate professor in the School of Nursing at the University of Minnesota and holds an adjunct faculty appointment in the School of Public Health. Her program of research is focused on health promotion among the vulnerable, including adolescent mental health promotion, and employs community-based participatory methods to develop, implement, and evaluate school-based, family-centric interventions for youth and their families. Garcia has worked as a public health nurse for nearly 20 years in settings ranging from teen clinics and detention centers to refugee camps in Rwanda and post-9/11 Red Cross disaster relief centers in Washington, DC. Garcia teaches courses focused on public health nursing and mixed/qualitative research methods and advises undergraduate and graduate students' programs in nursing and public health. She serves on the board of directors for the International Association of Forensic Nurses, and she is a former president of Zeta Chapter of the Honor Society of Nursing, Sigma Theta Tau International.

Marjorie A. Schaffer, PhD, MS, RN, PHN, is a professor of nursing at Bethel University in St. Paul, Minnesota. In 2010, Schaffer received the University Professor Award from Bethel University in honor of her scholarly work. A founding member of the Henry Street Consortium, she has taught public health nursing for more than 25 years. She has traveled to Norway as a Fulbright Scholar and to Norway and New Zealand as a Fulbright Specialist to consult and present on public health nursing. She has served as president of Chi-at-Large Chapter of the Honor Society of Nursing, Sigma Theta Tau International. She has coauthored articles on the Public Health Intervention Wheel and Henry Street Consortium. Schaffer has written more than 40 articles and book chapters and coauthored *Being Present: A Nurse's Resource for End-of-Life Communication*, also published by Sigma Theta Tau International.

Patricia M. Schoon, MPH, RN, PHN, is a clinical instructor for the University of Wisconsin Oshkosh and a doctoral student at the University of Minnesota. She is a founding member of the Henry Street Consortium and has taught nursing and public health for more than 35 years. She received the Minnesota Nurses Association Nurse Educator Award in 2005 for her work on Nurses Day on the Hill and has developed an online political advocacy tool kit. She was president of Chi-at-Large Chapter and faculty advisor for Zeta Chapter of the Honor Society of Nursing, Sigma Theta Tau International. Schoon has developed innovative programs in the community, including a foot-care clinic for the homeless and a faith-based program for older adults. She has coauthored articles on the Henry Street Consortium and is the author of two chapters, "Population-Based Health Care Practice" and "Power and Politics," in two current nursing leadership textbooks.

Contributing Authors

Maureen A. Alms, MSN, PHN (Chapters 9, 12), is a public health nurse consultant with the Minnesota Department of Health (MDH). She provides consultation and technical assistance regarding public health practice to promote and maintain a strong public health infrastructure. Prior to working at MDH, she was a PHN team leader for Mental Health in Goodhue County.

Linda J. W. Anderson, DNP, MPH, RN, PHN (Chapters 4, 8), is an associate professor of nursing and director of the prelicensure nursing program at Bethel University in St. Paul, Minnesota. She teaches public health nursing theory and clinical in both the preprofessional and degree-completion programs. Her current research interests include investigation of the public health nursing practice of faith community nurses and the development of faith community nurses as public health nursing preceptors for RN-to-BSN degree-completion students.

Christine C. Andres, BSN, PHN (Chapter 9, 11, 12), is the family health supervisor at Kanabec County Public Health in Mora, Minnesota. She is actively involved in efforts to protect and promote the health of the residents of Kanabec County. She is a preceptor for nursing students and involved in training and development for PHNs in Kanabec County.

Joyce Bredesen, DNP, RN, PHN (Chapter 5), is an associate professor of nursing at Metropolitan State University in St. Paul, Minnesota. She teaches public health nursing theory and clinical in both the prelicensure and degree-completion programs. Her current research interests include participatory research with Parkinson's disease as well as work with the homeless population within the community setting. Other research interests include utilization of women's healthcare during pregnancy for underserved populations.

Bonnie Brueshoff, DNP, RN, PHN (Chapters 6, 13), is the public health director for the Dakota County Public Health Department in West St. Paul and Apple Valley, Minnesota. She manages and provides leadership for a staff of 100 with a budget of $10 million. Brueshoff has spent the majority of her 34 years in nursing in public health and has a special interest in prevention and early-intervention programs and the development of public health leaders. She is a graduate of the Robert Wood Johnson Executive Nurse Fellows Program and the NACCHO Survive and Thrive Fellowship Program. She completed the University of Minnesota Doctorate in Nursing Practice program in September 2013.

Colleen B. Clark, MSN, RN, PHN (Chapter 10), is an assistant professor at Minnesota State University, Mankato. She teaches public health theory and clinical in the RN Baccalaureate Completion Program and has previously taught in nursing prelicensure programs. She has more than 35 years of experience in community and school health agencies.

Carol Flaten, DNP, RN, PHN (Chapter 7), is a clinical assistant professor at the University of Minnesota School of Nursing. Her public health nursing experience has included health promotion programs and disease-prevention and -control programs. Her scholarly work has included the application of quality improvement theory to maternal child health programs. She is currently involved in simulation and digital media strategies to enhance learning in undergraduate education. She enjoys partnerships with clinical agencies to facilitate student experiences in public health nursing.

Karen Goedken, MS, BSN, BA, PHN, and LTC retired, Army Reserve Nurse Corps (Chapter 12), has worked as a PHN for Hennepin County in a variety of positions, serving the disability community for more than 20 years. She spent 4 of those years on active duty with the military, again using her disability expertise to provide support to the Army Wounded Warrior program at the Pentagon and to the Army's Traumatic Brain Injury Task Force in 2007. Most recently, she helped Hennepin County develop a mentorship program for nursing students and integrated some of those students into an experimental health and wellness project with Minnesota Life College in Richfield, Minnesota.

Carol L. Hargate, PhD, CNP (Chapter 5), is an associate professor of nursing at Bethel University in St. Paul, Minnesota. Hargate maintains an active community-based pediatric nurse practitioner practice. She teaches public health nursing theory and clinical in both the preprofessional and degree-completion programs and serves as a community engagement coordinator. Her current research interests include community-engaged interprofessional practice, access to healthcare, and ways to address health disparities from a public health perspective.

Rose M. Jost, MEd, PHN (Chapters 5, 8), is recently retired from the City of Bloomington Division of Public Health, Bloomington, Minnesota. As the Family Health Manager, she was responsible for intensive home-visiting services to high-risk families, child care consultation, school health services, health promotion activities, and services for children with special needs. She has a lifelong interest in supporting nursing education. Currently, she serves on the Richfield, Minnesota, Advisory Board of Health and the Minnesota State Community Health Services Advisory Committee.

Madeleine Kerr, PhD, RN (Chapter 4) is an associate professor at the University of Minnesota School of Nursing. She has taught public health nursing for 30 years in Illinois, Michigan, and Minnesota. Her research focus is the prevention of occupational noise-induced hearing loss among construction workers.

Noreen Kleinfehn-Wald, MA, PHN (Chapters 3, 4, 10), is the team leader for disease prevention and control for Scott County Public Health in Shakopee, Minnesota. She has 31 years of experience in public health in two Minnesota counties, in inner-city settings, and in east Africa. She has primary responsibility for communicable disease investigation and management and immunization services and has a special interest in public health data analysis.

Cheryl H. Lanigan, MA, PHN (Chapter 3), is the director of quality improvement and analysis for Family Health at Minnesota Visiting Nurse Agency (MVNA) in Hennepin County, Minnesota. She coordinates nursing student and resident experiences at MVNA and manages the MVNA Interpreter Program.

Raney Linck, MSN, RN (Chapters 6, 8), is a nursing faculty member at the University of Minnesota School of Nursing as part of the VA Nursing Academic Partnership with the Minneapolis VA Health Care System. He has taught public health nursing theory and worked in hospice case management, home health, and chemical dependency treatment in addition to critical care and informatics. He publishes the blog *Digital Trends in Nursing* in association with *Reflections on Nursing Leadership* (RNL) magazine, published by the Honor Society of Nursing, Sigma Theta Tau International.

Karen S. Martin, RN, MSN, FAAN (Chapter 3), is based in Omaha, Nebraska, and has been a Health Care Consultant in private practice since 1993. She works with diverse providers, educators, and computer software companies nationally and globally. While employed at the Visiting Nurse Association of Omaha (1978–1993), she was the principal investigator of Omaha System research. She has been a visiting scholar and speaker in 20 countries, has served as the chair of numerous conferences, and is the author of more than 100 articles, chapters, and books and 70 editorials.

Bernita Missal, PhD, RN (Chapters 9, 11), is a professor of nursing at Bethel University, St. Paul, Minnesota, where she teaches Evidence Translation for Practice, Cultural Diversity in Health Care, and a population-focused theory course. Her current research interests focus on Somali immigrant mothers' support systems.

Table of Contents

About the Authors vii

Foreword xiii

Introduction xv

Part I: Foundational Concepts for Public Health Nursing Practice 1

1   Introduction to Public Health Nursing Practice 3

2   Evidence-Based Public Health Nursing Practice. 33

Part II: Entry-Level Population-Based Public Health Nursing Competencies 65

3   Competency #1: 67
Applies the Public Health Nursing Process to Communities, Systems, Individuals, and Families

4   Competency #2: 111
Utilizes Basic Epidemiological Principles (the Incidence, Distribution, and Control of Disease in a Population) in Public Health Nursing Practice

5   Competency #3: 141
Utilizes Collaboration to Achieve Public Health Goals

6   Competency #4: 165
Works Within the Responsibility and Authority of the Governmental Public Health System

7   Competency #5: 193
Practices Public Health Nursing Within the Auspices of the Nurse Practice Act

8   Competency #6: 221
Effectively Communicates With Communities, Systems, Individuals, Families, and Colleagues

9   Competency #7: 249
Establishes and Maintains Caring Relationships With Communities, Systems, Individuals, and Families

10 Competency #8: 273
Shows Evidence of Commitment to Social Justice, the Greater Good, and the Public Health Principles

11 Competency #9: 307
    Demonstrates Nonjudgmental and Unconditional Acceptance of
    People Different From Self

12 Competency #10: 329
    Incorporates Mental, Physical, Emotional, Social, Spiritual, and
    Environmental Aspects of Health Into Assessment, Planning,
    Implementation, and Evaluation

13 Competency #11: 353
    Demonstrates Leadership in Public Health Nursing With
    Communities, Systems, Individuals, and Families

14 Putting It All Together: 385
    What It Means to Be a Public Health Nurse

Part III: Appendixes 399

    A References.. 401
    B Resources 433
    C Comparison of Henry Street Entry-Level PHN Competencies
       to Other Public Health Practice Frameworks 451
       Index... 455

Foreword

Almost a decade ago, I was pleased to lead a group of public health nurses in Wisconsin in designing a project that aimed to connect nurse educators and practitioners to improve public health nursing practice and education in our state. For inspiration and best practices, we needed to journey no farther than our neighboring state of Minnesota. We purposefully took a "follow-the-leader" approach in adopting or adapting many collaborative education and practice improvement strategies pioneered in Minnesota for our Linking Education and Practice for Excellence in Public Health Nursing (LEAP Project). Throughout the 6 years of the LEAP Project, we often looked to public health nursing leaders in Minnesota for guidance, because they clearly understood the processes and challenges of academic-practice collaboration and of contemporary public health nursing practice and education. I clearly recall the "Minnesota-nice" generosity of the outstanding faculty and public health nurse members of the Henry Street Consortium in sharing their wisdom on academic-practice collaboration when we consulted with them during a groundbreaking international public health nursing conference held in St. Paul in 2011. In many ways, the Henry Street Consortium epitomizes the best of the best practices for academic-practice partnership and sustainable efforts toward improving public health education and practice.

Publication of the first edition of the *Population-Based Public Health Clinical Manual* (2011), authored by members of the Henry Street Consortium, was an important milestone. Its creation demonstrated that magic happens when public health nurses in academic and practice settings work collaboratively. The first edition offered a refined set of competencies for entry into contemporary, population-based public health nursing practice. The authors went on to provide clear, practical, evidence-driven content and activities for teaching and learning the knowledge, skills, and values required for becoming a public health nurse in the 21st century. This book was truly a gift to public health nursing faculty, students, and preceptors across the United States and beyond because of its accessible format, applicability to contemporary practice, and clarity of language. It clearly fulfilled the need for a practical guidebook to public health nursing practice for students and novice nurses.

The legacy of excellence continues with this second edition of that manual. As a former public health nurse and a current public health professor, I think it offers exactly what is needed for readers seeking to teach or learn population-based public health practice. I am impressed with the use of a scaffolding approach that leads students to compare and contrast new information and experiences about public health with what they have already encountered as students in acute care. I am enthused by the many opportunities for readers to apply and develop critical thinking skills, the essence of all knowledge professions. The highly regarded Public Health Intervention Wheel remains central to the second edition as a core component of the population-based approach. It is refreshing and important that the authors do not expect that students and novice nurses will only be able or asked to work with individuals or families but also provide case examples, stories, and learning activities that support public health nursing interventions provided at the community and systems levels. The case examples and stories included are representative of contemporary practice, while the suggested active learning strategies align with contemporary pedagogy. Past users of this manual will be pleased with the enhancements in the second edition's content on global health, new technologies, and emerging evidence for effective public health nurse–provided or –directed interventions.

Although it is clearly aimed at student nurses and nurses who are new to public health practice, I think this book could be used in at least two additional ways. First, faculty at the graduate level may find it useful in guiding curricular design for advanced practice public health nurses. Second, the examples that demonstrate the role of nurses as members of interprofessional teams practicing in public health settings could also be used in interprofessional health education activities and to help teach collaborative practice and leadership.

Collaboration between academia and practice, although increasingly common, remains challenging. The Henry Street Consortium is one of the finest examples of linking education and practice to improve public health nursing education and practice. The *Population-Based Public Health Clinical Manual, Second Edition,* is one of the best products I have seen that illustrates a successful and sustained academic-practice partnership. Although many community health textbooks are good, none is as clear, organized, practical, and relevant to population-based public health nursing clinical experiences as this one. Students, teachers, and preceptors will find it the best guidebook for the journey toward becoming a public health nurse.

Susan J. Zahner, DrPH, MPH, RN, FAAN
Vilas Distinguished Achievement Professor
University of Wisconsin–Madison School of Nursing
Immediate Past Chair,
PHN Section, American Public Health Association
Project Director, LEAP Project (2006–2012)
January 12, 2014

Introduction

What is your current favorite application (app) for your smartphone? Does it track your running time? Does it allow you to edit photographs? Does it help you manage your budget? Does it play white noise while you try to sleep? Wouldn't it be great if you could easily download an app that would give you all the tools you need to become a great public health nurse? One wonders how Lillian Wald, founder of public health nursing, would have used the technology that is at our fingertips when she walked the streets of New York City, caring for and living alongside families in crowded tenements. Such technological advances as smartphone apps have dramatically increased our access to knowledge, data, tools, and other people. However, although advances in technology might offer new ways to learn about and connect to things, information, and people, technology has limitations as to what it can provide. Other resources, such as textbooks, journal articles, and even nursing faculty members, also have limitations.

Developing competencies (i.e., skills, abilities, knowledge) that will help you become a great public health nurse takes more than mere access to or internalization of information and experiences from other people. These tools and resources are important, but more important is the individual—the hands, heart, and mind—using the tools to care and positively influence. Lillian Wald used the tools that were available to her, and when something wasn't readily available, she fought to gain access. She was driven by something deep and profound. She was grounded in the lived experiences of those she was working to serve. She acted with purpose that might have begun with caring but was fueled by the relationships she established with the sick, the impoverished, and the needy.

Nursing, especially public health nursing, can be very overwhelming. The needs of individuals, families, and communities can appear insurmountable. The idea for this book originated from a shared recognition by public health nursing faculty, agency staff, and preceptors that public health nursing courses and clinical experiences are difficult for students and faculty alike. It has been well established that clinical faculty struggle with finding enough enriching experiences for students. Often, one student is placed in a school-based experience, another student is placed with a local public health agency, and yet another might be placed in a correctional setting. On the one hand, this diversity in settings and opportunities facilitates chances for students to learn from one another as they share and reflect. On the other hand, this diversity also challenges faculty to ensure that all students are learning about and growing in all the core competencies. It can also be confusing for students who have difficulty adapting clinical learning expectations to diverse settings and who might not have a nursing instructor or public health nursing preceptor with them during their clinical experiences.

The Henry Street Consortium (HSC), a group of public health nursing faculty from diverse schools of nursing and local public health nurses employed in health departments, schools, parish settings, and nonprofit community agencies, has been meeting regularly since 2001 to support positive, rich learning experiences for public health nursing students. The HSC developed a set of entry-level public health nursing competencies that all participants agreed to use in developing curriculum and clinical learning experiences. These HSC competencies have been informed by key public health nursing standards and guidelines, including the Quad Council core competencies, the Scope and Standards of Public Health Nursing, and Essential Public Health Services (see Appendix C, at the end of the book). Companion documents have included clinical guidelines and a menu of potential learning activities based on the competencies and recognized public health nursing interventions. What had been missing, however, was a manual or guide for students and faculty to use in developing the skills necessary for effective entry-level public health nursing practice. We wanted to develop a manual that would speak to students in an understandable, meaningful way and that would also address student concerns about practicing nursing in the complex and often disorganized community environment. We needed to prepare future public health nurses for population-based practice. We hoped to motivate students to excel in their public health nursing clinical experiences and to engage in activities that facilitate learning and, in direct care, the health promotion of diverse individuals, families, communities, and populations. We sought to encourage students to think, think, think—to use their minds to grapple with moral and ethical dilemmas and complex health needs, disparities, and inequities.

This second edition retains the strengths of the original manual, including relevant case studies, evidence-based examples of the competencies in action, and numerous suggestions for reflection, application, and hands-on learning in your own clinical setting. Importantly, evidence examples have been updated with recent publications that demonstrate the growth in public health nursing evidence in the U.S. and globally. We have given attention to strengthening the global relevance of the manual, with specific focus on examples and activities that draw upon global public health problems and solutions (for example, inclusion of the United Nations Millennium Development Goals). New additions to most chapters include:

- Healthy People 2020 activities for each competency.

- Linkages to technological advances, including suggested activities that require students to identify or use apps to address public health nursing challenges and issues.

- Reflection questions that encourage ongoing attention to the public health nursing cornerstones.

- Up-to-date resources that students, nurses, and instructors can use to enhance learning.

For the Student Nurse:

- You have chosen a career as a nurse, and some of you might become public health nurses. This clinical manual has been developed to serve as a tool you can use as you develop competencies and experience what it means to be a public health nurse.

- The knowledge and skills you acquire in your public health nursing course will enhance your effectiveness as a nurse, regardless of your employment setting. This manual helps you identify the public health principles that guide care for individuals, families, communities, populations, and systems. You will recognize and gain appreciation for public health's promotion of health and well-being and the prevention of disease and illness. You will also become aware of public health nursing's overarching commitment to addressing health disparities and inequities with strategies that improve the well-being of individuals, families, communities, and systems.

- This manual guides you in learning what public health nurses are, what they do, and what makes a public health nurse effective. It leads you through the critical, or core, competencies that you need to develop.

For the New Public Health Nurse:

- This manual provides an opportunity to orient yourself to the core competencies you are expected to demonstrate as a new public health nurse.

- As part of an orientation process, the manual offers opportunities for reflection on a range of issues, challenges, and ethical dilemmas that you will likely experience in one way or another during your initial months of employment.

- Such competencies as assessment, collaboration, communication, and leadership are abilities that all new public health nurses should possess; this manual offers you the opportunity to work through some of these broader competencies using public health nursing case studies and evidence from the literature.

- Additional competencies focus on developing critical relational nursing abilities, such as establishing caring relationships, demonstrating nonjudgmental acceptance of others, committing to social justice principles, and holistically undertaking the nursing process of assessment, planning, intervention development, implementation, and evaluation.

- The collaboration of practicing public health nurses and public health nursing faculty to develop this manual has contributed to the high relevance of examples, practical applications, and discussion of each competency contained therein.

For Public Health Nursing Faculty/Preceptors:

- This manual is a tool to help ensure that your students are equally exposed to core competencies and a foundational level of knowledge with respect to public health nursing. For example, the initial chapters lay a critical foundation for public health nursing, and the subsequent chapters are individually devoted to a core competency. To help address this common difficulty of ensuring that all students receive the same foundational knowledge and skill development, regardless of clinical setting, clinical faculty might choose to assign a particular competency chapter to all students to ensure common ground. Other faculty might decide instead to assign different competencies to different students, depending on the scope of their individual clinical experience.

Organization of the Manual

This manual begins with a description of foundational public health nursing concepts. Each subsequent chapter is devoted to one core competency and organized according to its key characteristics. The elements of each competency chapter are outlined below.

Chapter Element	Description of the Element
Case Study	A new case study is included in each chapter to provide the reader with real-life scenarios experienced by student nurses or new public health nurses that address principles and challenges that are relevant to the core competency.
Notebook	A table at the start of each competency chapter lists the competency, its components, and useful definitions of key chapter concepts.
Evidence Examples	These examples provide the reader with summaries of research studies and other evidence-based practice sources that are relevant to the competency. These also offer a sense of the level of evidence available for each competency.
Activities	Activities interwoven throughout the text offer opportunities for readers to reflect and engage in key ideas that are being presented.
Ethical Considerations	This section of each competency chapter applies ethical principles to a common dilemma that public health nurses might face. Three ethical frameworks are used: rule ethics (principles), virtue ethics (character), and feminist ethics (reducing oppression).
Learning Examples	These are additional examples that demonstrate effective use of the competency in real practice that the reader can access as desired (e.g., additional articles, web-based resources).
Reflective Practice	This section provides a conclusion to the case study with additional questions for the reader to consider.
Key Points	This section summarizes the main ideas of each chapter.
Think, Explore, Do	These opportunities present the reader with ideas for continued learning applications for each competency. Course faculty might explore these opportunities and incorporate some into clinical assignments. For example, this section might suggest a health education project or a social marketing activity to help students learn about and experience the core competency.

In summary, this manual appreciates public health nursing tradition and encourages adoption of innovative, future-thinking practice. Lillian Wald, the founder of public health nursing, was not bound by the traditions or limitations of nursing practice in her era. She challenged, questioned, and acted. She perpetuated change and demanded that attention be given to the public health needs of children, families, and communities. She used every available asset and resource to combat poverty and disease, and when a resource didn't exist, she created one. She used evidence of the realities and challenges to inform her solutions and strategies.

Today's public health nurse should do no less and has a growing base of evidence upon which to advocate for the health of those being served—evidence that ranges from a child's story to the results of a randomized controlled trial. We hope this manual promotes greater appreciation of what is expected from public health nurses and what makes them effective. We hope the manual's emphasis on evidence-based practice facilitates greater efforts by public health nurses to document effectiveness while continuing to appreciate, not minimize, the value of diverse sources of evidence. The path toward becoming an effective nurse starts with you—with your interest and determination to embrace what it means to be a nurse and, for some of you, a public health nurse. A commitment to figuring out nursing, or public health nursing, will take you on a journey that teaches, models, informs, changes, and challenges.

How can you not grow when faced with so many opportunities? Well, you can choose to ignore, deny, or reject what is being offered. Some nurses are hesitant to adopt emerging intervention ideas or practices that deepen, challenge, or conflict with the way things have always been done. Other nurses critically embrace new ways of thinking, acting, and evaluating. Still others advance the discipline of nursing by continually questioning, examining, and reflecting on what nursing is, what it isn't, and how it is practiced. We encourage you to become a nurse who is able to critique, willing to challenge, ready to adopt or reject, and eager to curiously and creatively problem-solve. With a commitment to becoming this type of nurse, you will have the tools you need. This internal drive, along with externally available resources (e.g., faculty, experiences, readings, this manual), will contribute to your development into a successful and competent nurse. Finally, we hope this book finds its way into the tools that are within each of you—open hands, an open heart, and an open mind—tools that can never be replaced by a downloaded smartphone application.

FOUNDATIONAL CONCEPTS FOR PUBLIC HEALTH NURSING PRACTICE

INTRODUCTION TO PUBLIC HEALTH NURSING PRACTICE

Patricia M. Schoon

with Marjorie A. Schaffer and Carolyn M. Garcia

Abby will soon be starting her public health nursing clinical and is struggling with the idea of practicing nursing outside the hospital. She was at lunch with two of her classmates, Alberto and Sia. "I can't imagine myself out in someone's home, or in a school, or in a community center or public health agency. How will I be respected without scrubs or my uniform? Is it really true that one of the most important skills in public health is listening and that sometimes that is all that you do? I feel like I should be doing something."

Alberto responded, "My friend, Zack, had public health last semester. He said that it bothered him a lot at first that he had to listen and not tell his family what to do. He wanted to do more than listen—take a blood pressure or something. But after a while, he started to get comfortable. He said he really worked on his communication skills and got an 'A' for therapeutic listening."

Sia commented, "I worry about all of this too. I was talking with Jen, a friend of mine who took public health last year. She said that on her first home visit, she went with her public health nursing preceptor. I hope our preceptors will do the same thing."

Abby said, "I am really worried about being out alone. I wonder what the neighborhood where my family lives will be like and whether I will be safe."

Sia stated, "I already have my instructor's cell phone number on speed dial. We should get together with Jen and Zack and find out more about what they did to feel comfortable. I think they could give us some great advice."

ABBY'S NOTEBOOK

Useful Definitions

Client: A client (syn. patient) is the individual/family, community, population or subpopulation, or system that is the public health nurse's focus of care.

Community: A community can refer to (a) a group of people or population group; (b) a physical place and time in which the population lives and works; or (c) a cultural group that has shared beliefs, values, institutions, and social systems (Dreher, Shapiro, & Asselin, 2006, p. 23).

Health determinants: Health determinants are factors that influence the health of individuals, families, and populations. Health determinants can potentially have a positive (protective factors) or negative (risk factors) influence on health.

Social determinants of health: The social determinants of health are the conditions in which people are born, grow, live, work, and age. The distribution of money, power, and resources at the global, national, and local levels shape these circumstances. The social determinants of health are mostly responsible for health inequities—the unfair and avoidable differences in health status seen within and between countries (Modified from World Health Organization, 2013).

Health status: Health status refers to the level of health or illness and is the outcome of the interaction of the multiple health determinants. Health status indicators, also called global measures of population health, include birth, longevity, and death rates (mortality); illness (morbidity) patterns; perception of wellness and life satisfaction; level of independence; and functional ability.

Levels of prevention: The levels of prevention compose a health intervention framework applied to the stages of health and disease for individuals and groups (Stanhope & Lancaster, 2008). The levels of prevention are (a) primary—the prevention of disease and promotion of health; (b) secondary—early diagnosis and treatment; and (c) tertiary—limits negative effects of disease and restores function.

Population: A population is defined as the "total number of people living in a specific geographic area." A subpopulation (syn. group or aggregate) "consist[s] of people experiencing a specific health condition; engaging in behaviors that have potential to negatively affect health; or sharing a common risk factor or risk exposure, or experiencing an emerging health threat or risk" (American Nurses Association, 2013, p. 3).

Population-based practice: Population-based practice focuses on the population as a whole to determine its priority needs (Minnesota Department of Health, 2001).

Public health: Public health refers to all organized measures (whether public or private) to prevent disease, promote health, and prolong life among the population as a whole (WHO, n.d.).

Public health nursing: "Public health nursing practice focuses on population health through continuous surveillance and assessment of multiple determinants of health with the intent to promote health and wellness; prevent disease, disability, and premature death; and improve neighborhood quality of life. . . . Public health nursing practice emphasizes primary prevention with the goal of achieving health equity" (ANA, 2013).

System: A system is an institution or organization that exists within one or multiple communities.

Practicing Nursing Where We All Live

Public health nursing care is provided to individuals, families, communities, and populations through a population-based lens that enables nurses to view their clients within the context of the community in which the clients live. All aspects of the client's life are considered as the public health nurse carries out the nursing process. Public health nurses (PHNs) practice in their communities, where they can make a difference in the lives of their families, the people they serve, and their communities on a daily basis. The health of people in our families, neighborhoods, and communities affects us all both socially and economically. The health of our environment has a direct impact on the health of our families, friends, and neighbors. As you read this chapter, consider from both your personal and professional perspectives the concepts presented. As nurses, we are all citizens of the world and have civic and professional responsibilities to promote health and provide for a safe environment.

In the case study at the beginning of the chapter, Abby and her friends are concerned about providing nursing care in the community. It is difficult for nursing students to think about practicing nursing outside the acute and long-term care settings. Many of the skills that nursing students learn in the acute or long-term care setting (e.g., IV therapy, medication administration, tube care) are part of the delegated medical functions of nursing practice, which, by necessity, are priorities when caring for acutely ill individuals. In the community setting, most of what PHNs do is part of the independent practice of nursing (e.g., teaching, counseling, coordinating care), as the focus of public health nursing practice is primary prevention. Components of public health nursing can be practiced in any setting, although they are most often practiced in the community. Not all nursing practiced in the community can be described as public health nursing. For example, home care and hospice care, both very important areas of nursing, are practiced in the community and exhibit components of public health nursing but are not typically categorized as public health nursing. As you work through this manual and engage in nursing activities, think about how you are integrating the components of public health nursing into your nursing practice. Also, think about how you practice nursing where you live and what your civic and professional responsibilities are to promote the health of your community.

Public Health

As the practice of public health nursing includes components of public health and is a part of the broader field of public health, it is important to understand the nature and scope of public health practice. A definition of public health from the World Health Organization (WHO, n.d.) helps explain the nature of this practice:

> *Public health refers to all organized measures (whether public or private) to prevent disease, promote health, and prolong life among the population as a whole. Its activities aim to provide conditions in which people can be healthy and focus on entire populations, not on individual patients or diseases. Thus, public health is concerned with the total system and not only the eradication of a particular disease.*

Public health professionals monitor and diagnose the health concerns of entire communities and promote healthy practices and behaviors to ensure that populations stay healthy. The World Health Association uses the term "global public health" to recognize that, as a result of globalization, forces that affect public health can and do come from outside state boundaries and that responding to public health issues now requires paying attention to cross-border health risks, including access to dangerous products and environmental change (WHO, n.d.). PHNs need to take a global perspective about the nature of population health threats and issues when practicing in the community.

Why Is Public Health Important to Nursing?

In this chapter, you will read about how nurses practice public health nursing in the community, and you will consider how important nurses are to the health of communities at the local, national, and international levels. Since the time of Florence Nightingale, nurses have always been essential participants in improving and maintaining the health of individuals, families, and communities.

Emerging threats to public health require a dramatic shift in the focus of healthcare, public health, and public health nursing. The American Nurses Association (2013) has identified six 21st-century threats that form a context for the current and future directions of public health nursing practice. Nursing continues to expand its leadership role in healthcare in all settings, but in public health nursing that leadership role often takes place in the community, including in the public policy-making arena (ANA, 2003, 2013). A key principle to keep in mind is that PHNs must place more importance on goals related to the public good than goals for the benefit of individuals in the social and economic systems (see Chapter 10 for a discussion of social justice). Table 1.1 compares the emerging public health threats and related nursing leadership responsibilities.

Table 1.1   Emerging Public Health Threats and Nursing Leadership Responsibilities

Emerging Public Health Threats	Nursing Leadership Responsibilities
• Reemergence of communicable disease and increasing incidence of drug-resistant organisms • Environmental hazards • Physical or civic barriers to healthy lifestyles (e.g., food "deserts") • Overall concern about the structure and function of the healthcare system • Challenges imposed by the presence of modern public health epidemics, such as pandemic influenza, obesity, and tobacco-related diseases and deaths • Global and emerging crises with increased opportunities for exposure to multiple health threats (ANA, 2013, p. 2)	• Identifying health hazards and working to reduce and respond to them (ANA, 2013) Participation in: • Organizing, delivery, and financing of healthcare; • Developing health resources that are directed at helping individuals and communities manage their own healthcare needs; • Providing for the health of the public through use of preventive and environmental measures; • Participating in development of national policies and regulations (ANA, 2003, pp. 30–31).

"I still don't understand how we are going to practice nursing differently in this clinical setting than we did in the hospital setting," Albert sighed.

Sia responded, "What I remember from our public health theory class this morning is that taking care of people in their homes is different because we have to take into account the home environment and the community. Our instructor also talked about public health nurses having a responsibility to improve the health of the public at the local, national, and international levels. She mentioned that this idea can be an overwhelming for nursing students and suggested that we focus on what we could do to improve the health of individuals and families as a way to help improve the health of our community. She used the term 'glocal,' which means to think global, but act local."

Abby added, "Maybe we should read more about this in our textbook and look at some of the websites suggested."

"Good idea," said Sia.

Public Health Nursing

Public health nursing combines the theory and practice of nursing and public health. Public health nursing, like nursing practice everywhere, involves the interaction of the nurse and client; the health of the client; the influence of the home, healthcare, and community environment; and the nursing care provided. One of the unique features of public health nursing is that the client can be an individual or family, a group of people, or a whole community. The client could also be a system within the community (such as a school, church, or community health or social service agency). PHNs work to improve population health at the local, state, national, and international levels (ANA, 2013; American Public Health Association, 1996). Public health nursing goals are to promote and preserve the health of populations and the public, prevent disease and disability, and protect the health of the community as a whole.

Public health nursing practice is considered population-based, because it starts by focusing on the population as a whole to determine the community's priority health needs (MDH, Public Health Nursing Section, 2000, 2001; MDH, Center for Public Health Nursing, 2003). PHNs in a variety of work settings can carry out population-based practice. To be population-based, public health nursing practice should meet five criteria:

1. Focus on entire populations possessing similar health concerns or characteristics.

2. Be guided by an assessment of population health status that is determined through a community health assessment process.

3. Consider the broad determinants of health.

4. Consider all levels of prevention, with a preference for primary prevention.

5. Consider all levels of practice (individual/family, community, system) (MDH, 2001, pp. 2–3; MDH, 2003).

PHNs work in homes, clinics, schools, jails, businesses, religious organizations, homeless shelters, camps, hospitals, visiting nurse associations, health departments, and Indian reservations. Public health nursing is defined by its goals and not by its setting. Although public health nursing is considered a specialty area of practice (ANA, 2013), its standards include expectations for entry-level baccalaureate nursing graduates. Even at the entry level, PHNs are expected to function as change agents and to help shape the healthcare system to meet the public health needs of the 21st century. This leadership expectation for public health nursing practice is implicit in its definition and standards (ANA, 2013). The definition of public health nursing provided in the Definition of Public Health Nursing Practice sidebar reflects its population and prevention focus. Like ANA, the International Council of Nurses (2007) sees nursing as having a leadership role in social, technological, political, and health systems changes.

Definition of Public Health Nursing

"Public health nursing practice focuses on population health through continuous surveillance and assessment of multiple determinants of health with the intent to promote health and wellness; prevent disease, disability, and premature death; and improve neighborhood quality of life. These population health priorities are addressed through identification, implementation, and evaluation of universal and targeted evidence-based programs and services that provide primary, secondary, and tertiary preventive interventions. Public health nursing practice emphasizes primary prevention with the goal of achieving health equity" (ANA, 2013).

As students, you have already learned about nursing core concepts that also shape public health nursing, which include:

- Care and compassion;
- Holistic and relationship-centered practice;
- Sensitivity to vulnerable populations; and
- Independent nursing practice (Keller, Strohschein, & Schaffer, 2011).

This manual also introduces you to public health core concepts that also shape public health nursing, which include:

- Social justice;
- Population focus;
- Reliance on epidemiology;
- Health promotion and prevention;
- The greater good; and
- Long-term commitment to community (Keller et al., 2011).

Cornerstones of Public Health Nursing

The Cornerstones of Public Health Nursing (MDH, 2007) provide the foundation for population-based nursing practice (Keller et al., 2011). The Cornerstones reflect the values and beliefs that guide public health nursing practice, and they are also closely related to the ANA Principles of Public Health Nursing Practice (ANA, 2013), as represented in Table 1.2.

Table 1.2   Cornerstones of Public Health Nursing and Related ANA Principles of Public Health Nursing Practice

Cornerstones of Public Health Nursing	ANA Principles of Public Health Nursing Practice
Focuses on the health of entire populations	The client or unit of care is the population.
Reflects community priorities and needs	The primary obligation is to achieve the greatest good for the greatest number of people or the population as a whole (also related to the social justice Cornerstone).
Establishes caring relationships with communities, systems, individuals, and families	
Is grounded in social justice, compassion, sensitivity to diversity, and respect for the worth of all people, especially the vulnerable	A public health nurse is obligated to actively identify and reach out to all who might benefit from a specific activity or service.
Encompasses mental, physical, emotional, social, spiritual, and environmental aspects of health	Public health nursing focuses on strategies that create healthy environmental, social, and economic conditions in which populations may thrive.
Promotes health through strategies driven by epidemiological evidence	Optimal use of available resources and creation of new evidence-based strategies is necessary to assure the best overall improvement in the health of the population. Primary prevention is the priority in selecting appropriate activities.
Collaborates with community resources to achieve those strategies but can and will work alone if necessary	Public health nurses collaborate with the client as an equal partner. Collaboration with other professions, populations, organizations, and stakeholder groups is the most effective way to promote and protect the health of the people.
Derives its authority for independent action from the Nurse Practice Act	

Source for Cornerstones: Keller et al., 2011; MDH, Center for Public Health Nursing, 2007. Adapted from original, 2004, by the Center for Public Health Nursing.

Source for ANA Principles: ANA, 2013, pp. 8–9

These Cornerstones are reflected in PHNs' daily practice when they:

- Organize their workload and schedule based on priority health needs of clients and community;

- Take time to establish trust when visiting families in their homes;

- Carry out holistic assessments of individuals and families within the context of culture, ethnicity, and communities;

- Use evidence-based practice from nursing and public health sciences to select appropriate and effective interventions;

- Collaborate with other members of the healthcare team; and

- Make critical decisions about the needs of their clients and the selection, implementation, and evaluation of interventions based on their professional knowledge and professional licensure.

 ACTIVITY
Keep a log of your nursing activities. Reflect on how you have demonstrated the public health nursing Cornerstones in your clinical activities.

Abby is spending the day with her PHN preceptor. Her preceptor receives a referral to visit a family who just moved into the community and is homeless. The PHN knows that a health priority for her community and agency is to improve the health of homeless populations, particularly those in the population with young children. Recent data on the health needs of her county demonstrate that young children in homeless families have higher rates of malnutrition and developmental delays. Abby works with her PHN preceptor to modify her home-visiting plan for the day so that she can make an initial visit to this family at the local family homeless shelter. The family speaks Spanish but the PHN does not, so she arranges for an interpreter to accompany her on the visit to this family. The PHN has Abby call Social Services to find out whether the family's application for cash assistance and temporary housing in a family homeless shelter has been approved. The PHN also has Abby gather information about local homeless shelters and food banks to take to the visit and has her get some bus passes for the family to use when they go to different agencies to apply for assistance. After her busy day with her PHN preceptor, Abby discussed her visit to the homeless family with Alberto and Sia that evening. Their instructor has challenged them to identify the Cornerstones of Public Health Nursing found in their clinical visits that day.

BSN Preparation

The need for nurses to be prepared to both work in the community and to have the ability to practice entry-level public health nursing has become more urgent as healthcare moves from the acute care setting to the community and new models of healthcare and nursing practice emerge. The challenge of practicing in the community is influenced by the persistence of health disparities among all age groups and diverse populations, the aging of the population, and the continuous increase in healthcare costs. In addition, healthcare needs and diseases are not isolated by geographic boundaries but evolve within a global environment. Recognition of the need for nurses to have the ability to improve the health of populations by taking leadership roles within the healthcare system and in their communities and by partnering with other health professionals and community leaders has resulted in a renewed commitment to increase the proportion of nurses with baccalaureate degrees and to enrich the baccalaureate nursing curriculum to prepare nurses for the challenges that face them (Education Committee of the Association of Community Health Nurse Educators [ACHNE], 2010; Institute of Medicine, 2011; Robert Wood Johnson Foundation, 2013). ACHNE has identified 15 basic core knowledge competencies for baccalaureate nursing graduates that should be included in the baccalaureate nursing curriculum:

- Communication
- Epidemiology and biostatistics
- Community/population assessment
- Community/population planning
- Policy development
- Assurance
- Health promotion and risk reduction
- Illness and disease management
- Information and healthcare technology
- Environmental health
- Global health
- Human diversity
- Ethics and social justice
- Coordination and care management
- Emergency preparedness, response, and recovery

 ACTIVITY

Which knowledge areas have you already studied?

What are your knowledge and competency goals for your public health nursing clinical?

Scope and Standards of Public Health Nursing Practice

All professional nurses have a scope of practice regardless of their clinical areas of practice. A *scope of practice* refers to the boundaries of safe and ethical practice (see Chapter 7 for a discussion of the scope of practice of public health nursing) and depends on four components: educational preparation, credentials, state licensure law, and clinical or employer role description. A PHN's job description is a good measure of the nurse's scope of practice.

Professional nurses are also guided by standards of practice developed by their professional nursing organizations. One nationally accepted set of standards for public health nursing is the American Nurses Association (ANA) publication *Public Health Nursing: Scope and Standards of Practice* (2013); Table 1.3 lists these standards. Specific criteria for operationalizing these standards and measuring performance are included in the publication.

Table 1.3   Standards of Public Health Nursing Practice and Professional Performance

Standards of Public Health Nursing Practice

Standard 1. Assessment: The public health nurse collects comprehensive data pertinent to the health status of populations.

Standard 2. Population Diagnosis and Priorities: The public health nurse analyzes the assessment data to determine the diagnosis or issues.

Standard 3. Outcomes Identification: The public health nurse identifies expected outcomes for a plan specific to the population or issues.

Standard 4. Planning: The public health nurse develops a plan that prescribes strategies and alternatives to attain expected outcomes.

Standard 5. Implementation: The public health nurse implements the identified plan.

Standard 5A. Coordination of Care: The public health nurse coordinates care delivery.

Standard 5B. Health Teaching and Health Promotion: The public health nurse employs multiple strategies to promote health and a safe environment.

Standard 5C. Consultation: The public health nurse provides consultation to influence the identified plan, enhance the abilities of others, and effect change.

Standard 5D. Prescriptive Authority: Not applicable.

Standard 5E. Regulatory Activities: The public health nurse participates in the application of public health laws, regulations, and policies.

Standard 6. Evaluation: The public health nurse evaluates progress toward the attainment of outcomes.

Standard 7. Ethics: The public health nurse practices ethically.

Standards of Professional Performance

Standard 8: Education: The public health nurse attains knowledge and competence that reflect current nursing practice.

Standard 9. Evidence-based Practice & Research: The public health nurse integrates evidence and research findings into practice.

Standard 10. Quality of Practice: The public health nurse contributes to quality nursing practice.

Standard 11. Communication: The public health nurse communicates effectively in a variety of formats in all areas of practice.

Standard 12. Leadership: The public health nurse demonstrates leadership in the professional practice setting and the profession.

Standard 13. Collaboration: The public health nurse collaborates with the population and others in the conduct of nursing practice.

Standard 14. Professional Practice Evaluation: The public health nurse evaluates her or his own nursing practice in relation to professional practice standards and guidelines, relevant statutes, rules, and regulations.

Standard 15. Resource Utilization: The public health nurse utilizes appropriate resources to plan and provide nursing and public health services that are safe, effective, and financially responsible.

Standard 16. Environmental Health: The public health nurse practices in an environmentally safe, fair, and just manner.

Standard 17. Advocacy: The public health nurse advocates for the protection of the health, safety, and rights of the population.

Source: American Nurses Association, 2013, pp. 28–64.

 ACTIVITY

Review your preceptor's job description with your preceptor.

Share the list of the ANA practice standards for public health nursing.

Discuss how your preceptor's job description and nursing practice incorporates specific ANA standards.

Key Components of Public Health Nursing

The key components of public health nursing practice discussed in this manual include:

- Cornerstones of Public Health Nursing (MDH, 2007);
- The standards of public health nursing practice (ANA, 2013);
- Health determinants framework (U.S. Department of Health and Human Services, n.d.);
- Levels of prevention (Stanhope & Lancaster, 2008);
- Public health nursing process (ANA, 2013; MDH 2001); and
- Public Health Intervention Wheel (MDH, 2001).

The Cornerstones, health determinants framework, and levels of prevention are included in this chapter. The public health nursing process and Public Health Intervention Wheel are discussed in Chapter 2.

Three Core Public Health Functions and Ten Essential Services of Public Health

In the United States, PHNs and other public health professionals who work for governmental public health agencies have a scope of practice that is based on identified *core public health functions* and the *essential services of public health* (IOM, 1988).

Figure 1.1 demonstrates the relationship between the core functions and the essential services (Core Public Health Functions Steering Committee, 1995; U.S. DHHS, 2010) that formal government agencies and their staff must carry out.

The three core functions (Core Public Health Functions Steering Committee, 1995) in Figure 1.1, defined below, are very similar to the main functions of global public health identified by the World Health Organization (n.d.):

- **Assessment**—Community assessment of population health needs by monitoring and investigating levels of population health and illness
- **Policy Development**—Development of health policies, goals, plans, and interventions to meet priority community health needs
- **Assurance**—Measurement of outcomes of health policies, goals, plans, and interventions and the competency and adequacy of public health professionals to determine whether a community's priority health needs have been met in an efficient, effective, and timely manner

The Ten Essential Services of Public Health (Core Public Health Functions Steering Committee, 1995) in Figure 1.1 have been identified as those that need to be carried out by PHNs and other public health professionals to maintain the health of a community and its diverse populations. Table 1.4 outlines these essential services and provides examples of each.

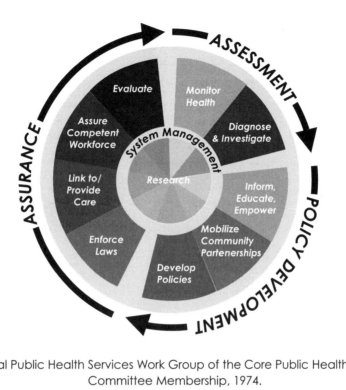

Figure 1.1   Essential Public Health Services Work Group of the Core Public Health Functions Steering Committee Membership, 1974.

Table 1.4   The Ten Essential Services of Public Health

Essential Service	Examples
1. Monitor Health	• Carry out community assessment to determine levels of health and illness in community and populations.
2. Diagnose and Investigate	• Check lead levels of preschool children, infants, and toddlers at risk for lead poisoning.
	• Offer diabetes screening in the Native American community.
3. Inform, Educate, and Empower	• Teach first-time parents how to care for their new baby.
	• Provide car seat education to new parents.
4. Mobilize Community Partnerships	• Develop a network of community services for elderly people within the community.
5. Develop Policies	• Work with county board members to develop a policy for playground safety in local communities.
6. Enforce Laws	• Report suspected child abuse or neglect.
	• Monitor compliance with immunization laws for schoolchildren.
7. Link to/Provide Care	• PHNs and Emergency Department staff develop a referral and follow-up system for homebound elderly who visit the Emergency Department and then return home.

continues

Table 1.4   The Ten Essential Services of Public Health   (continued)

Essential Service	Examples
8. Assure Competent Workforce	• Update public health nursing staff on the H1N1 virus. • Teach rural PHNs how to do well-water testing.
9. Evaluate	• Carry out evaluation studies to determine the effectiveness of public health nursing programs, such as home visiting to new families.
10. System Management & Research	• Determine needs for public health services and service gaps in the community. • Provide data to justify claims that tax dollars improve the public's health.

Source: Core Public Health Functions Steering Committee, 1995

"Well this is all very interesting. But I still don't have a clue how I am actually going to practice public health nursing," Albert sighed.

Sia responded, "I think there are levels of practice. Our instructor told us we would be practicing at the individual/family level of practice most of the time. There are some good web videos in the Resource section of our textbook. I suppose we could look at them. And there is additional information in the textbook itself."

Abby stated, "Great! But I think I want to spend more time actually doing something. I am going to spend a day with my preceptor tomorrow. Maybe I can apply some of what I have read and watched on the web."

Practicing Public Health Nursing

As a student, you will probably be spending most of your clinical hours working with individuals and families. However, the role of the PHN is broader; PHNs also spend time working with community groups and other members of the community team. Public health nursing is carried out at different levels of practice within society: individual/family, community, and systems (MDH, 2001, pp. 4–5).

Individual/Family Level of Practice

PHNs work with individuals and families to promote health and reduce risks. The family is the essential unit of all communities and societies. A family is defined as two or more people who identify themselves as a family, share emotional bonds, and carry out the functions of a family who share bonds of emotional closeness (Clark, 2008; Friedman, Bowden, & Jones, 2003). PHNs work with individuals and families in many different community settings (see Chapter 3 for information on home visiting and family assessment). Working with families in the community helps you understand the diverse socioeconomic, cultural, and environmental factors that influence the health, wellness, and disease of individuals and families. If you are working with an individual or family to help them adapt or change their values, health beliefs, or behaviors to improve their health status, then you are working at the individual/family level of practice.

Community Level of Practice

You initially identify the community when you begin to work with vulnerable individuals, families, and groups. A community can refer to: (a) "a group of people or population group; (b) a physical place and time in which the population lives and works; or, (c) cultural groups that have shared beliefs, values, institutions, and social systems" (Dreher et al., 2006, p. 23). If you are working with members of the community to help the community adapt or change its values, health beliefs, or behaviors to improve the members' health status, then you are working at the community level of practice.

PHNs work with two types of populations in the community: populations of interest and populations at risk (MDH, 2001, p. 2). Table 1.5 defines and provides examples of these populations.

Table 1.5   Populations Served by Public Health

Population	Examples
Population of Interest: Population who is essentially healthy but could improve factors that promote or protect health (MDH, 2001)	• Families who live in urban areas with little opportunity for exercise because of lack of parks, playgrounds, or bike paths • College students who have increased stress because of study needs and college debts and are looking for ways to reduce their stress level
Population at Risk: Population with a common identified risk factor or risk exposure that poses a threat to health (MDH, 2001)	• Children who are not immunized for major childhood illnesses, such as measles and chickenpox • Older members of a church congregation who live alone and are at risk for falls

Systems Level of Practice

A system is an institution or organization that exists within one or multiple communities. Key systems include healthcare systems, public health systems, schools, churches, government agencies, nonprofit organizations, and businesses. PHNs practice at the systems level when they work with providers and professionals like teachers, social workers, nurses, doctors, government officials, and members of the business community working for different agencies. If you are working with members of systems to help these systems adapt or change their values, health beliefs, or the way they conduct their business (behaviors) so that they can improve their capacity to meet the health needs of those they serve, then you are working at the systems level of practice.

The Relationships Between Individuals/Families, Communities, and Systems

Individuals, families, and systems are best understood within the context of the community in which you live. Individuals and families interact with, and are influenced by, their social and physical environments and the systems that influence their health. For example, families living in an inner-city neighborhood might not have access to a grocery store with fresh fruits and vegetables or transportation to the store. The neighborhood's characteristics influence family access to quality food and their nutritional well-being. Figure 1.2 shows an example of the interrelationships among families, communities, and systems.

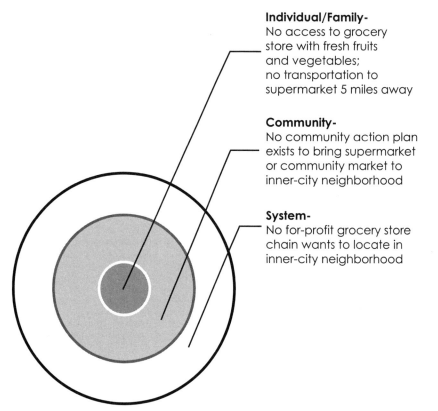

Individual/Family-
No access to grocery store with fresh fruits and vegetables; no transportation to supermarket 5 miles away

Community-
No community action plan exists to bring supermarket or community market to inner-city neighborhood

System-
No for-profit grocery store chain wants to locate in inner-city neighborhood

Figure 1.2. Interrelationships of Families, Communities, and Systems

To make a difference for these families and others in their inner-city neighborhood, PHNs might carry out the following interventions:

- Refer families who are eligible for food stamps and nutrition services to Women, Infants, and Children (WIC)—individual/family level of practice.

- Work with a community action council to make its members aware of a problem in their inner-city neighborhood and assist them with taking action to obtain bus service from the neighborhood to a shopping center or supermarket—community level of practice.

- Help form a coalition of nonprofit organizations and businesses to bring a cooperative store or other full-service grocery store to the neighborhood—systems level of practice.

Table 1.6 summarizes the three levels of PHN practice and provides examples of how public health nursing is carried out at these levels. These are all actions that you as a student or a newly practicing public health nurse can also take.

Table 1.6   Levels of Public Health Nursing Practice

Individual/Family Level	Examples
"Population-based, individual-focused practice changes knowledge, attitudes, beliefs, practices, and behaviors of individuals. This practice level is directed at individuals, alone or as part of a family, class, or group. Individuals receive services because they are identified as belonging to a population at-risk" (MDH, 2001, p. 5).	<ul><li>Make home visits to newborns and their parents.</li><li>Teach hand-washing to a first-grade class.</li><li>Assess for the presence of lead-based paint in a home with preschool children.</li><li>Develop a fall-prevention plan for an elderly person living alone.</li></ul>

Community Level	Examples
"Population-based, community-focused practice changes community norms, community attitudes, community awareness, community practices, and community behaviors. They (PHNs) are directed toward entire populations within the community or occasionally toward target groups within those populations. Community-focused practice is measured in terms of what proportion of the population actually changes" (MDH, 2001, p. 4).	<ul><li>Write a letter to the editor of a local paper to stress the value of home visits to parents of newborns.</li><li>Create a billboard about the hazards of lead-based paint.</li><li>Participate in a community "town hall" meeting to make the community aware of safety hazards for elderly people living alone.</li></ul>

Systems Level	Examples
"Population-based, systems-focused practice changes organizations, policies, laws, and power structures. The focus is not directly on individuals and communities but on the systems that impact health. Changing systems is often a more effective and long-lasting way to impact population health than requiring change from every single individual in a community" (MDH, 2001, pp. 4–5).	<ul><li>Meet with legislators to advocate for reimbursement for home visits with families of newborns.</li><li>Develop a hand-washing program at an elementary school.</li><li>Teach real-estate agents how to recognize lead-based paint in a home.</li><li>Develop a fall-prevention protocol for nurses working with the elderly in the community.</li></ul>

Health Determinants

Public health nurses consider the multiple factors that determine the health of their clients. Health determinants are factors that influence the health of individuals, families, and populations. Health determinants can have a positive or negative influence on health. Table 1.7 presents examples of protective and risk factors at all three levels of practice for communicable disease in childhood:

- Protective factors are health determinants that protect a person from illness and/or assist in improving the person's health.

- Risk factors are health determinants that contribute to the potential for illness to occur or to a decrease in health or well-being.

Table 1.7 Protective and Risk Factors for Childhood Communicable Diseases

Protective Factors by Level of Practice		
Individual/Family Level	**Community Level**	**Systems**
• Family has insurance that covers immunizations.	• 95% of children in the community are immunized (herd immunity).	• Immunizations are available at public health clinics, pharmacies, and medical clinics.
• Children are up to date on immunizations.	• Community billboards urge parents to immunize their children.	• Free or low cost immunizations are available to uninsured.
• Parents teach children proper hand-washing and to cover their mouths when coughing.	• Low-density housing and/or single-dwelling homes reduce contact between infected and noninfected children.	• Childcare center has effective infection prevention and control practices.

Risk Factors by Level of Practice		
• Family is uninsured.	• 45% of children in the community are immunized (no herd immunity).	• Immunizations are not available at the public health clinic.
• Family members are not aware of the need for immunizations.	• Some community groups oppose childhood immunizations.	• Funding for low-cost immunizations for the uninsured is lacking.
• Parents not aware of how to prevent the spread of infectious diseases.	• Many high-density housing and apartment complexes in the community place people living close together at greater risk.	• School district does not track students' immunization records.

Biological, behavioral, and environmental factors interact and contribute to the health and illness of individuals, families, and populations (ANA, 2013; Marmot & Wilkinson, 1999; U.S. DHHS, 2010; Zahner & Block, 2006). Individuals and families are able to influence or control many of their biological and behavioral health determinants but are not able to control many of the physical and social environmental determinants of health that occur at the community and systems levels. Health determinants shaped by social, economic, and political forces, including systems put in place to deal with illness, are called the social determinants of health (see Chapter 10 for further discussion on the social determinants of health). These social determinants of health affect population health in all nations of the world:

> The social determinants of health are the conditions in which people are born, grow, live, work and age. These circumstances are shaped by the distribution of money, power and resources at global, national and local levels. The social determinants of health are mostly responsible for health inequities—the unfair and avoidable differences in health status seen within and between countries. (WHO, 2013)

Health Status

PHNs use the community assessment process (see Chapter 3) and public health nursing process (see Chapter 3) to determine the health statuses of individuals, families, communities, and populations. *Health status* refers to the level of health or illness and is the outcome of the interaction of the multiple health determinants. Health status indicators are frequently represented by statistical measures, such as rates and percentages. Some common examples of population health status indicators are teen pregnancy rates, percentage of low-birth-weight babies, neonatal mortality rates, percentage of malnutrition in a group, and obesity rates. Rates and percentages of different population groups can be compared to determine similarities or differences in the health status of the different groups. Health status comparisons can also be applied at an individual level, such as identifying a child with malnutrition as having a lower level of health than a child who is not malnourished. Health status comparisons allow PHNs to determine their priorities for actions with specific individuals, families, communities, and populations.

This health determinants model is a comprehensive approach to assessing and intervening with clients in the community. Figure 1.3 illustrates a health determinants model. In this model, the social environment includes access to healthcare and health policy as aspects of health systems. PHNs can use it to organize and identify the complex contributors to the health status of specific individuals, families, and populations and to develop interventions to improve health. Health determinants, including protective and risk factors, exist at individual/family, community, and systems levels, so nursing interventions should address health determinants at all levels as needed. The health determinants identified in a social environment include social determinants of health (discussed in depth in Chapter 10). PHNs collaborate with their clients by building on their protective factors and helping them reduce their risk factors.

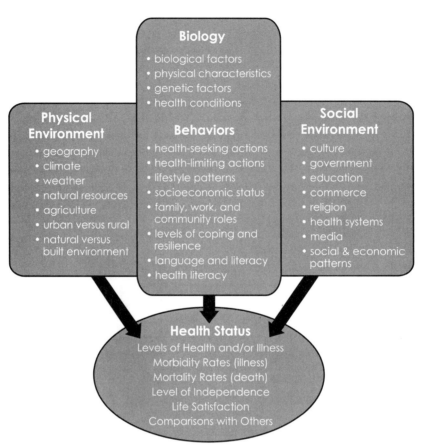

Figure 1.3. A Health Determinants Model for Individuals/Families, Communities, and Populations

ACTIVITY

Review the following Health Determinants Analysis Case Study:

Identify the health status indicators for this community.

Identify health determinants, including protective and risk factors that contribute to the health status of this community.

How would you work with community members to build on their protective factors and reduce their risk factors?

Case Study: Health Determinants Analysis

A community assessment in a small rural community determines that more than one-third of the adult residents are overweight or obese. The assessment reveals that 40% of the adults in this community report that they have high cholesterol, and 30% report that they have high blood pressure. The majority of adults admits to eating out at fast-food restaurants at least five times a week. This community contains many fast-food restaurants, and the most common foods sold in them are high in fat, sodium, sugar, and calories. This community has few outdoor recreational sites, such as bike and walking paths, and the county board has voted against increasing tax levies to provide those paths. The local hospital does provide evening and weekend health education classes on modifying diet and exercise to lead a healthier life. A coalition of healthcare clinics, the public health agency, and local businesses is working on a plan to increase healthy living resources in the community.

Levels of Prevention

The levels of prevention (i.e., primary, secondary, and tertiary) provide a framework that is often used to differentiate the stages of health and disease for individuals and groups (Stanhope & Lancaster, 2008). It is important to determine the health status of individuals/families, communities, and populations and to determine the level of prevention for specific health concerns to implement the appropriate interventions. Figure 1.4 provides an overview of the stages of health, the levels of prevention, and intervention approaches.

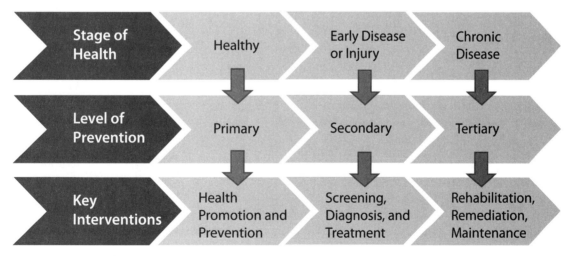

Figure 1.4. Stages of Health and Disease and Levels of Prevention

Although focus of public health nursing is primary prevention, public health nursing practice encompasses all three levels of prevention. In contrast, within the hospital setting, the focus of most nursing care is on ill patients and their family members, and nurses more often provide secondary and tertiary prevention but may also provide some primary prevention. Table 1.8 shows the definition of each level with examples.

Table 1.8   Prevention Continuum With Public Health Nursing Examples

Definitions	Examples
Primary prevention promotes health and protects against threats to it. It is designed to keep problems from occurring in the first place. It promotes resiliency and protective factors or reduces susceptibility and exposure to risk factors. Primary prevention occurs before a problem develops. It targets populations that are essentially well.	PHN Antepartal home visit: • Teaching parents the importance of taking a newborn home from the hospital in an approved car seat • Providing parents with information about approved car seats PHN Postpartum home visit: • Checking the car seat to determine that it is correctly installed • Monitoring the parents' use of car seat
Secondary prevention detects and treats problems in their early stages. It keeps problems from causing serious or long-term effects or from affecting others. It identifies risks or hazards and modifies, removes, or treats them before a problem becomes more serious. Secondary prevention is implemented after a problem has begun, possibly before signs and symptoms appear. It targets populations that share common risk factors.	PHN at WIC Clinic: • Using a growth chart to plot children's heights and weights • Identifying children who are outside established norms • Referring parents and children who are above 95th percentile or below 5th percentile to a primary care provider for assessment and to a nutritionist for nutritional education and counseling
Tertiary prevention limits further negative effects from a problem and aims to keep existing problems from getting worse. Tertiary prevention is implemented after a disease or injury has occurred. It alleviates the effects of disease and injury and restores individuals to their optimal levels of functioning. It targets populations that have experienced disease or injury.	School Nurse Beginning of the school year: • Identifying students with asthma and obtaining asthma plans • Working with teaching staff to reduce environmental asthma triggers in the school building During the school year: • Monitoring students with asthma for compliance with asthma plans and health statuses • Providing nebulizer treatments in the health office

Source: Levels of Prevention modified from MDH, 2001, p. 4

"Okay! Now I understand why public health nurses do what they do, but I am still not clear about what I am supposed to do!" Albert stated in an exasperated tone of voice.

Sia responded, "I guess we have to assess our clients' health status, identify their health determinants, and develop a plan of care that builds on their protective factors and reduces their risk factors. Now it makes sense that we would be mostly listening, teaching, and counseling. Did you know that the words listen and silent have the same letters? I guess we need to use silence to listen to our clients!"

Abby stated, "I really like all the secondary and tertiary prevention interventions that I do in the hospital setting, so I am afraid I am going to get bored working in the community. I can only sit and listen for so long. I like action!"

Albert reflected, "Our instructor says we can apply public health nursing in any nursing practice setting. Maybe I will think about how I can use everything I learn in my community clinical in my hospital practice. But, who knows—maybe I will decide to become a public health nurse!"

Sia asked, "I understand what we are supposed to focus on when we work with individuals and families, but I am not sure how identifying their health statuses and health needs fits in with the concept of population-based practice. I guess I need to talk to my preceptor about how our home visits fit in with the priority health needs of our community. How do I know whether what we are doing reflects what the community really wants public health nurses to do?"

Healthy People 2020 Healthy People, a program of the U.S. Department of Health and Human Services, has established science-based benchmarks and 10-year national objectives for improving the health of all Americans. Healthy People 2020 is the third set of national health priorities identified over the last three decades. Its vision is "a society in which all people live long healthy lives" (U.S. DHHS, n.d.). The mission and goals are displayed in Table 1.9. This national program seeks to involve all Americans by encouraging community and organizational collaboration, empowering individuals to make informed health decisions, and measuring the outcomes of prevention activities (U.S. DHHS, n.d.).

Table 1.9   Healthy People 2020 Mission and Goals

Mission—Healthy People 2020 strives to:	Overarching Goals
• Identify nationwide health-improvement priorities; • Increase public awareness and understanding of the determinants of health, disease, and disability and opportunities for progress; • Provide measurable objectives and goals that are applicable at the national, state, and local levels; • Engage multiple sectors to take action to strengthen policies and improve practices that are driven by the best available evidence and knowledge; and • Identify critical research, evaluation, and data-collection needs.	• Attain high-quality, longer lives free of preventable disease, disability, injury, and premature death. • Achieve health equity, eliminate disparities, and improve the health of groups. • Create social and physical environments that promote good health for all. • Promote quality of life, healthy development, and healthy behaviors across all life stages.

Source: U.S. DHHS, n.d.

A set of national health priorities titled Leading Health Indicators (LHIs) is included in Healthy People 2020 (National Center for Health Statistics, 2012; U.S. DHHS, n.d.). They include 42 health outcomes organized into 12 health topics. These priorities reflect the greatest unmet national health needs based on an analysis of Healthy People 2010 health outcome data. These LHIs are found in the sidebar on the facing page.

 ## WEB-BASED ACTIVITY

Go to the Healthy People web page (http://www.healthypeople/gov) and search for the LHIs.

Read about one of the LHI health outcomes that interests you.

Find the Healthy People 2010 statistical data that measured the achievement of that outcome.

What is the goal for the Healthy People 2020 outcome? Which statistic would demonstrate improvement of that outcome?

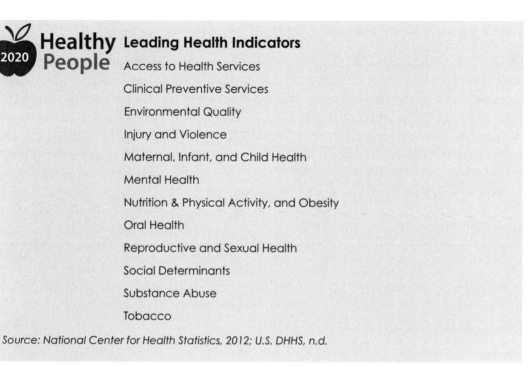

Healthy People 2020

Leading Health Indicators

Access to Health Services

Clinical Preventive Services

Environmental Quality

Injury and Violence

Maternal, Infant, and Child Health

Mental Health

Nutrition & Physical Activity, and Obesity

Oral Health

Reproductive and Sexual Health

Social Determinants

Substance Abuse

Tobacco

Source: National Center for Health Statistics, 2012; U.S. DHHS, n.d.

ACTIVITY

Explore the community health priorities of your state or local health department. Compare them with the LHIs.

Identify programs or activities in your clinical agency that are related to the LHIs.

Discuss with your preceptor how nurses are involved in these programs or activities.

How might you become involved as a citizen or as a nurse in working on one of the LHI priorities in your community?

Entry-Level Population-Based Public Health Nursing Competencies

This chapter has given you a lot to think about. Now it is time to focus on the entry-level public health nursing competencies that you can work to develop in your community clinical. This manual is going to help you focus on the entry-level competencies expected of baccalaureate nursing graduates and novice nurses entering public health nursing.

Henry Street Entry-Level PHN Competencies

The Henry Street Consortium (HSC, 2003) identified 11 entry-level population-based public health nursing competencies for baccalaureate nursing graduates and novice public health nurses. These competencies are consistent with national benchmark standards for entry-level public health nursing (ANA, 2013; Quad Council of Public Health Nursing Organizations, 2011) and are listed in Table 1.10. A consortium of practicing public health nurses and educators developed these simplified entry-level standards to facilitate the teaching and learning of public health nursing knowledge and skills in the clinical setting (Schaffer et al., 2011). Indices to measure the HSC competencies—which provide the organizing framework for this book—are found in Appendix C.

Table 1.10   Henry Street Consortium Entry-Level PHN Competencies

1. Applies the public health nursing process to communities, systems, individuals, and families.

2. Utilizes basic epidemiological principles (the incidence, distribution, and control of disease in a population) in public health nursing practice.

3. Utilizes collaboration to achieve public health goals.

4. Works within the responsibility and authority of the governmental public health system.

5. Practices public health nursing within the auspices of the Nurse Practice Act.

6. Effectively communicates with communities, systems, individuals, families, and colleagues.

7. Establishes and maintains caring relationships with communities, systems, individuals, and families.

8. Shows evidence of commitment to social justice, the greater good, and the public health principles.

9. Demonstrates nonjudgmental and unconditional acceptance of people different from self.

10. Incorporates mental, physical, emotional, social, spiritual, and environmental aspects of health into assessment, planning, implementation, and evaluation.

11. Demonstrates leadership in public health nursing with communities, systems, individuals, and families.

Source: Henry Street Consortium, 2003

 ACTIVITY

Review the competencies and their related activities in Appendix C. Make a list of activities within each competency that you would like to practice during your community clinical.

Talk with your preceptor about how you might practice these public health nursing activities.

Key Points

- Public health nursing combines the theory and practice of nursing and public health. It is a required component of baccalaureate nursing education.

- Public health nursing practice is guided by the national scope of practice standards.

- The goal of public health and public health nursing is to improve the health of the public at the local, national, and international levels.

- The Cornerstones of Public Health explain the beliefs and values of the clinical specialty of public health nursing practice.

- Public health nursing practice is population-based, focusing on the priority health needs of populations.

- Primary prevention is the focus of public health nursing, but PHNs also provide secondary and tertiary prevention interventions.

- PHNs work at all three levels of practice: individual/family, community, and systems.

- Emerging threats and challenges in health and healthcare require changes in and leadership from public health nursing.

- The HSC Entry-Level Public Health Nursing competencies, based on accepted national standards, provide a guide for baccalaureate nursing students to achieve the expected outcomes of baccalaureate nursing education.

Reflective Practice

Alberto takes a deep breath, closes his eyes as if in deep thought, and says, "Let's see if I have this straight. Public health nursing is part of my professional nursing practice. It can be practiced anywhere, because public health nursing is shaped by its goal, not by its setting, but it is most often practiced in the community. The goal of public health nursing is to improve the health of the public, the health of the communities in which we live. The client in public health nursing may be an individual, a family, the community, or a population within the community. To improve and protect the public's health, I need to assess the health status and identify the health determinants that affect the health status of individuals, families, communities, and populations. Then I need to intervene by helping my clients build on their protective factors and reduce their risk factors. The interventions I will use most often are teaching and counseling, but we will learn about more interventions as we read this manual and complete our community clinical. When I practice in the community, I will probably be partnering with other members of the healthcare team as well as community members. I need to demonstrate a set of entry-level public health nursing competencies to successfully complete my baccalaureate nursing education. The

Henry Street Consortium Population-Based Public Health Nursing Competencies focus on what I should be learning and practicing in my public health clinical activities. Whew! Do I have that right?"

Abby and Sia responded, "Yes. You've got it! You get an 'A' for the course!"

1. Think about what Alberto, Abby, and Sia have learned about public health nursing from their observations and discussions with their preceptors.

   _____

   _____

2. How will you analyze what you observe about public health nursing during your clinical experience?

   _____

   _____

3. How would you describe public health nursing practices you observe in your clinical to your classmates?

   _____

   _____

References

American Nurses Association. (2003). *Nursing's social policy statement, 2nd ed.* Silver Spring, MD: Nursesbooks.org.

American Nurses Association. (2013). *Public health nursing: Scope and standards of practice.* Silver Spring, MD: Nursesbooks.org.

American Public Health Association, Public Health Nursing Section. (1996). *Definition and role of public health nursing.* Washington, DC: Author. Retrieved from http://www.apha.org/membergroups/sections/aphasections/phn/about/defbackground.htm

Clark, M. J. (2008). *Community health nursing.* Upper Saddle River, NJ: Pearson.

Core Public Health Functions Steering Committee. (1995). *Public health in America: Core functions and essential services of public health.* Adopted 1994. Retrieved from http://www.health.gov/phfunctions/public.htm

Dreher, M., Shapiro, D., & Asselin, M. (2006). *Healthy places, healthy people: A handbook for culturally competent community nursing practice.* Indianapolis, IN: Sigma Theta Tau International.

Education Committee of the Association of Community Health Nurse Educators. (2010). Essentials of baccalaureate nursing education for entry-level community/public health nursing. *Public Health Nursing, 27*(4), 371–382. doi:10.1111/j.1525-1446.2010.00867.x

Essential Public Health Services Work Group of the Core Public Health Functions Steering Committee Membership: American Public Health Association; Association of Schools of Public Health; Association of State and Territorial Health Officials; Centers for Disease Control and Prevention; Environmental Council of the States; Food and Drug Administration; Health Resources and Services Administration; Indian Health Service; Institute of Medicine; National Academy of Sciences; National Association of County and City Health Officials; National Association of State Alcohol and Drug Abuse Directors; National Association of State Mental Health Program Directors; National Institutes of Health; Office of the Assistant Secretary for Health; Public Health Foundation; Substance Abuse and Mental Health Services Administration; U.S. Public Health Service Agency for Health Care Policy and Research. (1994). *Public health core functions and essential services.* Retrieved from http://www.cdc.gov/nphpsp/essentialservices.html

Friedman, M., Bowden, V., & Jones, E. (2003). *Family nursing: Research, theory, and practice, 5th ed.* Upper Saddle River, NJ: Prentice Hall.

Henry Street Consortium. (2003). *Population-based public health nursing competencies.* St. Paul, MN: Author. Retrieved from http://www.health.state.mn.us/divs/opi/cd/phn/henrystreet/docs/0303henryst_corecomp.pdf

Institute of Medicine. (1988). *The future of public health.* Washington, D.C.: National Academy Press.

Institute of Medicine. (2011). *The future of nursing—Leading change, advancing health.* Washington, D.C.: National Academy Press.

International Council of Nurses. (2007). *Vision for the future of nursing.* Retrieved from http://www.icn.ch/about-icn/icns-vision-for-the-future-of-nursing/

Keller, L. O., Strohschein, S., & Schaffer, M. A. (2011). The cornerstones of public health nursing. *Public Health Nursing, 28*(3), 249–260. doi:10.1111/j.1525-1446.2010.00923.x

Marmot, M., & Wilkinson, R. G. (1999). *Social determinants of health.* Oxford, UK: Oxford University Press.

Minnesota Department of Health, Center for Public Health Nursing. (2003). *Definition of population-based practice.* Retrieved from http://www.health.state.mn.us/divs/opi/cd/phn/docs/0303phn_popbasedpractice.pdf

Minnesota Department of Health, Center for Public Health Nursing. (2007). *Cornerstones of Public Health Nursing.* Adapted from original by Center for Public Health Nursing, 2004. St. Paul: Author. Retrieved from http://www.health.state.mn.us/divs/opi/cd/phn/docs/0710phn_cornerstones.pdf

Minnesota Department of Health, Division of Community Health Services, Public Health Nursing Section. (2001). *Public health interventions: Applications for public health nursing practice.* St. Paul, MN: Author. Retrieved from http://www.health.state.mn.us/divs/opi/cd/phn/docs/0301wheel_manual.pdf

Minnesota Department of Health, Public Health Nursing Section. (2000). *Public health nursing practice for the 21st century: Competency development in population-based practice.* National Satellite Learning Conference. St. Paul, MN: Author. Retrieved from http://www.health.state.mn.us/divs/opi/cd/phn/docs/0001phnpractice_learningguide.pdf

National Center for Health Statistics. (2012). *Healthy People 2010, final review.* Hyattsville, NY: U.S. DHHS. Retrieved from http://www.cdc.gov/nchs/data/hpdata2010/hp2010_final_review.pdf

Quad Council of Public Health Nursing Organizations. (2011). *Public health nursing competencies.* Retrieved from http://www.phf.org/resourcestools/Pages/Public_Health_Nursing_Competencies.aspx

Robert Wood Johnson Foundation. (2013). *Forum on the future of public health nursing, February 8, 2012—Proceedings and feedback: Summary report.* Retrieved from http://www.rwjf.org/content/dam/farm/reports/reports/2012/rwjf404144

Schaffer, M. A., Cross, S., Olson, L. O., Nelson, P., Schoon, P. M., & Henton, P. (2011). The Henry Street Consortium population-based competencies for educating public health nursing students. *Public Health Nursing, 28*(1), 78–90. doi:10.1111/j.1525-1446.2010.00900.x

Stanhope, M., & Lancaster, J. (2008). *Public health nursing: Population-centered health care in the community, 7th ed.* St. Louis, MO: Mosby.

U.S. Department of Health and Human Services. (n.d.). *Healthy People 2020: About Healthy People 2020: Leading health indicators.* Retrieved from http://healthypeople.gov/2020/default.aspx

U.S. Department of Health and Human Services. (2010). *Public health functions project: Public health in America statement.* Retrieved from http://www.health.gov/phfunctions

World Health Organization. (n.d.). *Public health.* Retrieved from http://www.who.int/trade/glossary/story076/en/

World Health Organization. (2013). *What are social determinants of health?* Retrieved from http://www.who.int/social_determinants/sdh_definition/en/index.html

Zahner, S. J., & Block, D. E. (2006). The road to population health: Using Healthy People 2010 in nursing education. *Journal of Nursing Education, 45*(3), 105–108.

EVIDENCE-BASED PUBLIC HEALTH NURSING PRACTICE

2

Patricia M. Schoon

with Carolyn M. Garcia and Marjorie A. Schaffer

Abby is talking with Jaime, an RN who has returned to school to get his baccalaureate nursing degree. She is struggling to understand the three levels of public health nursing practice. Abby asks, "How do you use the nursing process in your hospital work? Did you ever think you could use it for more than the patients you are caring for?"

Jaime replied, "It still seems kind of strange to me. But I am a member of the Quality Improvement Team. We just finished an audit to look at the incidence of patient falls to find out whether our unit is meeting the goals set by the hospital to reduce the patient fall rate. Our patient fall rate is still higher than the goal set by the hospital, so we decided that we need to hold an in-service on assessing patients for their fall risk and the different protocols we can use to reduce the number of patient falls. So, I guess if we think of my unit as a community, we are using the nursing process at more than one level."

Abby pondered, "I guess I can kind of see that you are using the nursing process to assess the fall rate. The idea of using the nursing process at the systems level still seems very strange to me."

Jaime thought about the idea of nursing at the systems level and finally said, "Maybe if I think of the nursing staff on my unit as part of the hospital system, then Quality Improvement Team members can assess what they know about fall risk and prevention and design a program just for our staff members to improve their skills in that area. What do you think?"

Abby sighed, "I kind of understand how I can use nursing process to assess the health needs of individuals, families, and communities, but I can't think how I would assess the health status of a system. Do systems have a health status?" Abby mused, "If a system, like a public health agency, doesn't have enough money to provide the health services that the community needs, then I guess it wouldn't be very healthy."

Jaime said thoughtfully, "Maybe we need to look at a community's health needs and determine whether specific community systems, such as hospitals, schools, educational systems, and public health agencies, have the resources to meet the priority needs of their community. If they don't have the resources, then maybe we can plan interventions to help them get the resources or services they need."

ABBY'S NOTEBOOK

Useful Definitions

Critical appraisal of literature: A systematic process you can use to examine and synthesize the research data presented in an article or a group of articles (Fineout-Overholt, Melnyk, Stillwell, & Williamson, 2010)

Evidence-based practice: "[A]n explicit process that enables clinicians to seek out best practices and make determinations regarding if and how these practices can be incorporated into patient care" (Poe & White, 2010, p. 3)

Public health nursing process: Integration of concepts of public health, community, and all three levels of the public health nurse's (PHN) practice (i.e., individual, community, and systems) into the nursing process (Minnesota Department of Health, 2003)

Public health interventions: Actions that PHNs take on behalf of individuals, families, systems, and communities to improve or protect their health status (MDH, 2001); PHNs commonly practice all 17 interventions

Several years ago, a nursing student about to graduate reflected on what she had learned. She said, "I get it. Nursing is about critical thinking!" Nursing is a knowledge profession. That means we think before we do (assessment and planning), while we do (modifying interventions), and after we do (evaluation). This chapter explains how to apply the nursing process to public health nursing practice and to identify and use interventions that support public health practice goals. You will learn how to apply what you already know about evidence-based nursing practice to your public health nursing practice. PHNs are accountable to their clients and to the public for practicing effectively and efficiently to achieve the best outcomes using the least amount of resources. This chapter discusses how PHNs use best practice information to improve their clients' health.

The Public Health Nursing Process

The public health nursing process integrates concepts of public health, community, and all three levels of public health nursing practice (i.e., individual, community, and systems) into the nursing process (i.e., assessment, diagnosis, planning, implementation, and evaluation; MDH, 2003). Critical thinking throughout the PHN process is essential in identifying and modifying the complex determinants of health that influence the health status of individuals, families, and communities. This application of the nursing process is reflected in the American Nurses Association's (ANA's) *Public Health Nursing: Scope* and *Standards of Practice* (2013), as illustrated in Figure 2.1. The application of the nursing process to all three levels of practice is discussed in Chapter 3.

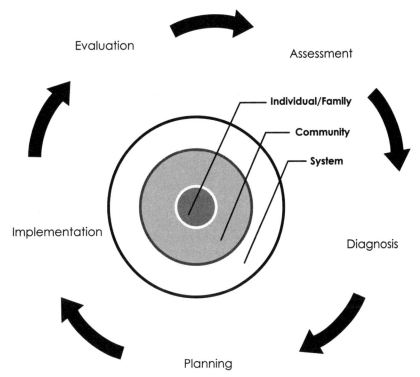

Figure 2.1. Nursing Process at Three Levels of Public Health Nursing Practice

Source: American Nurses Association's (ANA's) *Public Health Nursing: Scope* and *Standards of Practice* (2013)

PHNs often work with people in other professions as well as community members to achieve public health goals (see Chapter 5 for a discussion of interprofessional collaboration). Many of the interventions that PHNs use are also used by other professionals in the community. Whenever possible, PHNs work with other members of the community health team but will work alone if necessary.

> *Abby commented, "My PHN preceptor told me that we are going to make a joint visit with the social worker to a family where a baby has Failure to Thrive. My preceptor is going to focus on assessing the health status of the baby, and the social worker is going to focus on the family support system and resources in the community for the mother. It will be interesting to see how they work together."*

> *Jaime responded, "I am going to an interdisciplinary child abuse team meeting with my preceptor. It is a county-wide team made up of police, social workers, lawyers, and public health nurses. It seems like my preceptor is always working with other people."*

> *Abby concurred, "It really does seem that PHNs work with lots of other disciplines. My preceptor says that is the best way to deal with community-wide health problems."*

Public Health Intervention Wheel

Because PHN practice occurs at three levels, interventions must also be implemented at all three levels. *Public health interventions* are actions that PHNs take on behalf of individuals, families, systems, and communities to improve or protect their health status (MDH, 2001). A study of more than 200 public health nurses from a variety of practice settings identified 17 population-based interventions specific to public health nursing that are found at all three levels of public health nursing practice: individual/family, community, and systems (Keller, Strohschein, Lia-Hoagberg, & Schaffer, 1998, 2004).

These interventions are organized in the Public Health Intervention Wheel illustrated in Figure 2.2. The Public Health Intervention Wheel is evidence-based and represents what PHNs do (Keller et al., 2004). PHNs often use more than one intervention at more than one level of practice (individual and family, community, or system) to influence the multiple health risks affecting individuals, families, and populations.

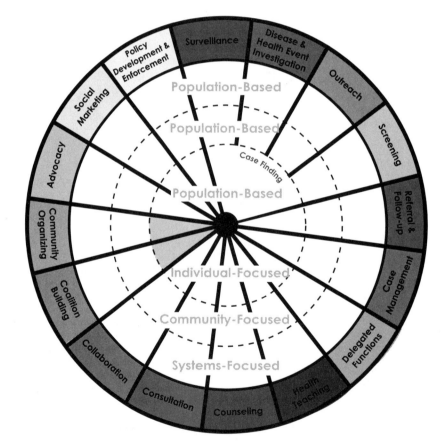

Figure 2.2. Public Health Intervention Wheel
Source: Minnesota Department of Health, Center for Public Health Nursing, 2001

The intervention wheel has 17 interventions divided into five wedges with 3 or 4 interventions each. Each group of wedges reflects a cluster of interventions. The cluster of interventions within each wedge often occurs either concurrently or consecutively. The three inner circles, called segments, represent the three levels of public health nursing practice (i.e., individual/family, community, and systems). All interventions except case finding are carried out at all three levels of practice. Case finding is only carried out at the individual/family level of practice, so it is placed inside the individual/family circle in the wheel diagram. Sixteen of the interventions are independent nursing actions that can be practiced under your state's Nurse Practice Act without a physician's orders. The seventeenth intervention, delegated functions, can include medical functions delegated by a medical professional, such as immunizations, which would require a physician's order. Nursing activities that the PHN delegates to another health team member, such as vision and hearing assessments, are part of the independent practice of nursing and usually reflect one of the other PHN interventions.

Definitions and examples of the 17 population-based public health interventions are outlined in Table 2.1. Interventions are organized within the five wedges on the Public Health Intervention Wheel. Nursing students can do all the intervention examples.

Table 2.1 Public Health Nursing Interventions at All Three Levels of Practice

PHN Intervention Definition	PHN Intervention Examples
Surveillance (Wedge 1) Surveillance describes and monitors health events through ongoing and systematic collection, analysis, and interpretation of health data for the purpose of planning, implementing, and evaluating public health interventions (MDH, 2001, p. 13).	• Investigate and report the incidence and prevalence of sexually transmitted infections in the local teen population (community level). • Work with a school nurse at an elementary school to develop a tracking program to identify the incidence and prevalence of student-on-student bullying before and after the implementation of an anti-bullying curriculum (systems level).
Disease & Health Event Investigation (Wedge 1) Disease and other health event investigation systematically gathers and analyzes data regarding threats to the health of populations, ascertains the source of the threat, identifies cases and others at-risk, and determines control measures (p. 29).	• Identify and follow up on cases of sexually transmitted infection in a high school population to identify sources of infection and provide treatment (individual/family level). • Gather information about radon levels in your community and determine high-risk geographical areas (community level).

continues

Table 2.1   Public Health Nursing Interventions at All Three Levels of Practice   (continued)

PHN Intervention Definition	PHN Intervention Examples
Outreach (Wedge 1) Outreach locates populations of interest or populations at risk and provides information about the nature of the concern, what can be done about it, and how services can be obtained (p. 41).	• Interview people at a family homeless shelter to determine who needs information about the location of local food shelves and WIC clinics (individual/family level). • Develop brochures for local grocery stores to hand out about nutritional needs for children and the location of local food shelves and WIC clinics (systems level).
Case Finding (Wedge 1) Case finding locates individuals and families with identified risk factors and connects them to resources (p. 55).	• Identify new immigrants from southeast Asia who might be at risk for tuberculosis (TB) (individual/family level). • Give at-risk immigrants information on where to receive TB screening (individual/family level).
Screening (Wedge 1) Screening identifies individuals with unrecognized health risk factors or asymptomatic disease conditions in populations (p. 63).	• Organize a blood pressure screening clinic at a community center (systems level). • Conduct blood pressure screening for African-American males (individual/family level).
Referral & Follow-up (Wedge 2) Referral and follow-up assists individuals, families, groups, organizations, and communities to utilize necessary resources to prevent or resolve problems or concerns (p. 79).	• Give an elderly person who is homebound information about how to contact a local Meals on Wheels program and then contact the individual a week later to see if he or she has successfully reached the Meals on Wheels program (individual/family level). • Work with Emergency Department (ED) nurses and home visiting nurses to develop and use a referral process for elderly individuals seen in the ED that need home healthcare services (systems level).
Case Management (Wedge 2) Case management optimizes self-care capabilities of individuals and families and the capacity of systems and communities to coordinate and provide services (p. 93).	• Work with parents of a newborn with Down's Syndrome to identify services in their community that they can use to help them (individual/family level). • Work with a PHN and school nurse to coordinate in-home and school health services for children with severe developmental delays (systems level).

PHN Intervention Definition	PHN Intervention Examples
Delegated Functions (Wedge 2) Delegated functions are direct care tasks a registered professional nurse carries out under the authority of a healthcare practitioner, as allowed by law. Delegated functions also include any direct care tasks a registered professional nurse entrusts to other appropriate personnel to perform (p. 113).	• Provide immunizations at a community flu clinic under standing orders from medical personnel (individual/family and systems levels). • Direct a peer counselor to work with a new diabetic to organize a grocery list and menu plans (individual/family level).
Health Teaching (Wedge 3) Health teaching communicates facts, ideas, and skills that change knowledge, attitudes, values, beliefs, behaviors, and practices and skills of individuals, families, systems, and/or communities (p. 121).	• Teach a class for teen moms about how to care for new baby (individual/family level). • Develop a program on childcare for new moms at a local high school (systems level).
Counseling (Wedge 3) Counseling establishes an interpersonal relationship with a community, system, family, or individual intended to increase or enhance their capacity for self-care and coping. Counseling engages the community, system, family, or individual at an emotional level (p. 151).	• Provide support for parents who are coping with providing care for their dying child at home (individual/family level). • Provide crisis management services to a community that has just experienced a devastating tornado (community level).
Consultation (Wedge 3) Consultation seeks information and generates optional solutions to perceived problems or issues through interactive problem-solving with a community, system, family or individual. The community, system, family or individual selects and acts on the option best meeting the circumstances (p. 165).	• Help a recently divorced father who has custody of his two children to problem solve balancing parenting and work responsibilities (individual/family level). • Consult with a peer-counseling group for diabetes management to help them develop strategies for working with individuals with diabetes in their community (community level).
Collaboration (Wedge 4) Collaboration commits two or more persons or organizations to achieving a common goal through enhancing the capacity of one or more of them to promote and protect health (p. 177).	• Partner with the nurse and social worker in an adolescent correction facility in developing a program to help inmates maintain contact with caring individuals in their family or friendship network (systems level). • Work with the county parks and playground department and local young parents group to develop a plan to provide more bike and walking paths for family use (community and systems level).

continues

Table 2.1   Public Health Nursing Interventions at All Three Levels of Practice   (continued)

PHN Intervention Definition	PHN Intervention Examples
Coalition Building (Wedge 4) Coalition building promotes and develops alliances among organizations or constituencies for a common purpose. It builds linkages, solves problems, and/or enhances local leadership to address health concerns (p. 211).	• Establish a network of agencies to work together to develop a community disaster plan (systems level). • Develop an alliance between local environmental groups, waste management, and recycling organizations to improve community recycling (community level).
Community Organizing (Wedge 4) Community organizing helps community groups identify common problems or goals, mobilize resources, and develop and implement strategies for reaching the goals they collectively have set (p. 235).	• Organize a group of renters from several low-income housing developments to work together to improve the safety of their buildings (community level). • Help organize a group of low-income housing services organizations, community homeless shelters, and county human services to develop strategies to provide a more streamlined program for placing homeless people in affordable housing (systems level).
Advocacy (Wedge 5) Advocacy pleads someone's cause or acts on someone's behalf, with a focus on developing the community, system, individual, or family's capacity to plead their own cause or act on their own behalf (p. 263).	• Help a client file an appeal for an insurance denial for home-care services when the client meets eligibility criteria stated in insurance policy (individual/family level). • Lobby legislators for support of community mental health programs (systems level).
Social Marketing (Wedge 5) Social marketing utilizes commercial marketing principles and technologies for programs designed to influence the knowledge, attitudes, values, beliefs, behaviors, and practices of the population of interest (p. 285).	• Create a video for teen parents on how to help their infants and toddlers meet developmental milestones (individual/family level). • Participate in a televised panel discussion about the effects of drug and alcohol use during pregnancy on the fetus (community level).

PHN Intervention Definition	PHN Intervention Examples
Policy Development & Enforcement (Wedge 5) Policy development places health issues on decision-makers' agendas, acquires a plan of resolution, and determines needed resources. Policy development results in laws, rules and regulations, ordinances, and policies. Policy enforcement compels others to comply with the laws, rules, regulations, ordinances, and policies created in conjunction with policy development (p. 313).	• Participate on a county task force to revise county human services guidelines for mandating reporting of suspected child abuse or neglect (systems level). • Talk to a church group about the need to support a bill for community nutrition programs for children living in poverty (community level).

Definitions from Minnesota Department of Health, Center for Public Health Nursing (2001)

ACTIVITY

Review the interventions and examples in Table 2.1. Try to identify the interventions that your preceptor and other public health/community health nurses are using alone or in combination with each other. Select a few interventions that you would like to use in your clinical and discuss how you might do so with your preceptor and/or instructor.

Jaime said, "I am going to a meeting with my PHN preceptor this afternoon about how the different county agencies and the school district are working together as a team to try to reduce smoking among high school students. I guess that would be an example of collaboration, but I am not sure which level of practice that would be."

Abby pondered, "I think maybe when PHNs work with agencies and school districts, they are practicing at the systems level. If they use an intervention like social marketing to let teens know about the availability of a smoking cessation program at their school, then they would be practicing at the community level."

Jaime responded, "Teens at risk for smoking are a vulnerable population within the community, and PHNs work with populations within the community. If the team's goal is to change the smoking behaviors of individual high school students, even if they were part of a group and PHNs carried out some health teaching in the classroom, I guess those actions would be at the individual/family level. This gets kind of confusing at times."

ACTIVITY

Review the public health nursing interventions and examples in Table 2.1.

Which other interventions besides social marketing and health teaching could be used for the smoking cessation program in the high school? Choose two interventions.

Which level of practice would you use with each intervention?

Which members of the interdisciplinary team at the high school could carry out these interventions?

How might the PHN or school nurse work with these team members?

How might their roles and responsibilities be the same or different?

PHNs take a comprehensive approach to dealing with public health problems in the community. They use multiple interventions to achieve primary, secondary, and tertiary prevention goals and, when possible, work with other members of the interdisciplinary team and members of the community. Table 2.2 outlines how primary, secondary, and tertiary interventions might be employed at all three levels of practice to reduce tobacco use in teens (see Chapter 1 for a discussion of primary, secondary, and tertiary prevention).

Table 2.2   Three Levels of PHN Practice and Three Levels of Prevention With Public Health Interventions

Individual/Family Level of Practice		
Primary Prevention	*Secondary Prevention*	*Tertiary Prevention*
Health Teaching • Conduct classroom teaching on the dangers of tobacco use and strategies to avoid it.	**Screening, Case Finding, Referral, and Follow-Up** • Conduct middle school and high school health behaviors screening, including for tobacco use. • Identify students at risk for tobacco use and those already using tobacco. • Refer students who smoke to the school smoking prevention and cessation team. • Follow up with the school nurse.	**Case Management and Collaboration** • The school nurse, physical education teacher, and school psychologist team up to work with teens using tobacco and to monitor and implement a smoking cessation program.

Community Level of Practice

Social Marketing and Outreach
- Staff a teen booth at the county fair and hand out brochures on the hazards of tobacco use and available tobacco prevention and cessation programs.

Screening, Referral, and Follow-up
- Hold health behaviors screening, including tobacco use, for teens and young adults at the county fair.

Case Management and Social Marketing
- Initiate a community-wide campaign on teen tobacco use and prevention.
- Create a social networking site for teens to provide peer support for smoking cessation.

Systems Level of Practice

Health Teaching/Provider Education
- Develop and present a program to teachers and school staff about the hazards of tobacco use and available smoking prevention and cessation programs.

Screening, Referral, and Follow-up
- Develop a health behaviors screening, referral, and follow-up program for middle school and high school students.

Case Management and Collaboration
- Develop a case management protocol for the school smoking prevention and cessation interdisciplinary team.

ACTIVITY

Read the fall prevention case study and answer the following questions.

Who do you think should be members of the task force for fall prevention?

Should interventions be aimed at individuals, communities, or systems?

Should your interventions be at the primary, secondary, or tertiary prevention level or a combination of intervention levels?

Which interventions would the task force be likely to use in developing and implementing the fall prevention program?

Case Study: Fall Prevention Program for the Elderly

Over the last year, the number of elderly patients seen in the Emergency Department (ED) at a local hospital for injuries related to falls increased by 50%. The hospital contacted the local Visiting Nurse Agency and asked staff members to join a task force to develop and implement a fall prevention program for elderly people living in the community. The hospital wanted to reduce the number of elderly patients with fall injuries seen in its ED by 50% over the next year.

Evidence-Based Practice

Public health nursing practice seeks to be evidence-based, which means that the interventions that PHNs use are selected because they have been demonstrated to be effective. Evidence-based practice is a problem-solving approach for clinical practice that includes (a) a systematic search for and critical appraisal of the most relevant evidence to answer a burning clinical question, (b) clinical expertise, and (c) the clients' preferences and values (Keller & Strohschein, 2009; Melnyk & Fineout-Overholt, 2005). The evidence-based practice problem-solving process includes five steps, also known as the "5 As" (Hopp & Rittenmeyer, 2012, pp. 84-88):

- **Ask:** To find the right answer, you need to ask the right question (p. 84).

- **Acquire:** Search for the answer by exploring all levels or evidence.

- **Appraise:** Critically evaluate the evidence and select the "best practice evidence."

- **Apply:** Make the evidence actionable by using the evidence to change your practice.

- **Assess:** Evaluate the outcomes of the change in practice in your clinical setting.

Abby wondered how PHNs knew what to do when they worked with their clients. She said, "The PHNs keep talking about evidence-based practice, but I am not sure exactly what that is."

Jaime responded, "Today, my PHN preceptor and I made a home visit to an elderly woman who lives alone. We did a fall risk assessment and a home safety check. I asked the PHN how she selected which risk assessment and home safety assessment tools to use. She told me that a committee of PHNs reviewed journal articles to find research reports on which assessment tools were effective for determining fall risks in older adults. They also looked at which home safety tools had been developed specifically for frail older adults living at home. Then they piloted the home safety assessment tools themselves and picked the one that best fit what their PHNs needed to know about the home environment. I think this is the way you do evidence-based practice, but I need to read more about it."

Abby commented, "One of the PHNs at my agency went to a fall prevention workshop given by an occupational therapist and a physical therapist at the local hospital. They taught the workshop participants how to screen older adults for fall risk and which types of interventions would help reduce fall risks, such as using assistive devices, installing good lighting, removing slippery rugs, and wearing nonskid slippers. Do you think this information could be considered evidence-based? The two therapists said they were reporting on what they had found worked best with their patients."

Jaime said, "I guess we could review the material on evidence-based practice in our textbooks and then talk more to our PHN preceptors."

"Good idea," said Abby. "Let's do it."

Using interventions that are known to be effective is important. PHNs are accountable to their clients (individuals/families, communities, and systems) and to the public to determine the effectiveness of an intervention and to justify the use of resources. PHNs have carried out research to demonstrate the effectiveness of many interventions provided to individuals, families, and communities. Although research for evidence-based practice might be limited in public health nursing, you should refer to it whenever it exists (Keller & Strohschein, 2009, from Brownson, Baker, Leet, & Gillespie, 2002). Table 2.3 provides examples of interventions that have been found to be effective (Quad Council of Public Health Nursing Organizations, 2007).

Table 2.3   Effectiveness of Selected Public Health Nursing Interventions

Individual/Family Level

Intervention	Results
Health teaching	• Statistically significant increases in the prevention of scald burns (Corrarino, Walsh, & Nadel, 2001)
	• Improved vaccination rates for infants born to women chronically infected with the hepatitis B virus (Corrarino, 2000)
Home visiting by PHNs or PHN-led interdisciplinary teams (Home visiting as an intervention includes the use of multiple interventions such as teaching, counseling, and case management.)	• Reduced child maltreatment reports involving mothers identified as perpetrators of child maltreatment (Eckenrode et al., 2000)
	• 90% of pregnant women with substance abuse problems who were not in treatment entered treatment, and 100% had full-term births (Corrarino et al., 2000)
	• Higher than average prenatal hemoglobin levels and higher rates of breast-feeding (Fetrick, Christensen, & Mitchell, 2003)
	• At-risk families demonstrated significant reductions in postnatal depression screening scores and improvement in parental roles after receiving home-visiting interventions (Armstrong, Fraser, Dadds, & Morris, 1999)
	• Significant increase in the use of primary care providers by indigent mothers as a regular source of sick care and better recall of health education information (Margolis et al., 1996)
Standardized home-visiting programs	• Long-term, sustained improvement in the lives of women and children (Izzo et al., 2005; Kitzman et al., 2010; Olds et al., 2010)
	• A program for building trusting relationships and coaching maternal-infant interaction resulted in improved maternal and child health (Kearney, York, & Deatrick, 2000; Olds et al., 2002)

continues

Table 2.3   Effectiveness of Selected Public Health Nursing
Interventions   (continued)

Case management and teaching	• Interventions to parents of children with asthma resulted in statistically significant cost reductions for hospitalizations and ED visits (Corrarino & Little, 2006)
	• Case management, monitoring, and teaching interventions provided to women covered by Medicaid who were at risk for delivering low-birth-weight infants, resulted in a low-birth-weight rate that was lower than that of commercial enrollees of the same insurer (Milbank Memorial Fund, 1998)
Community Level	
Surveillance	• PHNs collected critical surveillance information for emergency preparedness (Atkins, Williams, Silenas, & Edwards, 2005)
Coalition building	• PHNs developed statewide and local community partnerships and coalitions for influencing policy development and organizational redesign (Padget, Bekemeirer, & Berkowitz, 2004)
Systems Level	
Health teaching	• PHNs demonstrated need for head-lice treatment guidelines and then developed and disseminated them to healthcare providers (Monsen & Keller, 2002)

Source: Excerpted from Quad Council, 2007

Evidence-based practice—and nursing interventions—should be effective and efficient. Before using an intervention, look at the literature or consult with expert PHNs to identify specific interventions that can best meet your clients' unique needs and characteristics. Your own experiences as a nursing student can also guide your choice of which interventions you can carry out effectively:

- Effective interventions fit your client's situation and preferences and result in the desired outcomes.

- Efficient interventions require the least amount of resources and achieve the desired outcomes in the shortest period of time.

Questions you can ask to determine effectiveness and efficiency are listed in Table 2.4.

Table 2.4   Analyzing Effectiveness and Efficiency of Interventions

Determining Intervention Effectiveness	Determining Intervention Efficiency
• Is the intervention culturally and developmentally congruent with the client's status and situation? • Is the intervention acceptable to the client? • Does the outcome of the intervention demonstrate improvement of the client's health status?	• What are the costs of the intervention (money, time, people involved, and other resources) for the PHN, the other members of the health team, the agencies involved, and the client? • Are the costs of implementing the intervention justified by the health benefits for the client and the community?

PHNs need to have effective and efficient methods for collecting and analyzing data on client problems, interventions, and outcomes. The *Omaha System*, a management information system developed specifically for public health nursing, meets this challenge by providing an organized data-classification system that has been used extensively to demonstrate the effectiveness of interventions and provide credible evidence for best practices in public health nursing (Martin, 2005).

You can use several evidence-based practice models to help you in your search for credible evidence. The model we are using in this manual is based on the *Johns Hopkins Nursing Evidence-Based Practice Model* (JHNEBP; Dearholt & Dang, 2012), as it includes the social environmental determinants of systems and communities. The three cornerstones of professional nursing—practice, education, and research—are used as a framework for this model (Figure 2.3):

- **Practice:** Professional nursing practice is the basic component of all nursing activity that reflects what nurses know into what nurses do (Porter-O'Grady, 1984, in Dearholt & Dang, 2012; Dearholt & Dang, 2012, p. 34). The clinical questions and problems that need to be addressed come from nursing practice.

- **Education:** Education involves teaching and learning that results in the acquisition of the knowledge and skills of nursing practice. Education is a life-long process, involving formal and informal experiences.

- **Research:** Nursing research is the process of systematic inquiry that generates new knowledge so that the practice of nursing can be based on scientific evidence. Nursing research focuses on the four domains of nursing: person, environment, health, and nursing.

While research is an umbrella term that refers to all forms of scientific inquiry, it is only one method for generating knowledge for evidence-based practice. This is often confusing. The term *evidence* includes knowledge gleaned from both research and non-research. The levels of evidence at the core of the JHNEBP model include research and nonresearch. You will find examples from all levels of evidence in the remaining chapters of this manual. Although the levels of evidence are presented in a hierarchical manner in Figure 2.3, this illustration does not mean that lower levels of evidence should be discounted or that randomized controlled trials (RCTs) in experimental research should be considered the only credible and most meaningful forms of evidence in public health. It is important to thoughtfully consider and analyze information from all levels of evidence. For example, the use of qualitative research, particularly when studying culture and ethnicity, has led to significant understanding of how diverse populations and people view themselves and the world around them.

Healthy People 2020 identified 11 Leading Health Indicators as priority health concerns, one of which is Nutrition, Physical Activity, and Obesity. Go to the Healthy People 2020 website, click "Leading Health Indicators," and then click "Nutrition, Physical Activity, and Obesity." Read about the most recent data and population disparities on nutrition, physical activity, and obesity. Look for the links to the science-based *Dietary Guidelines for Americans* and the *Physical Activity Guidelines.* What evidence do you find that supports a healthy eating and physical activity program for you and your family?

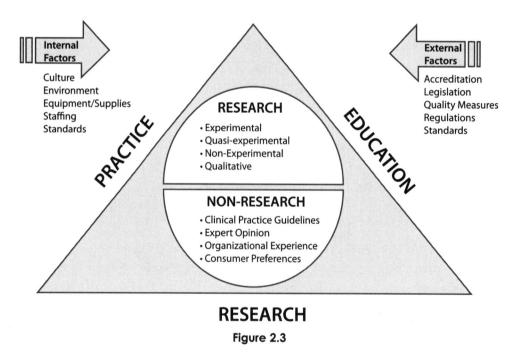

RESEARCH

Figure 2.3

Source: Dearholt & Dang, 2012, p. 34. Levels of evidence: Adapted from Johns Hopkins Nursing Evidence-Based Practice Model and Guidelines (Newhouse, Dearholt, Poe, Pugh, & White, 2007).

Just because "best practice" evidence is available does not mean that it will be adopted and used. Stephanie Poe and Kathleen White (2010) state that a strategic plan to develop the organizational infrastructure for evidence-based practice is necessary. Internal and external factors influence the successful implementation of evidence-based practice within an organization (Dearholt & Dang, 2012). The internal factors necessary to successfully institute evidence-based practice in an organization include:

- A culture that believes evidence-based practice will lead to optimal patient outcomes;
- Strong leadership support at all levels, with the necessary resource allocation to sustain the process; and
- Clear expectations that incorporate evidence-based practice into standards and job descriptions (Dearholt & Dang, 2012, p. 41).

Internal factors that have been identified as major barriers to the implementation of evidence-based practice include:

- Too much information available;
- Lack of time to review and analyze information;
- Practice constraints;
- Lack of infrastructure, leadership, and communication;
- Lack of incentives or rewards; and
- Nurses who lack the needed skills, knowledge, and confidence (Dearholt & Dang, 2012; Walsh, 2010).

Evidence of a supportive organizational environment includes:

- Access to nursing reference books and the Internet at staff workstations;
- Journals available in hard copy or online;
- A medical/nursing library;
- Knowledgeable library personnel to support staff and assist with evidence searches;
- Other resources for evidence-based practice; and
- Supportive leadership (Dearholt & Dang, 2012, pp. 176–177).

ACTIVITY

Explore the evidence-based practice infrastructure at your clinical agency. What are the facilitators and barriers for it in your clinical agency? Does your agency currently demonstrate any evidence-based practice activities? Which "best practice" examples are being used to justify changes in practice? How is your preceptor involved in this process?

This chapter presents an overview of evidence-based practice relevant to public health nursing practice. The term "best practices" is often used synonymously with evidence-based practice. However, they have different meanings. "Best practices" refers to using the best evidence available to provide the best care possible. A few points will be helpful to keep in mind as you think about and use evidence of "best practices" in your community health clinical:

- Experimental research using RCTs are considered unethical when placing an individual in the control group denies that individual treatment or interventions that have already been demonstrated to be effective.

- Public health/community health nursing agencies may be carrying out quasi- and nonexperimental research to determine the effectiveness of their programs and interventions. These activities may be a component of their ongoing quality improvement programs. Sometimes students participate in these research studies. If you are asked to participate, ask to see any informed consent or ethical guidelines that your agency is using.

- The policies and procedures of your public health/community agency and the professional practice standards guiding PHN practice may be considered clinical guidelines. Progress reports and annual agency reports may be considered organizational experiences.

- The knowledge and experiences of your preceptor and other PHN agency staff will be reflected in the practice you observe and the mentoring you receive. These represent expert opinions and clinical expertise.

- Clinical experiences may include both participant and nonparticipant observation. When you reflect on your observations of your preceptor or other public health/community health nurses interacting with clients by using PHN interventions, you are demonstrating nonparticipant observation. When you use these interventions yourself and reflect on your practice, you are demonstrating participant observation. Both types of experiences add to your clinical expertise.

- Community assessments that are carried out in collaboration with community members and client satisfaction surveys provide evidence of consumer preferences. See Chapter 3, Competency 1, for information on community assessments.

Table 2.5 provides some examples of best practices for public health nursing.

Table 2.5   Examples of Best Practices in Public Health Nursing by Level of Evidence

---

Level I: Experimental Research (Randomized Controlled Trial): The Nurse Family Partnership involving intensive structured home visiting by PHNs reduces repeat childbirths, improves the stability of partner relationships, facilitates children's academic adjustment to elementary school, and reduces childhood mortality from preventable causes (Kitzman et al., 2010; Olds, et al., 2004; Olds et al., 2010).

Level I: Systematic Reviews of RCTs: Professional organizations publish systematic reviews of medical and nursing research, such as *The Cochrane Database of Systematic Reviews*, published online by the Cochrane Collaboration, and *Worldviews on Evidence-Based Nursing*, a peer-reviewed journal published by Sigma Theta Tau International (Newhouse et al., 2007). The Joanna Briggs Institute provides an online listing of systematic reviews and meta-analysis specific to nursing practice. Systematic reviews of non-RCT research may be either Level II or Level III evidence.

Level II: Research—Quasi-Experimental: An educational program to improve the nutrition of homeless children living in a family homeless shelter improved mothers' nutritional knowledge, but this information did not result in mothers' being able to make changes in their children's nutrition, because the cafeteria food did not change (Yousey, Leake, Wdowik, & Janken, 2007).

Level III: Nonexperimental Descriptive Research: Disparities in TB risk factors and treatment outcomes between correctional inmate and noninmate populations were identified through analysis of national TB surveillance data. Inmates were found to have a higher rate of TB than noninmates and were less likely to complete treatment (MacNeil, Lobato, & Moore, 2005).

Level III: Nonexperimental Qualitative Research: Knowledge of community resources, sharing information, and support of colleagues were identified as increasing outreach effectiveness. Lack of knowledge about resources, not understanding the value of community assessment in identifying resources, and not understanding the intervention of outreach were identified as barriers to outreach (Tembreull & Schaffer, 2005).

Level IV: Clinical Practice Guidelines: The Centers for Disease Control and Prevention (CDC) has published immunization guidelines based on systematic reviews of the evidence (n.d.).

Level V: Expert Opinion and Organizational Experience: The ANA, the American Public Health Association (APHA), the Association of Community Health Nurse Educators (ACHNE), and the Association of State and Territorial Health Officials (ASTHO) are professional organizations that provide expert advice in public health and public health nursing. These associations also publish practice guidelines for nursing and public health.

You may be wondering whether there is a difference between research, evidence-based practice, and quality improvement. As all three processes overlap to some extent, this distinction is often confusing. Table 2.6 uses examples of breastfeeding studies to differentiate these three processes.

Table 2.6 Comparison of Evidence-Based Practice, Research, and Quality Improvement

Definitions	Examples
Research: *A systematic investigation that seeks to identify and generate new knowledge or contribute to existing knowledge. Research may study the client population, the nursing phenomena, diseases, and treatment or intervention outcomes.*	Research: *A descriptive study identified four significant predictors of breastfeeding attitudes: age, gender, number of breastfeeding observations in childhood, and breastfeeding beliefs (Vari et al., 2013).*

continues

Table 2.6   Comparison of Evidence-Based Practice, Research, and Quality Improvement   (continued)

Definitions	Examples
Evidence-based practice: *A life-long problem-solving approach to clinical decision-making involving a clinical question that is answered by researching "best practice" evidence, applying the evidence to practice, and evaluating outcomes. This activity's goal is to improve practice by moving existing knowledge into daily practice, not to generate new knowledge.*	Evidence-based practice: *A systematic review using CINAHL, PubMed, and Cochrane Library databases identified barriers to breastfeeding in the WIC population to make recommendations for guidelines for WIC clients (Hedberg, 2013). Evidence-based recommendations for public health to promote and support breastfeeding incorporated the views of professional and community stakeholders (Renfrew et al., 2008).*
Quality Improvement: *An ongoing process by individuals within an organization to improve systems, processes, and outcomes. This process measures change over time with the implementation of new or revised systems, processes, and interventions.*	Quality Improvement: *A breastfeeding program in a Korean community health center was evaluated using pre- and post-test rates of breastfeeding after staff training and an educational intervention were initiated (Kang, Son, Hyun, & Kim, 2005).* *The Best Start area-based intervention for increasing breastfeeding rates found that area-based interventions were effective and that quality community partnerships also had a positive influence on breastfeeding rates (Kelaher, Dunt, Feldman, Nolan, & Raban, 2009).*

Source: Based on Dearholt & Dang, 2012; Schaffer, Sandau, & Diedrick, 2012

Database and Internet Searches

The sources of evidence must be as credible as the evidence itself. That is why we search scientific databases. The online databases that provide the most relevant journal articles for nursing are CINAHL and PubMed. CINAHL is a proprietary database hosted by EBSCO, which means it is privately owned and available to members of subscribing institutions who pay a fee for remote access. PubMed is an open-source database and free to the public. Other credible sources include websites maintained by professional organizations and service providers and governmental websites, such as those run by the National Institutes of Health (NIH), the U.S. Surgeon General, and the CDC. The Cochrane Library is an international database of systematic reviews owned by the Cochrane Collaboration and is an open-source database that is free to use. The CDC Stacks, an excellent source for public health information, is a free digital repository of publications produced by the CDC.

The NIH provides guidelines for evaluating web-based health resources that will help you determine whether the website resource you have found is credible. One example of a credible website is a government program that reviews maternal-child health home-visiting program effectiveness, called *Home Visiting Evidence of Effectiveness (HOMVEE)*. Discussion of models and programs, whether they meet Department of Health and Human Services (DHHS) criteria, their target populations, and whether research shows positive effectiveness is found at the HOMVEE website.

See the Resource List for the website URLs.

Evidence of Best Practices

PHNs need to be critical consumers of public health and nursing research. They must use a deliberative problem-solving approach when making decisions about which evidence in the literature is strong enough to support a change in practice (Poe & White, 2010).

Much of the evidence for effective public health nursing comes from Evidence-Based Practice Levels III, IV, and V. It is often not ethical, possible, or practical to randomly place people in an experimental or a control group, especially if placement in either group could possibly have a negative effect on an individual's health or well-being. An increasing body of qualitative research in public health nursing exists. Understanding the context of the family, culture, and community; the meaning of events; and the impact of these factors on the clients' health behaviors and health status is often best achieved through the use of qualitative research methods. Public health nurses also learn a great deal from their practice experiences and those of their colleagues. Case study examples can be found in the literature, shared at professional conferences, or reported on the Internet. These anecdotal reports are also part of the practice evidence of public health nursing.

When you explore the scientific literature for best practice evidence, it is helpful to first identify your clinical question so that you are focused in your search. One helpful way to frame your clinical practice question is to use the PICOT approach by identifying the patient population (P), the intervention of interest (I), the comparison intervention (C), the outcome (O), and the timeframe (T) (Stillwell, Fineout-Overholt, Melnyk, & Williamson, 2010). For example, if you wanted to research the effectiveness of teaching parents about the "Back to Sleep" program to reduce the risk of Sudden Infant Death (SIDS), you might frame your PICOT question as outlined in Table 2.7.

Table 2.7   The PICOT Approach to Clinical Problem Solving

PICOT Question Elements	Examples
P = Patient population I = Intervention of interest C = Comparison intervention of interest O = Outcome(s) of interest T = Time it takes the intervention to achieve outcomes	P = Infants at risk for SIDS I = Teach parents to place infants on backs to sleep using "Back to Sleep" program C = No purposeful teaching about safe sleeping position of infants O = Percentage of babies sleeping on back T = Evaluate at 6 weeks and 3 months

PICOT Question: Will infants (P) whose parents are taught to place them on their backs to sleep using a "Back to Sleep" program (I), as opposed to infants whose parents received no purposeful teaching about safe sleeping positions for their infants (C), have a higher rate of sleeping on their backs than infants in control group (O) at 6 weeks and 3 months after receiving intervention (T)?

The "T" in PICOT may not be necessary to include when reviewing the literature, but it may be helpful to include "T" when you plan how and when you are going to evaluate the outcome of the intervention you have selected to implement in your clinical setting. Once you find a set of articles that report on the effectiveness of the intervention you are interested in, it is time to review them to determine their usefulness.

You may find it useful to conduct a rapid critical appraisal of the literature. A critical appraisal of the literature is a systematic process you can use to examine and synthesize the research data presented in an article or a group of articles (Fineout-Overholt et al., 2010). Generally, each article is reviewed, all the articles are compared and contrasted, and best practice evidence is identified based on the rigor and appropriateness of the literature. For each article you review, ask a few questions to complete a rapid appraisal. Table 2.8 includes questions that may be used for both research and nonresearch studies.

The next step is to compare and contrast the studies and reports you have appraised. Select the best studies or reports with the most credible evidence that fit your clinical situation and address your specific question. Then develop a set of recommendations for action based on the evidence.

PHNs in a county health department effectively used this critical appraisal process to develop a set of guidelines for pediculosis management-based best practices (Monsen & Keller, 2002).

Table 2.8   Critical Appraisal of the Literature Questions for Articles and Other Publications

Research-Based Literature	Non-Research-Based Literature
• Which type of research is presented?	• Which type of report is presented?
• What is the level of evidence of the research?	• What is the level of evidence?
• What is the purpose of the research?	• What is the purpose of this project?
• Who are the subjects of the research?	• Who are the subjects of this project?
• Is the purpose of the research clear?	• Is the purpose of the project clear?
• Are the research questions stated?	• Which question or concern is the author addressing?
• Are the research methods explained, and do they address the research questions?	• Are the project components explained, and do they address the questions or concerns?
• Are the results of the research presented in an understandable manner?	• Are the results of the project presented in an understandable manner?
• Are ethical guidelines addressed?	• Are any ethical issues addressed?
• Are the strengths and limitations of the research discussed?	• Are strengths and limitations of the project addressed?
• Are the recommendations made based on the findings of the study?	• Are recommendations made on the basis of the project?
• How useful are the study outcomes and recommendations to your clinical practice?	• How useful are the project outcomes and recommendations to your clinical practice?

Source: Based on work by Fineout-Overholt, Melnyk, Stillwell, & Williamson, 2010

Evidence Example: Best Practice Evidence Leads to Pediculosis Management Guidelines

Public health nurses in a county health department collaborated with epidemiologists, nursing students, and faculty to design and implement an effective population-based pediculosis management project. The focus of the project was the development of pediculosis treatment and prevention guidelines based on recognized best practices that were acceptable to both epidemiologists and practicing public health nurses. Guideline strategies had to meet two criteria: They had to be based on the life cycle of the louse, and they had to help reduce the barriers that families experienced in carrying out lice prevention and control measures. PHNs disseminated these guidelines to community providers and reinforced their use through consultation and educational sessions. Two critical changes occurred as a result of the project: First, community providers significantly changed their recommendations for the treatment of pediculosis after nursing intervention; and second, PHNs increased their population-based practice skills, continued to use those skills to address pediculosis, and extended those skills to additional population-based initiatives (Monsen & Keller, 2002, p. 201).

ACTIVITY

With your PHN preceptor, choose an intervention that the staff would like to have researched to identify any new best practice recommendations.

Look for evidence of best practices for the intervention you selected in the literature, analyze the evidence, and select the evidence you will use as potential best practices. Follow these steps:

- Determine which databases to use in your search.
- Carry out your literature search. Obtain help from the reference librarian if you are having difficulty with your keyword search.
- Select three to five journal articles to review. You may use articles that represent different levels of evidence.
- Carry out a rapid critical appraisal of each article.
- Compare and contrast the articles you have appraised. Are their findings and recommendations similar or different?
- Identify the articles that have the most credible evidence that best fits your clinical situation.

Translating Evidence Into Practice

One of the most difficult skills is knowing how to initiate the evidence-based practice process in a clinical setting. It is time to return to the "5 As" discussed earlier in the chapter (Hopp & Rittenmeyer, 2012): Ask, acquire, appraise, apply, and assess. Once you have completed the first three steps and have identified a best practice intervention, begin translating or applying the evidence into your clinical practice. Before you implement a change in your practice, you need to think about how you will evaluate the effectiveness of the change. Identify the outcome you would like to achieve.

Consider the PICOT question presented earlier: Will infants (P) whose parents are taught to place them on their backs to sleep using a "Back to Sleep" program (I), as opposed to infants whose parents received no purposeful teaching about safe sleeping positions for their infants (C), have a higher rate of sleeping on their backs than infants in control group (O) at 6 weeks and 3 months after receiving intervention (T)?

Think about how you would present your findings to your preceptor or clinical agency. Which recommendations would you make?

ACTIVITY

Use evidence-based practice in your public health nursing clinical. To find best practice evidence and think about how you might translate this evidence into practice, create a PICOT question. It might be helpful to outline the PICOT components first and then write your PICOT question. Remember that you are asking an evidence-based practice clinical question about an intervention, not a research question.

In Summary

PHNs need to make sure that their recommendations for change in practice are based on the best evidence and are appropriate and feasible for their client populations, their agencies, and their communities. Support and funding for PHN practice depends on documentation and dissemination of evidence that PHN practice makes a positive difference in the health of their communities. The example in Table 2.9 demonstrates the deliberative process one agency used to research and implement best practice interventions.

Table 2.9 Case Study: MVNA Evidence-Based Practice in Maternal/Child Health Home Visiting

Maternal-child health staff members of the MVNA (previously known as Minnesota Visiting Nurse Agency) wanted to improve the client outcomes for mothers and babies.

ASK: They asked, "What are the best practices for PHN home visiting to pregnant and parenting moms and their children that we are not already using?"

ACQUIRE: When they began to seriously consider implementing an evidence-based program, the Nurse Family Partnership (NFP) was the logical choice, as the MVNA was already using components of the model in its Pregnant and Parenting Teen Program. Staff members looked for research that compared long-term home-visiting models, including the NFP and Healthy Families America (HFA), for fidelity, impact, long-term outcomes, and cost. They also accessed the DHHS HOMVEE website, which publishes comparative data about evidence-based programs and those that meet its funding criteria; the HFA and the NFP both met these requirements. Staff at the MVNA also consulted with NFP and HFA national program experts and staff at the Minnesota Department of Health whose job is to support evidence-based programs in Minnesota.

APPRAISE: The MVNA focused on two programs that provided well-researched evidence of the efficacy of their maternal/child health programs.

Nurse Family Partnership (NFP): NFP, developed by Dr. David Olds (Kitzman et al., 2010; Olds et al., 2007; Olds et al., 2010), is a public health nursing home-visiting program based on more than 30 years of evidence from RCTs that demonstrate positive outcomes for young mothers and their children. The NFP provides PHN home visits to first-time pregnant young and at-risk women living in poverty, starting by the 28th week of pregnancy and continuing until the child is 2 years old. The NFP home-visiting model is client centered, building on the strengths of each family while delivering a comprehensive curriculum during pregnancy, infancy, and the toddler years. Because of their specialized knowledge, PHNs are able to establish trusting relationships and provide guidance and support for the emotional, social, and physical challenges these first-time moms face. The PHN home visitors make measurable, long-term differences in the lives of these families, including significant reductions in the areas of (a) substantiated child abuse and neglect, (b) arrests among the children, (c) convictions of mothers, (d) Emergency Department visits for childhood accidents and poisonings, and (e) behavioral and intellectual problems among children (according to data from NFP 15-year follow-up, more than 12 years after visits ended).

continues

Table 2.9   Case Study: MVNA Evidence-Based Practice in Maternal/Child Health Home Visiting   (continued)

Healthy Families America (HFA): HVA is a nationally recognized evidence-based home-visiting model designed to work with overburdened families who are at risk for adverse childhood experiences, including child maltreatment (Caldera et al., 2007). This program has been evaluated by HOMVEE and meets DHHS criteria for an "evidence-based early childhood home visiting service delivery model" (HOMVEE, n.d.). This home-visiting model is equipped to work with families who may have histories of trauma, intimate partner violence, and mental health and/or substance abuse issues. HFA home-visiting services begin prenatally or right after the birth of a baby and are offered voluntarily, intensively, and over the long-term (3 to 5 years after the birth of the baby). Home visitors use a curriculum (MVNA uses Growing Great Kids) as one means to provide guidance, information, and support to help parents to be the best parents they can be. The HFA is not exclusively a PHN home-visiting model.

APPLY: The MVNA staff members' appraisal of the published research, the HOMVEE comparative studies, expert consultations, and their own clinical experience using components of the NFP model convinced them to adopt both the NFP and the HFA models. The decision to implement the HFA was driven not only by the evidence but also a need to have an evidence-based program that could serve a slightly different population than the NFP, allowing the MVNA to offer evidence-based programming to mothers who are not first-time parents and do not necessarily enter the program early in their pregnancies. In addition, as part of the Affordable Care Act, federal monies were set aside to support evidence-based home visiting for young, low-income families. The MVNA created the Pregnant and Parenting Teen Program (PPTP) in 2000 that included four program pillars: (1) trusting relationship between teen mothers and PHNs through home visits; (2) outreach and coordination with schools, hospitals, clinics, and human service agencies; (3) a comprehensive and intensive maternal mental health curriculum; and (4) community support and caring through the provision of essential items needed for success in parenting (Schaffer, Goodhue, Stennes, & Lanigan, 2012, p. 218). The PPTP now includes both the accredited NFP and HFA programs.

ASSESS: The MVNA has not had the NFP and HFA programs in place long enough to identify any long-term outcomes separate from the outcomes it had already measured for the teens served at MVNA, but staffers are continually monitoring the models for fidelity. The agency's NFP data are inputted into the NFP national database, and the MVNA regularly receives feedback that compares its statistics with those of other NFP sites. In general, the agency compares well. The HFA does not offer the same opportunity for analysis, but the State of Minnesota is collecting data from all sites that have implemented the HFA and NFP models with money from the Affordable Care Act. This data collection is only 1 year old, and the data have not been released. However, PPTP outcome data collected from 2008 to 2010 has demonstrated progress toward goal achievement.

Sources: Lanigan, 2013; Schaffer, Sandau, & Diedrick, 2012

ACTIVITY

Think about an intervention you used to help a client achieve a specific outcome.

Evaluate the effectiveness of your intervention.

Did your client achieve the desired behavioral outcome?

Was your client satisfied with the outcome?

How did your intervention and client outcome compare with the evidence you found in the literature?

If your client did not achieve the behavioral outcome or the client's outcomes were inconsistent with best practices, review the best practice literature again. Look at all levels of evidence available. Consider consulting with a clinical expert.

If you follow through on these steps, you will be practicing nursing from an evidence-based practice framework. As a professional, you will be accountable for your own nursing practice, so you need to be aware of and use best practices. You will find that this manual presents many levels of evidence to justify using specific interventions.

Jaime commented, "I think I am going to do my intervention paper on ways to reduce smoking in high school students. I have to start looking for evidence-based practice articles. I wonder how I should go about that."

Abby said, "I have been working with the college reference librarian to research my topic. She suggested that I use three databases: CINAHL, PubMed, and the Cochrane Database of Systematic Reviews. I have found a few good articles in each database."

Jaime responded, "Great! I will try those databases, too! I know that both PubMed and the Cochrane Database are in the public domain and free to users. CINAHL is privately owned, and organizations have to pay for employees to use it. I don't think my hospital has a contract to access CINAHL."

Abby concluded, "Don't forget to write your PICOT question first!"

Key Points

- The public health nursing process guides the PHN's actions.

- PHNs work at all three levels of practice (individual/family, community, and systems).

- PHNs carry out 17 interventions unique to public health nursing; 16 of these interventions are practiced independently as part of professional nursing practice.

- Public health nursing practice is evidence-based.

- Evidence-based practice is a deliberative process starting with a practice question, followed by an appraisal of the evidence, and then a change in practice based on credible evidence. Remember the "5 As."

Reflective Practice

1. What do you think are the major differences between the nursing process and the public health nursing process?

   a. What will you do differently when following the public health nursing process?

   b. How will you prepare for this difference?

   _____

   _____

   _____

2. Which other disciplines will you work with most often in your public health clinical?

   a. What additional information do you need to know about the other health disciplines?

   b. How will you find out the information that you need?

   _____

   _____

   _____

3. Which public health nursing interventions have you used in previous clinical experiences?

    a. How will you carry out these interventions in your public health clinical?

    b. How will this experience be the same or different from what you have done before?

_____

_____

_____

4. Have you used an evidence-based practice approach in other nursing clinical experiences?

    a. What have you learned in reading this chapter that you did not know before?

    b. How will your past experiences and your new knowledge help you practice evidence-based public health nursing?

_____

_____

_____

5. Which types of best practice evidence related to a PHN intervention would you like to explore?

    a. What is your PICOT question?

_____

_____

_____

6. Refer to the Cornerstones of Public Health Nursing in Chapter 1. Which of the Cornerstones support the use of evidence-based practice in public health nursing?

_____

_____

_____

References

American Nurses Association. (2013). *Public health nursing: Scope and standards of practice.* Silver Spring, MD: Nursesbooks.org.

Armstrong, K. L., Fraser, J. A., Dadds, M. R., & Morris J. (1999). A randomized, controlled trial of nurse home visiting to vulnerable families with newborns. *Journal of Paediatrics and Child Health, 35*(3), 237–244.

Atkins, R. B., Williams, J. R., Silenas, R., & Edwards, J. C. (2005). The role of PHNs in bioterrorism preparedness. *Disaster Management Response, 3*(4), 98–105.

Brownson, R. C., Baker, E. A., Leet, T. L., & Gillespie, K. N. (Eds.). (2002). *Evidence-based public health.* New York, NY: Oxford University Press.

Caldera, D., Burrell, L., Rodriguez, K., Crowne, S. S., Rohde, C., & Duggan, A. (2007). Impact of a statewide home visiting program on parenting and on child health and development. *Child Abuse & Neglect, 31*(8), 829–852. doi:10.1016/j.chiabu.2007.02.008

Centers for Disease Control and Prevention. (n.d.). *Vaccines and immunizations.* Retrieved from http://www.cdc.gov/vaccines/

Corrarino, J. E. (2000). *Lessons learned: Successful strategies to implement a perinatal hepatitis B program.* Centers for Disease Control and Prevention Annual Hepatitis B Conference. San Diego, CA.

Corrarino, J. E., & Little, A. (2006). *Breathing easy: A public health nursing/community coalition success story.* American Public Health Association. 128th Annual Meeting. Boston, MA.

Corrarino, J. E., Walsh, P. J., & Nadel, E. (2001). Does teaching scald burn prevention to families of young children make a difference? A pilot study. *Journal of Pediatric Nursing, 16*(4), 256–262.

Corrarino, J. E., Williams, C., Campbell, W. S., 3rd, Amrhein, E., LoPiano, L., & Kalachik, D. (2000). Linking substance-abusing pregnant women to drug treatment services: A pilot program. *Journal of Obstetric, Gynecologic, and Neonatal Nurses, 29*(4), 369–376.

Dearholt, S. L., & Dang, D. (2012). *Johns Hopkins nursing evidence-based practice: Model and guidelines, 2nd ed.* Indianapolis, IN: Sigma Theta Tau International.

Eckenrode, J., GanzeI, B., Henderson, C. R., Jr., Smith, E., Olds, D. L., Powers, J., . . . Sidora, K. (2000). Preventing child abuse and neglect with a program of nurse home visitation: The limiting effects of domestic violence. *JAMA, 284*(11), 1385–1391.

Fetrick, A., Christensen, M., & Mitchell, C. (2003). Does public health nurse home visitation make a difference in the health outcomes of pregnant clients and their offspring? *Public Health Nursing, 20*(3), 184–189.

Fineout-Overholt, E., Melnyk, B. M., Stillwell, S., & Williamson, K. (2010). Critical appraisal of the evidence: Part I. *American Journal of Nursing, 110*(7), 47–52.

Hedberg, I. G. (2013). Barriers to breastfeeding in the WIC population. *American Journal of Maternal Child Health Nursing, 38*(4), 244–249. doi:10.1097/NMC.0b013e3182836ca2

Home Visiting Evidence of Effectiveness. (n.d.). *Healthy Families America: Evidence of program model effectiveness.* Retrieved from http://homvee.acf.hhs.gov/document.aspx?sid=10&rid=1&mid=1

Hopp, L., & Rittenmeyer, L. (2012). *Introduction to evidence-based practice: A practical guide for nursing.* Philadelphia, PA: F. A. Davis.

Izzo, C. V., Eckenrode, J. J., Smith, E. G., Henderson, C. R., Cole, R., Kitzman, H., & Olds, D. L. (2005). Reducing the impact of uncontrollable stressful life events through a program of nurse home visitation for new parents. *Prevention Science, 6*(4), 269–274.

Kang, N., Song, Y., Hyun, T. H., & Kim, K. (2005). Evaluation of the breastfeeding intervention program in a Korean community health center. *International Journal of Nursing, 42,* 409–413. doi:10.1016/j.ijnurstu.2004.08.003

Kearney, M. H., York, R., & Deatrick, J. A. (2000). Effects of home visits to vulnerable young families. *Journal of Nursing Scholarship, 32*(4), 369–376.

Kelaher, M., Dunt, D., Feldman, P., Nolan, A., & Raban, B. (2009). The effect of an area-based intervention on breastfeeding rates in Victoria, Australia. *Health Policy, 90,* 89–93.

Keller, L. O., & Strohschein, S. (2009, April). *E₂ evidence exchange: Your public health nursing e-source.* Public Health Nursing Faculty Conference. Otsego, MN.

Keller, L., Strohschein, S., Lia-Hoagberg, B., & Schaffer, M. (1998). Population-based public health nursing interventions: A model for practice. *Public Health Nursing, 15*(3), 207–215.

Keller, L., Strohschein, S., Lia-Hoagberg, B., & Schaffer, M. (2004). Population-based public health interventions: Practice-based and evidence-supported. *Public Health Nursing, 21*(5), 453–468.

Kitzman, H. J., Olds, D. L., Cole, R. E., Hanks, C. A., Anson, E. A., Arcoleo, K. J., . . . Holmberg, J. R. (2010). Enduring effects of prenatal and infancy home visiting by nurses on children: follow-up of a randomized trial among children at age 12 years. *Archives of Pediatrics & Adolescent Medicine, 164*(5): 412–418. doi:10.1001/archpediatrics.2010.76.

Lanigan, C. (2013). *Case Study: MVNA Evidence-Based Practice in Maternal/Child Health Home Visiting.* Unpublished manuscript for MVNA, Minneapolis, MN.

MacNeil, J., Lobato, M., & Moore, M. (2005). An unanswered health disparity: Tuberculosis among correctional inmates, 1993 through 2003. *American Journal of Public Health, 95*(10), 1800–1805.

Margolis, P. A., Lannon, C. M., Stevens, R., Harlan, C., Bordley, W. C., Carey, T., . . . Earp, J. L. (1996). Linking clinical and public health approaches to improve access to healthcare for socially disadvantaged mothers and children. A feasibility study. *Archives of Pediatric & Adolescent Medicine, 150*(8), 815–821.

Martin, K. S. (2005). *The Omaha System: A key to practice, documentation, and information management, 2nd ed.* Omaha, NE: Health Connections Press.

Melnyk, B. M., & Fineout-Overholt, E. (Eds.). (2005). *Evidence-based practice in nursing and healthcare: A guide to best practice, 1st ed.* Philadelphia, PA: Lippincott Williams and Wilkins.

Milbank Memorial Fund. (1998). *Partners in community health: Working together for a healthy New York.* New York, NY: Milbank Memorial Fund.

Minnesota Department of Health, Center for Public Health Nursing. (2001). *Public health interventions.* St. Paul, MN: Author. Retrieved from http://www.health.state.mn.us/divs/cfh/ophp/resources/docs/wheelbw.pdf

Minnesota Department of Health, Center for Public Health Nursing. (2003). *The nursing process applied to population-based public health nursing practice.* St. Paul, MN: Author. Retrieved from http://www.health.state.mn.us/divs/cfh/ophp/resources/docs/nursing_process.pdf

Monsen, K., & Keller, L. O. (2002). A population-based approach to pediculosis management. *Public Health Nursing, 19*(3), 201–208.

Newhouse, R. P., Dearholt, S. L., Poe, S. P., Pugh, L. C., & White, K. M. (2007). *Johns Hopkins evidence-based practice model and guidelines.* Indianapolis, IN: Sigma Theta Tau International.

Olds D. L., Kitzman, H. J., Cole, R. E., Hanks, C. A., Arcoleo, K. J., Anson, E. A., . . . Stevenson, A. J. (2010). Enduring effects of prenatal and infancy home visiting by nurses on maternal life course and government spending: Follow-up of a randomized trial among children at age 12 years. *Archives of Pediatrics & Adolescent Medicine, 164*(5): 419–424. doi:10.1001/archpediatrics.2010.49

Olds, D. L., Kitzman, H., Cole, R., Robinson, J., Sidora, K., Luckey, D. W., . . . Holmberg, J. (2004). Effects of nurse home-visiting on maternal life course and child development: Age 6 follow-up results of a randomized trial. *Pediatrics, 114*(6), 1550–1559.

Olds, D., Kitzman, H., Hanks, C., Cole, R., Anson, E., Sidora-Arcoleo, K., . . . Bondy, J. (2007). Effects of nurse home visiting on maternal and child functioning: Age 9 follow-up of a randomized trial. *Pediatrics, 120,* e832–e845, 2006–2111.

Olds, D. L., Robinson, J., O'Brien, R., Luckey, D. W., Pettitt, L. M., Henderson, C. R., Jr., . . . Talmi, A. (2002). Home visiting by paraprofessionals and by nurses: A randomized, controlled trial. *Pediatrics, 110*(3), 486–496.

Padget, S. M., Bekemeirer, B., & Berkowitz, B. (2004). Collaborative partnerships at the state level: Promoting systems changes in public health infrastructure. *Journal of Public Health Management Practice, 10*(3), 251–257.

Poe, S. S., & White, K. K. (2010). *Johns Hopkins nursing evidence-based practice: Implementation and translation.* Indianapolis, IN: Sigma Theta Tau International.

Porter-O'Grady, T. (1984). *Shared governance for nursing: A creative approach to professional accountability.* Rockville, MD: Aspen Systems Corporation.

Quad Council of Public Health Nursing Organizations. (2007, February). The public health nursing shortage: A threat to the public's health. Endorsed by the Quad Council of Public Health Nursing Organizations, American Nurses Association, Congress on Nursing Practice & Economics.

Renfrew, M. J., Dyson, L., Herbert, B., McFadden, A., McCormick, F., Thomas, J., & Spiby, H. (2008). Developing evidence-based recommendations in public health—Incorporating the views of practitioners, service users, and user representatives. *Health Expectations, 11,* 3–15. doi:10.1111/j.1369-7625.2007.00471.x

Schaffer, M. A., Goodhue, A., Stennes, K., & Lanigan, C. (2012). Evaluation of a public health nurse visiting program for pregnant and parenting teens. *Public Health Nursing, 29*(3), 218–231. doi:10.1111/j.1525-1446.2011.01005.x

Schaffer, M. A., Sandau, K. E., & Diedrick, L. (2012). Evidence-based practice models for organizational change: Overview and practice applications. *Journal of Advanced Nursing, 69*(5),1197–1209. doi:10.1111/j.1365-2648.2012.06122.x

Stillwell, S. B., Fineout-Overholt, E., Melnyk, B. M., & Williamson, K. M. (2010). Evidence-based practice: Step by step. *American Journal of Nursing, 110*(5), 41–47.

Tembreull, C., & Schaffer, M. (2005). The intervention of outreach: Best practices. *Public Health Nursing 22*(4), 347–353.

Vari, P., Vogeltanz-Holm, N., Olsen, G., Anderson, C., Holm, J., Peterson, H., & Henly, S. (2013). Community breastfeeding attitudes and beliefs. *Healthcare for Women International, 34*(7), 592–606. doi:10.1080/07399332.2012.655391

Walsh, N. (2010). Dissemination of evidence into practice: Opportunities and threats. *Primary Healthcare, 20*(3), 26–30.

Yousey, Y., Leake, J., Wdowik, M., & Janken, J. (2007). Education in a homeless shelter to improve the nutrition of young children. *Public Health Nursing, 24*(3), 249–255.

ENTRY-LEVEL POPULATION-BASED PUBLIC HEALTH NURSING COMPETENCIES

COMPETENCY #1:
Applies the Public Health Nursing Process to Communities, Systems, Individuals, and Families

3

Patricia M. Schoon
with Karen S. Martin, Noreen Kleinfehn-Wald, and Cheryl H. Lanigan

Cherise and Zack were listening to Shannon, their public health nurse (PHN) preceptor, tell them about the clients they were about to visit for the first time. Shannon told them about the halfway home for young adults with emotional and behavioral disorders. This home has 25 residents, ages 18 to 25, who live in congregate housing, sharing housekeeping, laundry, and cooking duties. The residents have been admitted from hospitals, chemical dependency treatment centers, local jails, homeless shelters, and homes where family caretakers had become overwhelmed. Cherise was assigned to work with a young woman who had been admitted from a homeless shelter the previous weekend. Cherise asked, "How will I do a family assessment when I don't know anything about my client's family? She doesn't even live with them! Her family is still living at the homeless shelter."

Zack responded, "I am more concerned about the community assessment we have to do for the halfway house. Is a halfway house a community? I am confused."

Cherise said, "Well, I guess the first thing we do is go and visit with them. We need to get them to trust us if we are to help them. Then we can look around and figure out whether they are a community, a population, or both!"

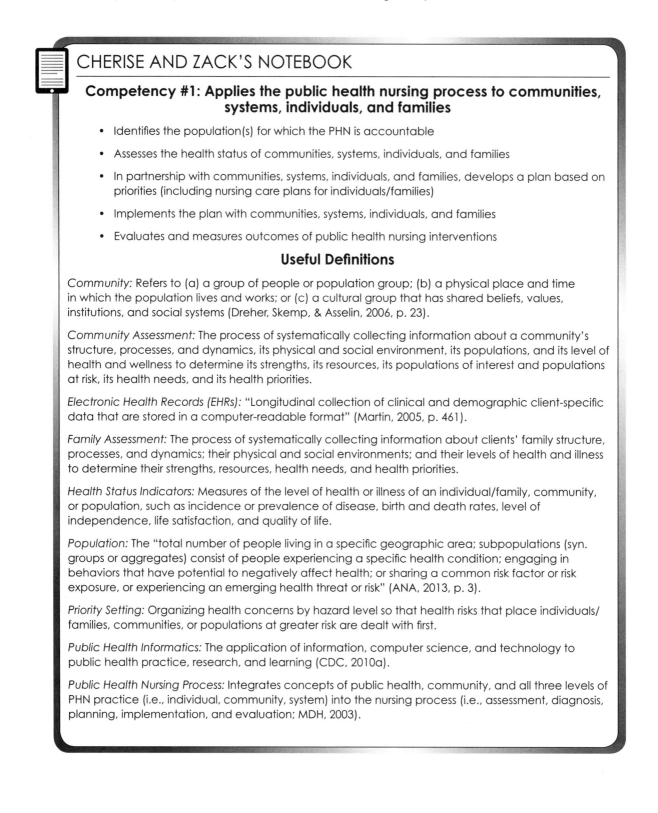

CHERISE AND ZACK'S NOTEBOOK

Competency #1: Applies the public health nursing process to communities, systems, individuals, and families

- Identifies the population(s) for which the PHN is accountable

- Assesses the health status of communities, systems, individuals, and families

- In partnership with communities, systems, individuals, and families, develops a plan based on priorities (including nursing care plans for individuals/families)

- Implements the plan with communities, systems, individuals, and families

- Evaluates and measures outcomes of public health nursing interventions

Useful Definitions

Community: Refers to (a) a group of people or population group; (b) a physical place and time in which the population lives and works; or (c) a cultural group that has shared beliefs, values, institutions, and social systems (Dreher, Skemp, & Asselin, 2006, p. 23).

Community Assessment: The process of systematically collecting information about a community's structure, processes, and dynamics, its physical and social environment, its populations, and its level of health and wellness to determine its strengths, its resources, its populations of interest and populations at risk, its health needs, and its health priorities.

Electronic Health Records (EHRs): "Longitudinal collection of clinical and demographic client-specific data that are stored in a computer-readable format" (Martin, 2005, p. 461).

Family Assessment: The process of systematically collecting information about clients' family structure, processes, and dynamics; their physical and social environments; and their levels of health and illness to determine their strengths, resources, health needs, and health priorities.

Health Status Indicators: Measures of the level of health or illness of an individual/family, community, or population, such as incidence or prevalence of disease, birth and death rates, level of independence, life satisfaction, and quality of life.

Population: The "total number of people living in a specific geographic area; subpopulations (syn. groups or aggregates) consist of people experiencing a specific health condition; engaging in behaviors that have potential to negatively affect health; or sharing a common risk factor or risk exposure, or experiencing an emerging health threat or risk" (ANA, 2013, p. 3).

Priority Setting: Organizing health concerns by hazard level so that health risks that place individuals/ families, communities, or populations at greater risk are dealt with first.

Public Health Informatics: The application of information, computer science, and technology to public health practice, research, and learning (CDC, 2010a).

Public Health Nursing Process: Integrates concepts of public health, community, and all three levels of PHN practice (i.e., individual, community, system) into the nursing process (i.e., assessment, diagnosis, planning, implementation, and evaluation; MDH, 2003).

Thinking and Doing Population Health—Nursing Process Leads the Way

PHNs work with individuals and families wherever they find them in the community and in whatever condition they find them. The priority for public health nursing is health promotion and disease prevention, but PHNs also work with individuals and families who have chronic health conditions to help them achieve their health potential and, whenever possible, manage their own lives and healthcare needs. Cherise and Zack's clinical is in a halfway house with young adults who have emotional and behavioral disorders and are currently unable to live by themselves or manage their own healthcare needs. They are going to need to discover their clients' potential for self-care and wellness to help them reach that potential. Instead of using a problem-based approach, they need to use a strengths-based approach as they carry out the public health nursing process. Because their clients live in the community, they need to find out as much as they can about the community's support systems, resources, and resource gaps.

Partnering With Individuals, Families, and Communities

PHNs need to understand the context of the lives of the people in the community in which they work. PHNs must know and understand the history, culture, and lifestyle of individuals, families, populations, or the entire community. For example, in a postclinical seminar, students were discussing the stresses and crises of the families they were visiting. They stated that they did not understand how these families could function with so much stress. One of the students, a recent immigrant, said she thought these families were fairly well off—they had housing, food, and were safe in their homes. The country she had emigrated from was in turmoil. She had seen family members murdered, their cattle slaughtered, homes burned, and people without food or clothing. These people, she thought, had truly stressful lives. The other students reflected on her comments and came to realize that people view the world from their own experiences. Understanding and appreciating the lived experiences of people is important. Knowing about and understanding each other helps promote the opportunity for people to work together in a mutually respectful manner that can build on each other's strengths.

PHNs work in partnership with individuals, families, and communities. Partnerships are mutual relationships based on trust. PHNs establish trust with individuals, families, and communities by respecting their rights to make their own health decisions and by adapting the nursing practice to fit the lived experiences and daily lives of those individuals, families, and communities. PHNs direct their efforts to meet the priority health needs their clients identify. Public health nursing practice includes the "3 Es":

- **Egalitarian (equal)** relationships with individuals, families, and communities

- **Enhancement** of individual, family, and community strengths, resilience, and resources

- **Empowerment** of individuals, families, and communities to advocate for and manage their own healthcare needs

Data Collection, Data Management, and the Public Health Nursing Process

Data compose the engine that drives the problem-solving process in nursing practice. Therefore, you need to have a system and process for data collection and management in place at the beginning of the nursing process. For this reason, we are discussing data before we discuss the components of the public health nursing process. Many public health and community agencies use EHRs and automated health information systems (HIS). Although more than one HIS exists, a system specifically created for public health nursing is useful as an example. The Omaha System, a standardized terminology initially developed for practitioners in the community, provides a problem-solving approach based on the nursing process (see Evidence Example below). The Omaha System is the foundation of the HIS that interdisciplinary team members at many health departments and other community provider sites regularly use. This HIS allows PHNs to collect and analyze data throughout the nursing process on individuals, families, and populations. The automated system facilitates aggregating data on individuals and families into larger data sets of populations so that patterns can be discerned within populations. This aggregation of data also allows PHNs to look at outcome data for specific programs and interventions. The Omaha System allows PHNs to collect their own evidence-based practice data, analyze those data, and generate meaningful information that can be used to improve the quality of the care they provide.

Evidence Example: *The Omaha System*

The Omaha System, developed by the Visiting Nurse Association of Omaha, Nebraska in 1975, enables healthcare providers to analyze and exchange client-centered coded data. It was designed to be relatively simple, hierarchical, multidimensional, and computer-compatible and to be used by interdisciplinary practitioners to guide their practice and document and communicate information about clients from admission to discharge. It exists in the public domain (no fee or license) and is intended for use across the continuum of care. It is based on a conceptual model that reflects the pivotal position of the individual, family, and community; the partnership with practitioners; and the value of the problem-solving approach. In other words, the Omaha System encourages critical thinking and operationalizes the nursing process. The problem-solving approach complements the strengths-based approach that focuses on building developmental assets and increasing the health of youth and communities (Martin, 2005; Martin, Monsen, & Bowles, 2011; Omaha System, 2010).

The Omaha System consists of three components:

1. *Problem Classification Scheme* (client-centered assessment that engages individuals, families, and communities)—The Problem Classification Scheme is a hierarchy that includes domains; individual-, family-, and community-centered problems; modifiers; and signs/symptoms.

2. *Intervention Scheme* (plans, pathways, care activities, and service delivery terms to improve safety, quality, and effectiveness)—The Intervention Scheme is a hierarchy of interventions that includes categories, targets, and client-specific information.

3. *Problem Rating Scale for Outcomes* (evaluation that provides usable information for measuring and reporting client progress across time)—The Problem Rating Scale for Outcomes consists of knowledge, behavior, and symptom status concepts and Likert-type rating scales.

WEB-BASED ACTIVITY

Complete this activity with your clinical group.

Go to the Minnesota Omaha System Users Group website (http://omahasystemmn.org/data.php) and select the "An Introduction to the Omaha System" video presentation. Watch this 7-minute flash video presentation.

Go to the Omaha System website (http://www.omahasystem.org) and click "Case Studies." Everyone should read the *Influenza* case study and one other case study about a client in a community setting. Compare and contrast the two case studies. Discuss the following topics:

1. How are they different, and how are they the same?

    -   their domains, modifiers, signs, and symptoms

    -   their interventions, targets, and client-specific information

    -   use of the problem rating scale to measure knowledge, behaviors, and symptoms

2. Select one of your own clients and organize your client data and status using the Omaha System components.

3. How might you use the Omaha System to analyze data about a group of clients to demonstrate that nursing interventions make a difference in population health outcomes?

EHRs and HIS provide ways to collect, store, analyze, and share information. Community and population data can be gathered from a variety of sources. When you collect data about your clients or combine data from a group of clients, these are considered primary data, because you gathered the information yourself. If you share the data you collected with someone else, the information is still your primary data, but it is secondary data for those who receive it. Secondary data are data gathered by others. PHNs collect and use primary data when they aggregate their client data to look at program and service outcomes. PHNs also collect primary data through key-informant interviews and focus groups. PHNs access and use secondary data when they gather health statistics data compiled by their agency or county, state, and national agencies, such as the U.S. Department of Health and Human Services (DHHS) and state health departments. PHNs often compare their primary data with secondary data about the same health problem or interventions to compare the outcomes of their programs with the outcomes of other programs at the local, state, and national levels.

Home Visiting and the Nursing Process

PHNs carry out assessments as part of the nursing process most often in a community setting, such as a home, a school, or a clinic. Most of the information is gathered through observation and listening. When in the home setting, PHNs are guests of the family members and need to follow their lead regarding communication methods; timing, length, and place of visit; and roles of the nurse and family members. To assess the family, PHNs must first establish a trusting relationship with family members based on mutual respect and understanding (Eriksson & Nilsson, 2008; McCann & Baker, 2001). Answering questions about personal family matters and health situations requires families to disclose information they generally do not share with strangers, so the development of a trusting relationship needs to precede or occur simultaneously with the interviewing process. Andrew Gardner (2010) found that one way to engage clients and help them feel comfortable was to start by being open and friendly; this approach seems obvious but can be challenging for nurses learning to be professional, maintain boundaries, and create an environment conducive to effective nursing practice. An appropriate level of openness certainly can facilitate a connection and mutual understanding, but this is sometimes a difficult balancing act, as friendship often occurs within the professional context of the nurse-client relationship. The initial visit to a family is critical in establishing the nurse-client trust relationship (see Evidence Example).

Evidence Example: Public Health Nurses' Views of a Good First Meeting

Swedish researchers (Jansson, Petersson, & Uden, 2001) used focus groups to determine what public health nurses believed constituted a good first home visit with parents of newborns. A good first visit is considered key to developing an effective relationship with parents. Three criteria were identified:

1. **Creating trust** through good contact/reciprocal relationships, listening, being a guest, having an equal role with parents, and having time, privacy, and peace and quiet

2. **Creating a picture of the family's life situation** by getting a holistic impression of the family, seeing them in their home environment, getting a picture of what the clients are like, and taking in, consciously and unconsciously, the mood and a variety of information about the family

3. **Creating a supportive climate** by confirming and affirming parents' feelings, abilities, and responsibilities and increasing their responsibilities while providing a safety net

Source: Jansson, Petersson, & Uden, 2001

Home-visiting programs may include one or more visits to a client. PHNs follow some families for months and years, depending on their health risks and needs. So you should not feel as though you have to get everything done in one visit. Table 3.1 demonstrates how a PHN would use the nursing process in making a series of home visits. The orientation phase might take one to three visits on average. The working phase might require multiple visits over a period of months or years.

Table 3.1 How the Nursing Process Occurs in Home Visits

Home-Visiting Components	Nursing Process
Orientation Phase	**Assessment and Diagnosis**
• Introduction	• Individual and family assessment
• Determine purpose of visit and visit activities with client	• Strengths-based assessment—protective factors identified
• Engage in social conversation	• Resources identified
• Assessment	• Health risks and active health problems identified
• Identify and state client's problems	• Unmet health needs identified

Working Phase: Identification
- Client asks questions and identifies nurse as someone who can help.
- Client identifies problems.
- Nurse provides health teaching, support and counseling, follow-up assessment, referral, and advocacy.

Working Phase: Mutual Relationship
- Client uses nurse as resource and accesses community resources.
- Nurse engages client in mutual problem solving.

Resolution and Termination
- Problems are solved or ongoing but stable.
- Client becomes independent of nurse or continues to need support.
- Relationship ends when client no longer needs nurse or no longer participates in plan (moves or refuses participation in plan or visits).

Planning and Implementation
- Mutual planning, priority setting, goal setting
- Primary interventions used are health teaching, counseling, referral and follow-up, and advocacy.

Implementation
- Primary interventions used are case management, health teaching, counseling, collaboration, and consultation.

Evaluation
- Evaluation of outcomes: outcomes met, partially met, or not met
- Replan—change in goals, outcomes, and/ or interventions
- New priorities or emerging problems identified and nursing process continues

Adapted from McNaughton, 2005

PHNs carry equipment they need to complete assessments on individual family members. For example, common equipment used on maternal/child health visits includes a baby scale, blood pressure cuffs, a stethoscope, paper tape measures, disposable thermometers, developmental screening tools, growth grids, and a thermometer for determining the temperature of bath water.

PHNs often carry laptops and smartphones to access information and enter family data into EHRs during their home visits. Due to a federal mandate, all health providers, including health departments, are expected to have EHRs by 2014 (Martin et al., 2011). PHNs use automated or paper guidelines or clinical pathways specific to individual client and family situations. For example, public health agencies have screening, assessment, and monitoring databases for newborns, infants, children, antepartum, post-partum, and family clients. PHNs collect admitting data on each client during their initial visits to their clients. They monitor and record health changes at each visit.

Public Health Nursing Assessment

Public health nursing assessment is a systematic deliberative and holistic process of collecting data about a client (individual, family, community, or system) that leads to an understanding of the client's health determinants, health status, and priority health concerns and needs. PHNs also need to carry out strengths-based assessments so that intervention plans for health concerns and problems are based on the clients' abilities to manage their own healthcare needs. Strengths-based assessments identify clients' abilities, resources, and resilience as well as health needs.

Individual/Family Level of Practice

The family is the focus of care when PHNs work at the individual/family level of practice. The family is the primary unit of society and is responsible for carrying out the functions that allow family members to survive and thrive. In a health sense, the family is a unit of care (Hunt, 2013). Families come in many shapes and sizes and in different stages of development. Family composition is varied and changeable in contemporary society (Kaakinen, Gehaly-Duff, Coehlo, & Hanson, 2010).

Family assessment is a holistic process in which all the factors that influence a family's level of health and wellness are considered. You need to identify the health determinants (protective factors and risk factors) for individuals and families who have similar characteristics. For example, postpartum depression is one of the most common forms of depression and places new mothers and other family members at risk for harm. Knowing this, a PHN would include a postpartum depression screening as part of the assessment of a pregnant or postpartum client. If a mother is experiencing postpartum depression, an assessment of the children to determine their own health and safety would be appropriate. Families who live in poverty are more likely to have inadequate nutrition than families with adequate incomes, so a PHN would include a family nutritional assessment when working with poor families. Table 3.2 outlines the components of family assessment typically included in a comprehensive family assessment.

Table 3.2   Components of a Comprehensive Family Assessment

Family Composition, Structure, and Household			
Names	**Age**	**Sex**	**Relationship**

Family Type and Structure: single, dyad, multiple members
Living arrangements: household members, type and condition of housing
Hint: Collaborate with family members in creating their family genogram, a graph of family structure and relationships (see Resources for online tutorials on family genograms)

Family Culture and Lifestyle

- Racial and ethnic background

- Birthplace of family members

- Culture

- Spirituality, religion

- Family beliefs, values, goals

- Lifestyle patterns, including caregiving and caretaking

- Communication and decision-making patterns

Hint: Use your observational skills as well as your interviewing skills in identifying family culture and lifestyle.

Family Developmental Stage and Life Cycle

- Identify the family developmental stage and life cycle

    - Forming and exploring partnerships

    - Stabilized partnership, childbearing, childrearing

    - Career diversity and lifestyle change, launching center for children

    - Middle years, middle-aged parenting

    - Aging, reconstituted families (based on concepts from Clark, 2008, and Kaakinen et al., 2010)

Hint: Identify family developmental tasks, needs, and developmental transition points. Are family members able to meet developmental needs and cope with crises and transitions?

Basic Family Functions

- Relational Support: Meet the emotional, nurturing, and support needs of family members.

- Socialization: Instill attitudes and values, educate members to fulfill family and societal roles and responsibilities, and provide for formal education of members.

- Reproduction: Ensure survival of family and society through birth, adoption, and caregiving.

- Economic: Provide financial resources sufficient to meet family needs.

- Provision of Basic Needs: Provide for food, shelter, clothing, safety, communication, transportation, and healthcare (adapted from Clark, 2008, p. 326).

Hint: Are family members able to carry out their role functions and fulfill family needs? Have roles changed to carry out family functions? What type of assistance is needed?

Health of Family Unit

- Communications: Communications and feelings are open, direct, honest, and shared.

- Self-Esteem and Caring: Sense of self-worth, responsibility, compassion, and love are expressed and shared.

- Rules and Freedom: Rules are known, clear, and flexible and allow for individual freedom.

- Community Connections: Family is linked to community and actively involved in community activities and groups; family and community members share mutual respect and friendship (adapted from Hunt, 2013).

Hint: Create a family ecomap, a pictorial representation that identifies connections with extended family, friends, and community organizations and the strength of those connections (see Resources for online tutorials on constructing ecomaps).

continues

Table 3.2 Components of a Comprehensive Family Assessment (continued)

Family Resilience

- Balancing needs and resources, stability, and flexibility
- Cohesion and support in good times and bad
- Shared beliefs, values, and goals
- Shared family routines, rituals, experiences, and tasks of daily living
- Open communication and collaborative problem-solving
- Successful history of coping with multiple stressors
- Sense of hope, confidence, and optimism
- Effective management of monetary and other resources
- Support network (includes concepts from Hunt, 2013; Kaakinen et al., 2010)

Hint: Ask about a past family or health crisis. How did the family members respond to that crisis? Do they believe that they managed the situation positively?

Family Health Management

Health History
- Current health problems and concerns
- Relevant medical diagnoses, medications, and treatments
- Preferences and compliance with medications and treatments
- Current health and social services providers

Healthy Lifestyle and Health-Seeking Behaviors
- Nutrition, exercise, sleep and rest, immunizations
- Emergency plans (household and community disasters)
- Cultural health beliefs and practices
- Seeking knowledge, resources, and assistance for health and illness needs

Healthcare Management Abilities
- Health literacy (knowledge about and ability to access and understand healthcare)
- Healthcare resources (insurance, access to providers, available caregivers)
- Caregiving patterns and abilities
- Management of therapeutic regime
- Effective coping abilities and crisis management

Hint: You may already have collected some of these data. Affirm your understanding of known data with family members.

Environment

Home Interior and Exterior
- Physical adequacy, safety, and comfort
- Living area
- Kitchen
- Bedrooms and bathroom
- Number of stories and steps
- Maintenance and structural safety
- Phone and other forms of communication
- Use of products that pose a hazard to those living in the household.

Hint: Use your observational skills!

Immediate Neighborhood
- Physical environment, adequacy, and safety
- Maintenance of sidewalks, roads, pedestrian crossings, public spaces
- Transportation
- Weather patterns
- Social environment and safety
- Adequate shopping and service resources
- Potential or actual environmental hazards (chemical, biological, physical)

Family Health Summary and Analysis

Family Assessment Summary
- Major family protective factors
- Major family risk factors
- Summary statement of family resilience and ability to manage own healthcare

Health Status Summary
- Priority health problems or concerns
- Family's current health priorities
- Family's current health goals

Hint: Summarize your findings with the family before you move on to developing a family care plan.

Whether an individual lives alone or with others, the same family functions are relevant. If you are working with an individual who lives alone or whose extended family lives elsewhere, you still need to use the same family assessment approach. Sometimes a complete family assessment is not needed or impossible to collect. In that case, the PHN would select the assessment components that relate to the specific family health problem or priority concern (see Table 3.3).

Table 3.3 Focused or Problem-Specific Family Assessment

- Family composition, structure, and household
- Current health problems and/or health threat
- Risk factors and protective factors related to current health problem
- Access to and use of healthcare services
- Appropriateness of existing healthcare services
- Health literacy
- Ability to manage family healthcare needs and resources
- Unmet healthcare needs and family health priorities

Public Health Nursing Diagnoses

PHNs may use the classification system for nursing diagnosis developed by the North American Nursing Diagnosis Association (NANDA) when working with individuals, families, populations, and communities (Scroggins, 2008). For example, 65 NANDA nursing diagnoses relevant to public health nursing, such as ineffective breastfeeding, were used to develop 65 family health documentation forms by one county public health agency (Parris et al., 1999). A nursing diagnosis adapted for public health would include the components outlined in Table 3.4.

Table 3.4 Nursing Diagnosis Components for Public Health

Nursing Diagnosis Components	Examples
Diagnostic Concept	Coping, family process, homelessness, hope or hopelessness, health-seeking behaviors
Subject	Individual, family, population, community
Judgment (descriptor or modifier of concept)	Readiness for impaired, compromised, altered, delayed, disturbed
Location	Site or place
Age	Biological stage (e.g., neonate, adolescent, older adult), individual or family developmental stage
Time	Acute, chronic, intermittent, continuous

Status	*Actual family health problem:* observable signs and symptoms of ineffective family unit; signs and symptoms of illness in one or more family members
	Wellness or health promotion focus: motivation to increase family well-being and health; responses to level of wellness imply readiness for enhancement or improvement
	Family at risk: exposure to risk factors that cause increased family vulnerability, illness, injury, or condition; psychological, physiological, genetic, chemical, environmental (physical or social)

Modified from Scroggins, 2008

When possible, a strengths-based diagnosis (wellness or health promotion diagnosis) should be developed. A strengths-based diagnosis leads to interventions that enhance potential for self-care and independence. Examples of strengths-based family diagnoses include the following:

- Readiness for enhanced family coping related to child with significant developmental delays, parental grieving, and anxiety, as evidenced by parents enrolling child in early childhood education program, parents seeking counseling, and parents stating that they were adapting their expectations of child to child's potential

- Potential for enhanced health-seeking behaviors related to inadequate family nutrition, loss of father's job, and lack of transportation, as evidenced by parents signing up for county food-assistance program, finding local food shelves on bus line, willingness to use meat substitutes for protein and powdered milk

Cherise has been introduced to her client, Nicole, a 23-year-old homeless woman who is shy, talks in monosyllables, and does not make eye contact. She responds to many questions by telling Cherise to ask her mother when her mother visits in the afternoon. Cherise returns in the afternoon to visit with Nicole and her mother.

ACTIVITY

If you were Cherise, how would you go about completing a family assessment with Nicole and her mother? Consider role-playing this interview with some of your classmates.

How would you establish a trust relationship with Nicole and her mother?

Where and how would you interview Nicole and her mother?

How would you provide for privacy and confidentiality?

What types of family information would you want to collect from Nicole and her mother?

The PHN continues the nursing process by moving into identification of the individual's or family's health priorities and mutual goal-setting. After goals have been established, a plan of action is developed with the individual or family.

Cherise meets with Nicole and her mother to complete a family health assessment. Nicole's mother states that things had been going well until both she and her husband lost their jobs and their health insurance and Nicole went off her meds. She and her husband are looking for jobs and an apartment. She says that they were very determined to keep their family together, but Nicole was not doing well in the homeless shelter, so the halfway house seemed like a good option. Nicole's current health problems include lack of health insurance, lack of a mental health provider, lack of medication to control her mental health problems, and several broken teeth and visible dental caries. The homeless shelter has a health clinic, and the halfway house has a social worker. Cherise, Nicole, and her mother decide that their priority is finding a mental health provider and a way to get medications for Nicole. Nicole cries when her mother leaves, stating, "I want to go with my mother. I am so lonely here."

ACTIVITY

Cherise wants to focus on Nicole's family's protective factors and strengths. She wants to enhance their ability to regain their independence. Cherise decides to write a strengths-based diagnosis. How might you help her develop her nursing diagnosis and intervention plan? Consider the following questions:

1. What are Nicole's and her family's strengths or protective factors?

2. What are their risk factors?

3. What wellness strength-based diagnosis might you develop?

4. Which public health nursing interventions might you use? See Chapter 2.

Healthy People 2020 One of the Leading Health Indicators in Healthy People 2020 is Environmental Quality. Go to the Healthy People 2020 website to find out what the major environmental health risks are for children, adults, and the elderly. How would you assess the existence of environmental risk factors for individuals/families and communities? What progress has been made on reducing some of these risk factors over the last decade? What are the targets for 2020?

Community Level of Practice

PHNs assess communities to determine their levels of health and wellness. These assessments are carried out in partnership with the community. One community partnership approach often used is the participatory community action research model (Kelly, 2005). In this approach, community partners are involved in the entire process of assessment, planning, implementation, and evaluation. Many geographic communities, such as cities, counties, and states, conduct a community assessment on a periodic basis, commonly every 2 years. They do this to monitor changing health conditions of the populations in their communities and to establish community priorities for health goals, funding, and actions. The governmental agencies conducting the assessment partner with other community organizations and members to ensure that the diversity of the community and all points of view are reflected in the assessment. PHNs are part of the team that collects and analyzes the community data.

It is important to conduct a strengths-based assessment as part of the community assessment process. PHNs work to enhance community strengths so that communities can be as independent as possible in solving their own healthcare problems and managing their own healthcare needs. Chapter 5 discusses the formation of community partnerships and building on community assets to strengthen the community's ability to manage its own healthcare needs.

> *After they visited their clients in the halfway house, Cherise said to Shannon, "I have never heard of halfway homes for adults with emotional and behavioral disorders. Who thought to build a home for them?"*

> *Shannon responded, "The public health department carries out a community assessment periodically to determine the priority health problems of the people living in the community. We want to know what the major health needs are and which needs are met and which are unmet. We also look at the assets or resources of the community to determine the community's capacity to manage its own healthcare needs and solve its own problems. Then we prioritize and decide which services to offer, what the funding should be, and how to allocate resources to our different programs. During the last community assessment process, we found out that 10% of adults in our community had chronic mental health problems and that many are on medications to control their symptoms. Many of our public health nurses provide case management services in the home to try to keep our clients stable and on their psychotropic medications. When we analyzed our caseloads, we found that we were not providing services to young adults with mental health problems."*

The population data collected in public health includes population health status, health differences or health status gaps between populations (health disparities), and health determinants (causes of health and illness within the population). See Chapter 1 for health determinant discussion. Health status data are considered the "vital signs" of the population and include the following:

- Mortality (death rates) data

- Life Expectancy (average years lived for someone born in specific year)

- Years of Potential Life Lost (life expectancy – age of death = YPLL)

- Morbidity (illness rates) data

- Health behaviors data (e.g., smoking, exercise, obesity, use of seat belts)

- Health and life satisfaction data (how satisfied one is with current health and lifestyle)

- Functional health data (ability to live independently and manage own healthcare needs)

These population "vital signs" are called global health status measures. Table 3.5 outlines the process that PHNs use in community assessment.

Table 3.5   Community Health Assessment Process

Organize

- Create a planning team and select the assessment/planning process.
- Identify who needs and wants to be involved.
- Set meeting dates/times and create a communications plan.

Plan Assessment in Partnership

- Agree on leadership and the decision-making process.
- Review background documents and establish team process and assessment ground rules.
- Create a work plan and timeline.

Gather and Analyze Assessment Data

- Compile data from a variety of sources.
- Summarize and analyze data to answer initial questions raised during the assessment.
- Refer to partners and staff to add additional meaning to the data.
- Ask additional questions and gather additional data (as needed).

Document and Communicate Findings

- Prepare print and/or web-based documentation of Community Health Assessment findings.
- Share key findings with decision-makers and the public.
- Deliver to the local health department the 10 most important community health issues.

Modified from Minnesota Department of Health, n.d.

A comprehensive community assessment tool based on the determinants of health (see Chapter 1) that includes all the data to be collected is outlined in Table 3.6. The community assessment project you participate in as a student may include many of these components. Remember that all data sources, both primary and secondary, must be documented.

Table 3.6   Community Assessment

Part 1: Determinants of Health

Section I. Biology

Unit of Analysis	Data
Geographic Area: Population by Census Track, Community, County, State, Country Population at Risk by Common Characteristic (e.g., ethnic, cultural or religious group, age or developmental stage, common health risk [potential or actual])	• Population at last census • Population density • Population changes in the last decade • Demographics: Age, race, gender • Physical characteristics • Genetic factors • Health conditions

Section 2. Behaviors

Socioeconomic Characteristics	• Employment (employed versus unemployed) • Income levels • Poverty level • Education levels • Language literacy
Lifestyle Patterns	• Living arrangements (type of housing, people in household, relationship of people in household) • Homelessness • Family, work, and community roles • Religious affiliations or memberships • Patterns of social conformity or nonconformity (lawfulness, antisocial behaviors, lawlessness)
Health Behaviors	• Health-seeking actions • Health-limiting actions • Coping and resilience • Health literacy

continues

Table 3.6   Community Assessment   (continued)

Section 3. Physical Environment	
Natural Environment (created by nature)	<ul><li>Geography (terrain, climate, weather, natural resources)</li><li>Air and water quality</li><li>Recreation</li></ul>
Built Environment (created by humans)	<ul><li>Urban versus rural, suburban</li><li>Transportation (roads, bridges, public and private transportation services)</li><li>Transportation access (ground, airports, waterways)</li><li>Governmental and protective services (police, fire, emergency response)</li><li>Public and handicapped access and accommodation</li><li>Leading industries and worksites</li><li>Educational facilities</li><li>Shopping (food, clothing, other)</li><li>Agriculture</li><li>Water, sanitation, waste management, and recycling services</li><li>Vector control (insects, rodents, large animals, ticks and fleas)</li><li>Air and water quality or contamination control</li><li>Housing stock (type, age, condition, availability)</li><li>Recreational facilities</li><li>Parks, playgrounds, athletic fields</li></ul>
Section 4. Social Environment	
History of Community	<ul><li>Pattern of settlement</li><li>Immigration and migration patterns</li><li>Key events</li></ul>
Culture and Ethnicity	<ul><li>Diversity in community</li><li>Festivals and celebrations</li></ul>

Political and Social Climate	• Conservative, liberal, independent, libertarian
Religious Institutions	• Denominations and membership
	• Calendar of holidays and events
	• Community and volunteer services
Commerce and Workplace	• Businesses, retail and shopping, banks, business community organizations
	• Workplace (worker organizations, unionization, workplace safety and hazards)
	• Distance from place of residence to workplace and commuting patterns
Education	• Public, private, secular
	• Variety of programs
	• Cost and access
Libraries and Public Information Access	• Library locations, hours, services, Internet access
Communication	• Public and private information and communication sources
	• Mail and courier services (public, private)
	• Telephone (landlines, mobile, access, emergency services, telephone chains)
	• Television, radio, print media, Internet
	• Newsletters, billboards, bulletin boards
Law Enforcement Services and Patterns (formal and informal)	• Police and special police services, animal enforcement, private security, neighborhood watch patrols, vigilante groups
Community Support Systems and Social Services (formal and informal)	Social services (e.g., food and clothing banks, homeless shelters, adult day care, child care)
	• Nonprofit community service organizations
	• Neighborhood organizations
	• Pattern of emergency services responses (type, frequency, availability, response time)

continues

Table 3.6 Community Assessment (continued)

Section 4. Social Environment	
Disaster Planning and Management	• Preparation for both natural and man-made disasters • Preparation, response, and recovery plans • Identifying and acquiring needed resources (material and human)
Health Services	• Public, private, for profit, nonprofit mix in community • Range of services (acute care, primary care, specialty care, home care, hospice, community clinics and home visiting, long-term care, occupational and rehabilitation services) • Access, cost, and quality of services
Health Services Access—Assessing the "7 As of Access" (Truglio-Londrigan & Lewenson, 2013, p. 93)	• Is the individual, family, or population *aware* of its needs and the services available in the community? • Can the individual, family, or population gain *access* to the services it needs? • Are services *available* and convenient for the individual, family, or population in terms of time, location, and place for use? • How *affordable* are the services for the individual, family, or population? • Are the services *acceptable* to the individual, family, or population in terms of choice, satisfaction, and congruency with cultural values and beliefs? • How *appropriate* are the services for the individual, family, or population? • Are the services *adequate* in terms of quantity or degree for the individual, family, or population?
Section 5. Policy and Interventions	
Laws, Regulations, Ordinances	• Existing health, safety, social service laws, regulations, and ordinances that affect health access and health delivery

Political Structures and Processes	• Elected and appointed officials (access and availability of officials and staff) • Political process cycle (elections, legislation, regulatory process and implementation, budgeting and allocation of funds, evaluation) • Lobbying groups and efforts • Coalitions and community organizing activities for social and political change • Community forums or public meetings
Current Health and Safety Issues	• Emerging, long-term • Identified community priority • Public consensus or disagreement on solution • Current actions or lack of action • Available funding or lack of funding

Part 2: Analysis of Population and Community Health Status

Section A. Health Statistics

Birth and Death Rates	General and by age, gender, ethnicity, causes
Accidents and Injuries and Deaths Related to Accidents and Injuries	General and by age, gender, ethnicity, location, type • Accidental • Intentional • Homicide and suicide
Communicable Disease Rates (top 10)	General and by age, gender, ethnicity, location
Immunization Rates	General and by age, gender, ethnicity, location

See Chapter 4 for discussion of health statistics.

continues

Table 3.6 Community Assessment   (continued)

Section 5. Policy and Interventions	
Noncommunicable Disease Rates (top 10)	General and by age, gender, ethnicity, location • Medical diseases • Mental health • Acute illnesses • Chronic diseases • Disabilities
Health Risk Behaviors	General and by age, gender and ethnicity (e.g., smoking or chewing, drinking, drug use, obesity, drinking and driving, sexual behaviors and unprotected sex, use of seatbelts and helmets, interpersonal abuse, participation in antisocial or illegal behaviors)
Level of Independence	Adult population by age, gender, location, illness, and disability
Life Satisfaction	By age, gender, location, socioeconomic status, illness, and disability
Section B. Determining Community Health Priorities	
Comparison of Populations	• Compare health risks and health status categories by key populations in community (age, gender, socioeconomic status, ethnicity, culture, location, health conditions). • Identify populations at risk and populations of interest.
Identify Key Health Concerns	• Analyze by incidence, prevalence, patterns of increase, and severity. • Analyze potential for harm to community as a whole. • Compare with Healthy People 2020 goals and priorities or existing community goals and priorities.

| Identify Community Health Priorities and Establish Goals | • Establish community health priorities with community members. |
| | • Align community health priorities with Healthy People 2020 goals and priorities or existing community goals and priorities. |

Source: Modified from Truglio-Londrigan & Lewenson, 2013

Windshield Survey

The *windshield survey* is a first look at a community through a car's windshield. Observers are asked to use their senses (sight, hearing, and smell) to learn about a community as they drive, walk, or use public transportation to get around the community. They then make observations about the physical and social environments and the natural and built environments. The windshield survey is sometimes referred to as a familiarization survey, because it helps establish the community context of care for PHNs. It can also be an initial step to a more comprehensive community assessment by raising awareness of issues for further exploration. Table 3.7 includes a list of questions you might ask yourself to help guide your windshield survey and analyze your findings.

Table 3.7   Windshield Survey—Snapshot of Community Assessment

Windshield Survey

The first steps of a windshield survey require identifying the community boundaries and determining whether you will conduct the survey by car, by public transportation, or partially on foot to determine feasibility of your possible travel routes. It is best to conduct the survey in pairs or as a group. As you drive or ride through the community, pay careful attention to as many characteristics of the community as possible. You may wish to take photos or videotape your windshield survey. Make sure that you are only taking photos of people in public places. Be sensitive to the privacy of others; avoid taking pictures of people, particularly those who are vulnerable, where they could be identified.

1. Which resources/assets do you see available in the community? Resources may include libraries, clinics, thriving local businesses, and other features that may provide support to community members.

2. Which types of services for families do you see in the community?

3. Are there other organizations, such as youth centers, churches, or Head Start programs, that might provide activities for children/families?

4. Where do people live in the community? Is the housing primarily single-family housing or apartments? What is the condition of the housing?

5. What types of jobs are available in the community? Would these jobs likely be held by people in the area?

6. Where do people shop? Which types of stores are available: locally owned or chain stores?

continues

Table 3.7 Windshield Survey—Snapshot of Community Assessment (continued)

Windshield Survey

7. How do people get around in the community? Is public transportation available?

8. What do you notice about ethnic diversity in the community? Which age range seems predominant?

9. What is the geographic environment? Which types of opportunities are available for exercise? Are parks available? Is there green space?

10. Which options are available for eating out?

11. What did you learn about the health status of population groups in the community that augments published population health data?

12. Where can people go for healthcare services?

13. Based on your observations, what would you identify as assets in this community?

14. Overall, how did you feel about being in the community (e.g., safe, comfortable, uneasy)?

Reflection and Analysis Questions

- What is the story of each photo you have taken? What do the photos tell you about the life and health of the community?

- What are the community's outstanding assets? Is there a relationship between these assets and the health of the community?

- What appear to be the community's major challenges? Is there a relationship between these challenges and the health of the community?

- What do you see as the most striking characteristic about the community? Would this characteristic influence your approach to providing care to the community?

- What did you find to be the most unexpected? Would the unexpected be an asset or a challenge to providing care to the community?

Source: Modified from Hargate, 2013

Other types of windshield surveys may also be carried out, such as:

- Environmental hazard surveys, which involve surveying both the natural and built environment of a community to identify potential or actual chemical, biological, physical, human (social and behavioral) hazards; and

- Walkabout and walkability surveys, which provide an opportunity to assess areas not easily accessible by car (e.g., neighborhood sidewalks and paths, parks, playgrounds, campuses, malls) to identify potential hazards as well as healthy living spaces.

At times, PHNs and community agencies want to determine the health status of a subpopulation or aggregate. This assessment can be conducted just like the community assessment, but with a more limited scope (see Evidence Example).

Evidence Example: Elementary School Health Assessment

Public health nursing students at a local college conducted a mass health screening of all students in a K–6 charter elementary school serving mainly African-American and Hispanic students. The health screening included assessments of height, weight, BMI, vision and hearing, dental, immunization compliance, and nutrition and activity levels. Data were collected on individual students so that students with health needs could be referred to the appropriate health providers for further assessment and interventions. The major finding was that 80% of the students had unmet dental needs, with 20–30% of the students having emergency dental needs. The health determinants that influenced the dental health status of these students included:

Personal–Behavioral

- Lack of family dentist
- Lack of awareness of resources
- Dental insurance
- Opportunities for free dental care
- Lack of transportation (no car available)
- 95% of families living in poverty
- Families at survival level with dental health a low priority
- Lack of toothbrushes and toothpaste
- Lack of knowledge about how to brush teeth
- English as a second language
- Parents unable to take children to dentist appointments during normal Monday to Friday business hours
- Parental concern about their children's health

Environmental–Physical

- The weather is cold with frequent rain and snow for 6 months of the year.
- City buses are not accessible from many of the neighborhoods in which the children live.
- Urban environment is dangerous for children out alone, so children would not be able to walk to the dentist on their own.

Environmental–Social

- Government financial resources for dental services for the poor are very limited.

- A voluntary dental organization provides free dental service to children twice a year.

- A local neighborhood clinic with ties to the school provides dental care, but only during Monday to Friday daytime hours.

- The poverty level is dense.

- Few dental clinics exist in older and poorer neighborhoods.

These findings led to the establishment of a dental health priority for the school.

Source: Schoon, 2010

 ## ACTIVITY

Review the summary of the school health assessment in the previous Evidence Example.

Which health determinant protective factors were found?

Which health determinant risk factors were found?

Which of these health determinants could be modified?

Zack asked Shannon, "What did you do when you found out that you weren't seeing many young people with mental health problems?"

Shannon responded, "We conducted some key-informant interviews with the doctors, nurses, and social workers who were already working with this group. We also talked with the local police chief and the county attorney. We found that young adults with mental health problems often tend to fall through the cracks because, for the most part, they have not been diagnosed with a major psychiatric diagnosis, such as schizophrenia or bipolar or borderline personality disorder. Their problems are often perceived to be antisocial or criminal rather than medical, and many of them wind up in jail for drug use, disorderly conduct, assault, and other behaviors that people find frightening. So the county decided to fund a demonstration project with a 25-bed halfway house for young adults with emotional and behavioral disorders who were living on the streets, in jail, or in and out of the hospital."

Zack commented, "So the young adults living in the halfway house can be considered a community or a subpopulation. I guess we would need to modify the community assessment process somewhat, but I am not sure what we really need to find out."

Shannon responded, "The public health agency staff need to know the residents' health status and their unmet health needs. We also need to know whether the halfway house is able to provide the services needed and whether any services are needed that can't be provided. We could use your help in collecting that information."

ACTIVITY

Zack is concerned about the community assessment that he and his fellow classmates will be conducting at the halfway home for young adults with emotional and behavioral disorders. How might he modify the community assessment process to fit the population and setting of the halfway house?

PHN Assessment at the Systems Level of Practice

Systems can be assessed to determine their ability to respond to public health priorities in the community. Systems that PHNs interact with on an ongoing basis include healthcare systems; public and governmental agencies; schools and school systems; community health and social service agencies; local and state governments, including elected and appointed officials; insurance companies; and faith-based organizations. PHNs assess systems to identify the extent to which they can meet community health needs and, if they can't, to identify the additional resources that are needed. In the case study about the halfway house, healthcare systems and providers were assessed to determine whether they could provide the needed healthcare services for the residents.

Identifying and Setting Health Priorities

PHNs employed in governmental public health agencies are accountable to the public for the health priorities they select, the populations they serve, and the services they provide (see Chapter 6). PHNs consciously make the connection between the health needs of the community as a whole and the health needs of individuals and families within the community. The priority health needs identified through the community assessment process help PHNs determine the most vulnerable and underserved populations in their communities and target those with greatest need for services.

PHNs also identify health priorities in the community by identifying health and illness patterns among their individual clients and families by aggregating data on all the families whom their agency serves. PHNs look at multiple interacting health determinants, including the social determinants of health, to identify population health patterns and causes when working with individual clients and community partners (Meagher-Stewart, Edwards, Aston, & Young, 2009). PHNs also conduct research to identify health concerns in known vulnerable populations. For example, a study of early care and education programs identified the following health needs of the centers and enrolled children: hygiene and hand-washing; sanitation and disinfection; supervision; and safety of indoor and outdoor equipment (Alkon, To, Mackie, Wolff, & Bernzweig, 2009). PHNs can determine community health priorities by reviewing the community assessment data to determine which health problems have the greatest potential for harm and have effective interventions. Questions to consider when establishing health priorities are listed in Table 3.8.

Table 3.8   Determining Community Health Priorities

1. What are the incidence and prevalence of major diseases, health risk behaviors, and health concerns in the community (e.g., heart disease, teen pregnancy, drinking and driving, smoking, depression, influenza)?

2. What are the major causes of death and disability in the community (e.g., heart attacks, stroke, cancer, dementia, car accidents, and homicide)?

3. Which populations in the community are most affected by these health problems?

4. What are the major health risks in the community (e.g., obesity, air pollution, homes with lead-based paint, seasonal flooding, homelessness, lack of health insurance)?

5. Which health needs are met by community resources?

6. Which health needs are not met?

7. Are affordable and effective interventions available for these health needs?

8. Who is responsible for meeting these health needs?

PHNs are ever-vigilant community watchers who are often the first to notice when a new health concern emerges or when a service gaps exists in the community. An example of a health concern identified by a PHN intake nurse, explored by agency staff, and taken to a group of community partners for a systems-level intervention is found in the Evidence Example below.

Evidence Example: Determining Population Needs in a Rural/Suburban County

The intake nurse at the public health agency was responsible for logging referrals and conversations of significant public health concern. The agency she worked at was small and lacked an on-site physician or walk-in clinic services. It was a 50-mile drive into a larger metropolitan community where low-cost clinics were available. An analysis of her monthly log included calls from uninsured adults with a variety of acute and chronic healthcare conditions. Her findings demonstrated a trend of increasing numbers of working adults lacking access to care. The intake nurse compiled a brief report summarizing 2 months of log entries and presented it to her public health director.

At the next community partner meeting with local medical clinics and hospitals, the director shared the summary provided by the intake nurse and inquired whether the hospital had data on unnecessary patient visits to the emergency department (ED). The group decided to form a committee and to consult with other community partners, such as the local community action program director and the director of one of the largest faith-based clinics in the metro area. This committee, led by the public health director, met numerous times to discuss options for serving their community. One option that they investigated was the establishment of a nursing center, which they proposed to hospital administration. The hospital agreed to fund the part-time center for 1 afternoon a week for 2 years.

The nursing center was located adjacent to the area employment and training center and was staffed by a PHN. Services focused on simple screening measures, referrals, and health promotion. The committee met every 4 months to review data for clients visiting the nursing center and identified a need for physician services, primarily for obtaining refills of medications to prevent an exacerbation of existing medical conditions. One medical clinic offered to see such patients free of charge if they were screened first at the nursing center. About a year later, another healthcare provider purchased a mobile health unit for doing mammography outreach. The committee approached this provider about using the mobile unit for seeing patients in a community setting. It took extensive organizing by the public health department, but eventually the mobile unit visited several community sites each month with a physician on board. These services were the direct result of systems-level collaboration and the determination to advocate for those lacking access to healthcare.

Source: Kleinfehn-Wald, 2010

Nursing diagnoses for populations are often written as risk diagnoses. These risk diagnoses have four components, as outlined in Table 3.9.

Table 3.9   Public Health Population Risk Diagnosis

Components	Example
Health risk	**Increased risk of** infection (pertussis)
Population at risk	**Among** nonimmunized or partially immunized infants and children in (specify geographic area, community, or county)
Modifiable risk factors	**Related to** contact with nonimmunized children and adults who may have pertussis, health beliefs opposing childhood immunizations, knowledge deficit about benefits of immunization, lack of access to health resources
Bio-statistical data (for geographic area, community, city, county, state, national)	**As evidenced by** lack of herd immunity (80–90% immunization) in preschool population (state immunization rate) in (geographic area or city, county, state, county) with (insert number of cases) reported cases of pertussis in the last month in infants and children ages (insert age range)

Because public health nursing is interdisciplinary and occurs within the context of the community, PHNs may decide not to develop their community nursing diagnosis using a nursing taxonomy (e.g., NANDA). The language PHNs use must be clear and understandable to community members and to the interdisciplinary team. Instead, PHNs often identify the public health concern or priority using population health terminology instead of the nursing diagnosis format. For example, PHNs might state their community diagnosis as a public health problem, such as an increase in SIDS deaths or lack of community resources for the mentally ill, and still use the format presented in Table 3.9. However, a nursing diagnosis could be used if it were understandable to all parties involved. An example of a wellness community diagnosis follows:

> Potential for enhanced community coping in Nightingale City following natural disasters related to community-wide planning process, availability of community mental health resources, and state funding for recovery as evidenced by publication of state and county plans, list of mental health providers available for crisis intervention and counseling, and availability of funding for rebuilding damaged housing units

Public Health Nursing Planning and Implementation Process

When working with families in the community, the PHN partners with the families in determining priorities, establishing goals, and developing an intervention plan. The plan should be congruent with and integrated into the family's culture, lifestyle, and daily routine and be within the family's potential to achieve. The plan should enhance the family's potential for self-care and autonomy. As in the traditional nursing care plan, the family care plan outcomes should be realistic, understandable, measurable, behavioral, achievable, and time-specific so that the effectiveness of the plan and the nursing interventions can be determined.

When the PHN is working with the community, the planning process, like the assessment process, involves an interdisciplinary team and key community members. After the team has established priorities and formulated clear statements of the health priorities to be addressed, it is time to determine goals. Community goals are based on community values, beliefs, and the willingness of community members and elected and appointed officials to make changes; the resources available; and a consensus of what is achievable in the given time frame. Specific outcomes are then established. An example of a goal and an outcome for a community follow. Be aware that sometimes the words *goal* and *outcome* are used interchangeably.

- Goal: Reduce obesity in our community.
- Outcome: Reduce obesity in adults in our community by 10% by 2020.

The DHHS created goals for Healthy People 2020 that are based in part on the level of achievement of Healthy People 2010 goals (Reinberg, 2010; U.S. DHHS, 2010). See the following Evidence Example.

Evidence Example: Healthy People 2020 Goals

A news conference by the DHHS related that Healthy People 2020 goals would be more modest than the 2010 goals. Only 19% of Healthy People 2010 goals were met, and progress was made on only 52% of them. Some, like obesity, have become worse since 2000 (a rate of 25% in 2000 increased to 34% in 2010). Examples of some of the new goals for 2020 are:

- Reducing obesity by 10%;

- Reducing the number of smokers by 21%;

- Reducing the number of deaths from heart attack by 20%; and

- Reducing the number of cancer-related deaths by 10%.

Source: Reinberg, 2010

You might notice that the goals for 2020 include measurable outcomes that are time specific and stated as a percentage. These measurable outcomes, called *health status indicators*, were determined by reviewing existing population health outcomes, comparing specific population outcomes with outcomes from other populations, and analyzing evidence from the literature on acceptable outcomes. For example, scientific evidence suggests that obesity is a risk factor for many diseases, so reduction of obesity within a population would be a positive health outcome. At the same time, outcomes need to be realistic. Because U.S. obesity rates increased from 25% to 34% between 2000 and 2010, a 10% reduction in obesity over the next decade might be reasonable, whereas a 25% reduction might be unreasonable.

 ## WEB-BASED ACTIVITY

Go to the Healthy People 2020 website and search for Healthy People 2020 goals.

Review the evidence on the Healthy People 2020 website or evidence in online databases related to the goal you have selected.

Does the evidence support the goal as being reasonable and achievable?

Sometimes intermediate indicators of health outcomes are set when the goal interval is long, such as a decade. For example, it might be a good idea to gather data periodically during the years between 2010 and 2020 to determine whether the interventions selected to achieve the 2020 outcomes are actually being implemented and whether they appear to be working. If the obesity rate has increased or stayed the same by 2015, a change in interventions might be needed.

Selecting and Implementing Best Practice Interventions

After the health status indicators or measurable outcomes have been determined, PHNs select the interventions based on best practice evidence (see Chapter 2). Once best practice interventions have been identified, PHNs present their findings to other staff and administration to receive endorsement of the selected intervention approach. PHNs use the 17 interventions in the Public Health Intervention Wheel (Keller, Strohschein, Lia-Hoagberg, & Schaffer, 2004; MDH, 2001) as an intervention template. (The 17 interventions of the Public Health Intervention Wheel are discussed in Chapter 2.) These interventions are interdisciplinary in nature; many health and helping professions use similar interventions. For example, health educators and social workers use health teaching and counseling as part of their discipline-specific practices, as do PHNs.

Each intervention selected has to fit the individual or family, population or community, situation, and health concern. Evidence of the effectiveness of a specific strategy should provide direction about what to do, how to do it, and how often. For example, the Advisory Committee on Immunization Practice (ACIP) recommends that all people ages 6 months and older receive an annual influenza vaccination (CDC, 2010b). However, not all children have ready access to this vaccine. The following Evidence Example demonstrates that flu shots administered to children and adults in the home setting allow PHNs to increase the level of immunity in families living in poverty.

Evidence Example: In-Home Influenza Immunizations

The MVNA family health nursing staff knew that MVNA had been providing flu shots at public clinics and at contracted corporate sites for more than 13 years but had not extended the program to in-home services. Staff members wanted to be able to give flu shots to family members of newborns and high-risk infants. They were concerned because new moms were getting flu shots before coming home with the baby, leaving the other family members (siblings and extended family) unprotected and putting the infants, who could not receive the influenza vaccine until 6 months of age, at risk. Many family members did not have health insurance. The family health nursing staff brought this unmet health need to the attention of MVNA program managers. The family health managers, flu program managers, and MVNA administration developed a plan to purchase the needed coolers to transport the vaccine and to provide the nurses with the training necessary to give the shots and complete the documentation for billing. MVNA found donors who were willing to underwrite the cost of the flu shots for family members who were uninsured. MVNA family health nursing staff members report that they have given more than 400 flu shots to members of families with new infants in their homes since the start of the program.

Source: Lanigan, 2010

When working with families, PHNs select interventions that will enhance the families' capacity for problem solving and self-care. Health teaching, counseling, consultation, and case management are interventions commonly used to build on and enhance the families' strengths and encourage them to manage their healthcare needs. PHNs employ mutual problem-solving strategies with clients to foster self-efficacy. They use advocacy to facilitate the individuals' and families' ability to access health and social resources. They also use advocacy when populations are found to be at risk for a specific health hazard. The case study in the following Evidence Example illustrates how a small group of PHNs advocated effectively for an individual, a family, and an entire community.

Evidence Example: Advocating for All

I received a referral on a 9-month-old boy with a diagnosis of meningitis secondary to active tuberculosis (TB). His parents, a young Hispanic non-English-speaking couple, had two children and another on the way. The entire family reacted positively to Mantoux tests I administered. I arranged an appointment at the local clinic for the family, complete with transportation and interpreters. The father had active infectious TB, which prevented him from returning to his job at the meat-packing plant and caused him to lose his insurance. I assisted the family in applying for medical assistance and other services.

I involved other PHNs in advocating for the health of the man's coworkers and community. The meat-packing plant employed more than 1,000 people who spoke 12 languages. We worked with the managers, who were worried more about losing production than worker exposure to TB, to convince them that exposure to TB was a serious problem and that they could cooperate with public health and not lose production. They allowed us to offer free Mantoux tests during work time to any employee who wanted to be tested. Out of more than 700 employees who participated, 70 tested positive. Many of the employees with positive Mantoux tests lacked access to healthcare. We negotiated reduced clinic fees and secured community grant funds to pay for X-rays and treatment for infected persons who were uninsured and without resources.

Source: Condensed from "Getting Behind the Wheel" Case Study, Minnesota Department of Health, 2006

Your public health nursing goal directs your actions toward individual/family, community, or systems intervention levels. PHNs often work at more than one level simultaneously. In analyzing the Evidence Example, we can identify goals and interventions at all three levels. Table 3.10 demonstrates the relationship between the client, goal, and interventions provided. (See Chapter 1 for a discussion of intervention levels and Chapter 2 for public health nursing interventions.)

Table 3.10   Public Health Nursing Goals Direct PHNs Toward Three Levels of Interventions

Goal: Identify workers with positive Mantoux results and provide them with follow-up medical options. Client: Individual/family	Screening: Administer Mantoux tests to individual workers at the meat-packing plant. Referral and Follow-Up: Refer workers with positive Mantoux results to community clinics. Teaching: Provide face-to-face teaching to individual workers with positive Mantoux results about the importance of follow-up medical care.
Goal: Prevent additional cases of infectious TB. Client: Community	Disease and Health Event Investigation: Monitor incidence of infectious TB in the community; identify those at risk for exposure; identify those with new positive Mantoux results; and provide community with results of the investigation.

continues

Table 3.10 Public Health Nursing Goals Direct PHNs Toward Three Levels of Interventions   (continued)

Goals: Carry out mass Mantoux screening at meat-packing plant; ensure access to medical care for uninsured workers. Client: Multiple Systems	Advocacy: Work with plant managers to convince them that TB is a hazard to workers and company. Collaboration: Partner with managers to arrange clinic services. Advocacy: Negotiate reduced clinic fees and secure community grant funds to pay for X-rays and treatment for infected persons who are uninsured and without resources.

Zack is working on the community assessment of the halfway house residents. He notices that many of the residents have unmet dental health needs. The residents all receive toothbrushes, toothpaste, and dental floss when they are admitted to the halfway house. The staff reports that almost all the residents brush and floss daily and are very concerned about having their teeth fixed. The staff members believe that improving the dental health and "smile potential" of the residents will improve their self-esteem. Zack thinks that providing accessible dental services for the residents will also help improve their sense of self-efficacy. He thinks dental services will make the residents feel more in charge of their lives. He wonders whether it would be a good idea to have the county mobile dental clinic visit the halfway house on a monthly basis.

ACTIVITY

When Zack considers having a mobile dental clinic visit the halfway house, which PHN intervention level is he practicing?

Which level(s) of prevention would be accomplished through the mobile dental clinic?

How could Zack involve the residents in setting up and managing the dental clinic visits?

Public Health Nursing Evaluation

Before you implement interventions, you need to determine your evaluation measures. You want to measure the outcomes of your interventions. Evaluation is an ongoing process in public health nursing. After you implement your interventions, you need to regularly reassess the progress you are making toward goal achievement. Evaluation data can tell you whether your interventions are effective and whether your clients have met, partially met, or not met expected outcomes. If outcomes have been met, you can choose to continue interventions or to cease interventions. If outcomes have not been met or have only been partially met, you need to discover why this is the case. Unmet outcomes could stem from inadequacies in the assessment of the client's readiness or ability to change, the reasonableness and achievability of the stated outcome, the measure used to evaluate the outcome, or the appropriateness or effectiveness of the interventions used. Interventions not only need to be specific to the health determinants but also need to fit the characteristics of the clients (i.e., culture, ethnicity, developmental level, language literacy). Evaluation and reassessment take thought, time, and effort. After you have evaluated the reason your outcomes have not been achieved, you need to revise your plan and interventions.

ACTIVITY

Write an outcome for dental health for the residents of the halfway house.

Zack has proposed the use of a mobile dental clinic. Think of the Public Health Intervention Wheel. List the interventions that would be involved in setting up and delivering dental services using the mobile clinic.

Determine how you would evaluate the effectiveness of the mobile dental clinic based on the outcome you developed.

The beginning of this chapter discusses the importance of HIS and EHRs in data management and the evaluation of public health nursing interventions and client outcomes. These electronic records provide an efficient and effective means for measuring individual client and family health outcomes and program outcomes. The Omaha System has been used effectively as a quality improvement strategy to promote excellence in client care; improve and ensure data quality; and increase the use of data analysis and reporting capacity (Monsen et al., 2006). The Omaha System has also been used to demonstrate how aggregation of data can be used within and across programs and agencies (Monsen et al., 2010). See the Evidence Example for a discussion of this study.

Evidence Example: Comparing Maternal Child Health Problems and Outcomes Across PHN Agencies

An exploratory descriptive study analyzed maternal child health data from four public health nursing agencies to determine the needs of maternal child health clients and to demonstrate outcomes of services provided. The four agencies developed and implemented a formal standardized data-comparison process using structured Omaha System data. The Omaha System problems addressed most often by the four agencies were Growth and Development; Antepartum/Postpartum; Caretaking/Parenting; Family Planning; Income; Mental Health; Residence; Abuse; Substance Use; and Neglect. Significant improvements were demonstrated in 84% of the problems addressed, with the greatest improvements noted in the categories of Antepartum/Postpartum and Family Planning. The smallest improvements were noted in the areas of Neglect and Substance Use. Although there were some differences by agency, statistically significant improvements were consistent across all four (Monsen et al., 2010).

Although a few program evaluation studies use electronic record systems, most program evaluations in public health nursing are still carried out by traditional research methods. Table 3.11 presents an example of a comprehensive program utilizing multiple public health nursing interventions to reduce repeat teen pregnancy. A global measure of the pregnancy rate was the health outcome used to measure the interventions' effectiveness.

Table 3.11   The Pregnancy-Free Club

Interventions	Outcome
Advocacy, Case Management, Collaboration, Community Organizing, Consultation, Counseling, Health Teaching, Policy Development, Screening, Referral and Follow-Up	A public health agency, school, and local hospital collaborated in the development of a Pregnancy-Free Club to reduce repeat pregnancies among adolescent students. Following program initiation, the repeat adolescent pregnancy rate declined from 25% to 7.2% over a period of 9 years (Schaffer, Jost, Peterson, & Lair, 2008).

Putting It All Together

PHNs understand the relationships that exist between individuals and their physical and social environments. They understand the complexity of individual and family developmental needs. PHNs work within the community and the multiple systems that influence the health and wellness of individuals, families, and populations. They use a holistic public health nursing process to assess the complex factors that influence health and wellness. They weave a tapestry of interventions that provides a safety net for vulnerable individuals, families, and populations. The teen parenting program example (see the Evidence Example below) demonstrates the effectiveness of public health nursing practiced within the community.

Evidence Example: Public Health Teen Parent Program

In one metropolitan county, PHNs providing home-visiting services to teens and their babies recognized that most teen parents were living in poverty, with their primary source of income being federal assistance, including cash and food stamps. In 2003, the rate of high school graduation or GED (General Education Development alternative measure) completion for teen parents was 34%. A study of teen parents showed that 50% of human service dollars spent in most counties in the state was expended on families with teens who had given birth. Public health nursing, human services, and workforce services implemented a system of service delivery that promoted positive prenatal and postpartum outcomes, and positive parental attachment and interaction. They used TANF (Temporary Assistance for Needy Families [pregnant women and families with one or more dependents]) System requirements as a method to improve high school graduation or GED completion rates among teen parents. An analysis of agency data found that the benefit of PHN services to teens was limited by teen parents' acceptance of nursing services, yet at the same time the literature reported the significant benefit of long-term, relationship-based services for teen parents. In this new model, public health nursing became a mandatory service for teen parents receiving TANF funding, and they assumed responsibility for monitoring school attendance and working with teens to improve it. PHNs also provided health assessments, teaching, and other interventions to improve the health status and well-being of the teen family. In 2009, 64.3% of teen parents enrolled in the program graduated from high school or completed a GED. At their exits from the program, the teen parents indicated that, based on their relationships with their PHNs, they knew they could rely on their PHNs for accurate information, health assessments, and teaching, advocacy, referrals, and case management.

Source: Cross, 2010

Ethical Application

Community assessment involves collecting data on individuals. These data are then aggregated to provide for confidentiality and anonymity. However, when the group size is small or the members of the group are easily identified, ethical issues related to privacy rights can arise.

> *Zack is collecting health data from the residents of the halfway house as part of his community assessment project. After analyzing the resident data, he will identify strengths of and health needs for the halfway house residents, work with them to identify their health priorities, and recommend interventions. The residents all have severe mental health disorders and are unable to live independently in the community. These residents are all considered vulnerable adults. Zack is concerned about ethical issues related to informed consent, confidentiality, and autonomy.*

Use the ethical framework in Table 3.12 to determine how you would handle this situation if you were working with Zack.

Table 3.12   Ethical Application of the Nursing Process in Public Health Nursing

Ethical Perspective	Application
Rule Ethics (principles)	• Respect the rights of individuals related to privacy, autonomy, and self-determination. • Critique selected actions and interventions for possible unintended harmful consequences that might occur for diverse populations in a community. • Select interventions that promote justice through reducing health disparities.
Virtue Ethics (character)	• Maintain the dignity and confidentiality of individuals, families, populations, and communities when assessing their health needs. • Be honest in communicating the purpose of selected interventions to individuals, families, populations, and communities. • Be an advocate for assessing the public health needs of vulnerable populations.
Feminist Ethics (reducing oppression)	• Include voices of vulnerable populations in community assessments and in setting priorities for action. • Emphasize the contribution of the assets that communities and diverse populations bring to resolving public health concerns.

Table based on work by Volbrecht (2002) and Racher (2007)

Key Points

- PHNs are accountable to the individuals, families, and communities in which they live and work to take action to maintain or improve their health status.

- PHNs work in partnership with individuals, families, communities, and systems.

- The public health nursing process is used to assess and intervene with individuals, families, communities, and systems.

- PHNs collect demographic and health determinant data when carrying out family and community assessments.

- PHNs use a strength-based approach when working with individuals, families, and communities.

- PHNs use the community assessment process to assess and intervene with specific populations and subpopulations or aggregates.

- PHNs use the 17 interventions of the Public Health Nursing Intervention Wheel (MDH, 2001) to provide nursing services to individuals, families, communities, and systems.

- PHNs use EMRs and HIS to assist them in assessing and monitoring their clients' health status, evaluating their clients' progress, and determining the effectiveness of interventions and programs.

Learning Examples for Practicing the Public Health Nursing Process

Students learn best when clinical activities are meaningful and directed at actually making a difference in peoples' lives. When students combine working with vulnerable populations community organizations, conducting community assessments, and intervening with individuals and families, they have the opportunity to develop public health nursing competencies at all three levels of PHN practice: individual/family, community, and systems. Review the following examples of student experiences and think about how the students used their public health nursing process skills at all three levels of practice.

PHN Clinical in Nicaragua

- Students from the United States worked with vulnerable families in Nicaragua, providing care to families, working in clinics, providing health-related teaching to community groups, completing a community assessment, and holding a health fair.

- Students learned about community health in a developing country, became more aware of social justice issues, and developed skills in cultural competency (Ailinger, Molloy, & Sacasa, 2009).

Population-Focused Analysis Project (PFAP)

- Students working in small groups selected a vulnerable population to study.

- They researched the population by using literature in print and on the web and by carrying out key-informant interviews.

- Outcomes included 45-minute presentations to peers, a poster session, and an advocacy letter written to elected officials, policy makers, or newspapers (Eide, Hahn, Bayne, Allen, & Swain, 2006).

Combining Community Assessment and Change Projects to Make a Difference

- Students working in teams chose a community or population to assess and carried out a change project.

- Students learned that they could create meaningful positive change in a community's health and assume leadership roles to promote positive change (Mansfield & Meyer, 2007).

Partnering With Faith Communities

- Students working in teams carried out community assessments and provided interventions to populations within faith communities.

- Students benefited from applying their skills in real community situations, developing their cultural awareness and competence related to faith communities, strengthening their critical thinking and communication skills, and learning how to work effectively in groups (Otterness, Gehrke, & Sener, 2007).

Establishing a Foot Care Clinic in a Homeless Shelter

- Students completed a needs assessment in a large urban homeless shelter and found that the major unmet health need was foot care.

- The next semester, students and faculty piloted a holistic foot care clinic offered on a monthly basis. The foot care clinic continues and is offered every month during the academic year (Schoon, Champlin, & Hunt, 2012).

Reflective Practice

1. Carrying out the nursing process with families in the home setting presents many challenges. PHNs need to be able to partner with the family, focus on members' immediate needs and priorities, establish realistic goals, and implement interventions over time in a way that builds on family strengths and enhances members' capacity for self-care. Review the following case study and think about what you would do if you were working with this family. Then answer the questions at the end of the case study.

"Getting Behind the Wheel"—Case Management Story

I received a referral for a 22-year-old and her 2-month-old baby. At my initial home visit, the baby appeared overweight and overfed. The young mom had started him on rice cereal in a bottle at 2 weeks. Every time he cried, she gave him a bottle, even though he often struggled and tried to pull away from the nipple. I talked to her about feeding the baby and my concern about his weight, but she responded, "Once he starts moving around, the weight will come off."

By 4 months of age, the baby weighed 27 pounds. By now I was very concerned and called both the nurse and the doctor at the clinic, but no action was taken. Next, I arranged a joint home visit with a nutritionist from WIC (Women, Infants, and Children Program). Both of us counseled the mom to feed the baby only when he was truly hungry.

Two weeks later, I returned to do an NCAST (Nursing Child Assessment Satellite Training) feeding interaction and videotaped the mom feeding the baby. We later watched the tape together and talked about hunger cues and how the baby did not appear to be hungry. The young mother listened but continued to feed the baby whenever he fussed or cried. It was as though she had no other way to comfort him other than to feed him. I was also becoming concerned about the baby's development as he exhibited several delays in fine-motor and language skills when I tested him.

At this point, I started visiting every 2 weeks and placed a family health aide in the home for 2 hours, 1 day a week. The aide's assignment was to role-model appropriate parenting and feeding habits. I also arranged to get a high chair for feeding the child through a nutrition program grant. Currently, I continue to coordinate services from the clinic, nutritionist, and family health aide. At the present time, the baby's weight has stabilized, and he has not gained any more weight.

Source: MDH, 2006

2. Which family protective factors and risk factors can you identify that influenced the baby's nutrition and growth and development?

_____

_____

3. How would you establish mutual priorities with the mother?

_____

_____

4. What would be an appropriate family nursing diagnosis?

_____

_____

5. Which behavioral outcomes would you like to achieve?

_____

_____

6. Which nursing interventions would you use to achieve these outcomes?

_____

_____

7. How would you determine the effectiveness of your interventions?

_____

_____

 ## Application of Evidence

1. Which basic family functions (Clark, 2008) are you trying to strengthen?

_____

_____

2. Which additional family-assessment data would you like to collect for each of these functions?

_____

_____

3. Which strategies would you use to ensure a good first meeting (Jansson et al., 2001)?

_____

_____

4. Which activities would you carry out in each phase of home visiting (McNaughton, 2005)?

_____

_____

Refer to the Cornerstones of Public Health Nursing in Chapter 1.

1. Which cornerstones support partnering with community members to identify community health priorities and develop plans to improve population health?

_____

_____

 Think, Explore, Do

Activity 1: Obesity Prevention

1. Divide the class into small groups. Each group should select one of the following populations:

   - Preschool children

   - Elementary school children

   - Middle school children

   - Adolescents in high school

   - Adult females (different ethnic groups)

   - Adult males (different ethnic groups)

2. Review literature and Internet sources to identify known causes (health determinants) of obesity in the population you have selected.

3. Review literature to identify effective interventions for obesity prevention in the population you have selected.

4. Select an intervention you would like to use with your client population.

5. Discuss how you would implement this intervention.

Activity 2: Electronic Medical Records (EMRs) and Health Information Systems (HIS)

1. Find out whether your clinical agency has an electronic data-management system for clients and services.

2. If yes, talk with your clinical preceptor about the EMRs and HIS at the community agency. Ask about how the system is organized. Find out how your preceptor inputs data, uses the system to monitor client progress, and evaluates the effectiveness of interventions. Find out whether the agency is aggregating individual client data to evaluate program outcomes.

3. If not, talk with your preceptor about the paper records system in use at the community agency. Review a client folder to see how data are organized. Ask your preceptor how the paper records are used to monitor client progress.

Activity 3: Shadowing Your PHN Preceptor

1. Talk with your preceptor about his or her job description and responsibilities.

2. Spend a day shadowing your preceptor. Identify:

    a. Your preceptor's client population;

    b. The PHN interventions your preceptor uses;

    c. The levels of interventions you observe; and

    d. The prevention levels you observe your preceptor using.

References

Ailinger, R. L., Molloy, S. B., & Sacasa, E. R. (2009). Community health nursing student experience in Nicaragua. *Journal of Community Health Nursing, 26,* 47–53. doi:10.1080/07370010902805072

Alkon, A., To, K., Mackie, J. F., Wolff, M., & Bernzweig, J. (2009). Health and safety needs in early care and education programs: What do directors, child health records, and national standards tell us? *Public Health Nursing, 27*(1), 3–16. doi:10.1111/j.1525-1446.2009.00821.x

American Nurses Association. (2013). *Public health nursing: Scope and standards of practice.* Silver Spring, MD: Nursesbooks.org.

Centers for Disease Control and Prevention. (2010a). *Definition of public health informatics.* National Center for Public Health Informatics. Retrieved from http://www.cdc.gov/ncphi/about.html

Centers for Disease Control and Prevention. (2010b). *CDC's Advisory Committee on Immunization Practices (ACIP) recommends universal annual influenza vaccination.* Retrieved from http://www.cdc.gov/media/pressrel/2010/r100224.htm

Clark, M. J. (2008). *Community health nursing.* Upper Saddle River, NJ: Pearson/Prentice Hall.

Cross, S. (2010). *Public health teen parent program.* Unpublished manuscript Ramsey County Public Health. St. Paul, MN.

Dreher, M. C., Skemp, L. E., & Asselin, M. (2006). *Healthy places—Healthy people.* Indianapolis, IN: Sigma Theta Tau International.

Eide, P. J., Hahn, L., Bayne, T., Allen, C. B., & Swain, D. (2006). The population-focused analysis project for teaching community health. *Nursing Education Perspectives, 27*(1), 22–27.

Eriksson, I., & Nilsson, K. (2008). Preconditions needed for establishing a trusting relationship during health counseling: An interview study. *Journal of Clinical Nursing, 17*(17), 2352–2359.

Gardner, A. (2010). Therapeutic friendliness and the development of therapeutic leverage by mental health nurses in community rehabilitation settings. *Contemporary Nurse, 34*(2), 140–148.

Hargate, C. (2013). *Windshield survey.* Unpublished manuscript, Bethel University. St. Paul, MN.

Hunt, R. (2013). *Introduction to community-based nursing.* Philadelphia, PA: Wolters Kluwer Health/Lippincott Williams and Williams.

Jansson, A., Petersson, K., & Uden, G. (2001). Nurses' first encounters with parents of new-born children: Public health nurses' views of a good meeting. *Journal of Clinical Nursing, 10,* 140–151.

Kaakinen, J. R., Gedaly-Duff, V., Coehlo, D. P., & Hanson, S. M. H. (2010). *Family health care nursing: Theory, practice and research, 4th ed.* Philadelphia: F. A. Davis.

Keller, L. O., Strohschein, S., Lia-Hoagberg, B., & Schaffer, M. A. (2004). Population-based public health interventions. *Public Health Nursing, 21*(5), 453–468.

Kelly, P. J. (2005). Practical suggestions for community interventions using participatory action research. *Public Health Nursing, 22*(1), 65–73.

Kleinfehn-Wald, N. (2010). *Determining population needs in a rural/suburban county.* Unpublished manuscript from Scott County Public Health. Shakopee, MN.

Lanigan, C. (2010). *In-home influenza immunizations.* Unpublished manuscript from Minnesota Visiting Nurse Association. Minneapolis, MN.

Mansfield, R., & Meyer, C. L. (2007). Making a difference with combined community assessment and change projects. *Journal of Nursing Education, 46*(3), 132–134.

Martin, K. S. (2005). *The Omaha System: A key to practice, documentation, and information management, 2nd ed.* Omaha, NE: Health Connections Press.

Martin, K. S., Monsen, K. A., & Bowles, K. H. (2011). The Omaha System and meaningful use: Applications for practice, education, and research. *CIN: Computers, Informatics, Nursing, 29*(1), 52–58. doi:10.1097/NCN.0b013e3181f9ddc6

McCann, T. V., & Baker, H. (2001). Mutual relating: Developing interpersonal relationships in the community. *Journal of Advanced Nursing, 34*(4), 530–537.

McNaughton, D. B. (2005). A naturalistic test of Peplau's theory in home visiting. *Public Health Nursing, 22*(5), 429–438.

Meagher-Stewart, D., Edwards, N., Aston, M., & Young, L. (2009). Population health surveillance practice of public health nurses. *Public Health Nursing, 26*(6), 553–560. doi:10.1111/j.1525-1446.2009.00814.x

Minnesota Department of Health. (n.d.). How to: Community health assessment. Retrieved from http://www.health.state.mn.us/divs/opi/pm/lphap/cha/howto.html

Minnesota Department of Health. (2001). *Public health interventions: Application for public health nursing practice.* St. Paul, MN: Author.

Minnesota Department of Health, Center for Public Health Nursing Practice. (2003). *The nursing process applied to population-based public health nursing practice.* Retrieved from http://www.health.state.mn.us/divs/opi/cd/phn/docs/0303phn_processapplication.pdf

Minnesota Department of Health, Office of Public Health Practice. (2006). *A collection of "Getting Behind the Wheel Stories" 2000–2006.* Retrieved from http://www.health.state.mn.us/divs/opi/cd/phn/docs/0606wheel_stories.pdf

Monsen, K. A., Fitzsimmons, L. L., Lescenski, B. A., Lytton, A. B., Schwichtenberg, L. D., & Martin, K. S. (2006). A public health nursing informatics data-and-practice quality project. *CIN: Computers, Informatics, Nursing, 24*(3), 152–158.

Monsen, K. A., Fulkerson, J. A., Lytton, A. B., Taft, L. L., Schwichtenberg, L. D., & Martin, K. S. (2010). Comparing maternal child health problems and outcomes across public health nursing agencies. *Maternal and Child Health Journal, 14*(3), 412–421. doi:10.1007/s10995-009-0479-9

Omaha System. (2010). *Omaha System website.* Retrieved from http://www.omahasystem.org

Otterness, N., Gehrke, P., & Sener, I. M. (2007). Partnerships between nursing education and faith communities: Benefits and challenges. *Journal of Nursing Education, 46*(1), 39–44.

Parris, K. M., Place, P. J., Orellana, E., Calder, J., Jackson, K., Karolys, A, . . . Smith, D. (1999). Integrating nursing diagnoses, interventions, and outcomes in public health nursing practice. *Nursing Diagnosis, 10*(2), 49–56.

Racher, F. (2007). The evolution of ethics for community practice. *Journal of Community Health Nursing, 24*(1), 65–76.

Reinberg, S. (2010). *U.S. government sets new health goals for 2020.* Retrieved from http://consumer.healthday.com/Article.asp?AID=646932

Schaffer, M. A., Jost, R., Peterson, B. J., & Lair, M. (2008). Pregnancy-free club: A strategy to prevent repeat adolescent pregnancy. *Public Health Nursing, 25*(4), 304–311. doi:10.1111/j.1525-1446.2008.00710.x

Schoon, P. (2010). *Elementary school health assessment.* Unpublished manuscript.

Schoon, P. M., Champlin, B., & Hunt, R. (2012). Developing a sustainable foot care clinic in a homeless shelter within an academic-community partnership through curricular integration and faculty engagement. *Journal of Nursing Education, 51*(12), 714–718. doi:10.3928/01484834-20121112-02

Scroggins, L. M. (2008). The developmental processes for NANDA international nursing diagnoses. *International Journal of Nursing Terminologies and Classifications, 19*(2), 57–64.

Truglio-Londrigan, M., & Lewenson, S. B. (2013). *Public health nursing: Practicing population-based care.* Sudbury, MA: Jones and Bartlett.

U.S. Department of Health and Human Services. (2010). *Introducing Healthy People 2020.* Retrieved from http://www.healthy-people.gov/2020/about/default.aspx

Volbrecht, R. M. (2002). *Nursing ethics: Communities in dialogue.* Upper Saddle River, NJ: Pearson/Prentice Hall.

COMPETENCY #2
Utilizes Basic Epidemiological Principles (the Incidence, Distribution, and Control of Disease in a Population) in Public Health Nursing Practice

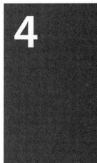

Carolyn M. Garcia

with Noreen Kleinfehn-Wald, Linda J. W. Anderson, and Madeleine Kerr

Elizabeth had worked as a public health nurse (PHN) doing home visits on the maternal child health team for approximately a year. One day as she was having lunch with her co-workers, someone mentioned that an outbreak of pertussis had occurred in an adjacent county. In fact, there were 42 cases! Two days later, Elizabeth's supervisor asked whether she could help the Disease Prevention & Control (DP & C) team investigate 10 probable cases of pertussis.

DP & C nurses operated the immunization clinic and worked with infectious disease issues, such as tuberculosis. Other than these activities, Elizabeth knew very little of what their day-to-day work was like. Her supervisor explained that disease investigation was case management work. She would not be required to do any additional home visits but would need to plan on a limited amount of time to place phone calls, review records, and work with community partners, such as school nurses. Elizabeth agreed to take the additional assignment and arranged to receive orientation from the lead nurse. During this briefing, the lead nurse explained the state's data-privacy laws, the state health department's infectious disease reporting requirements for pertussis, and the report form that needed to be completed by the healthcare provider or the lab associated with the clinic for each suspected or confirmed case. This was a lot of new information!

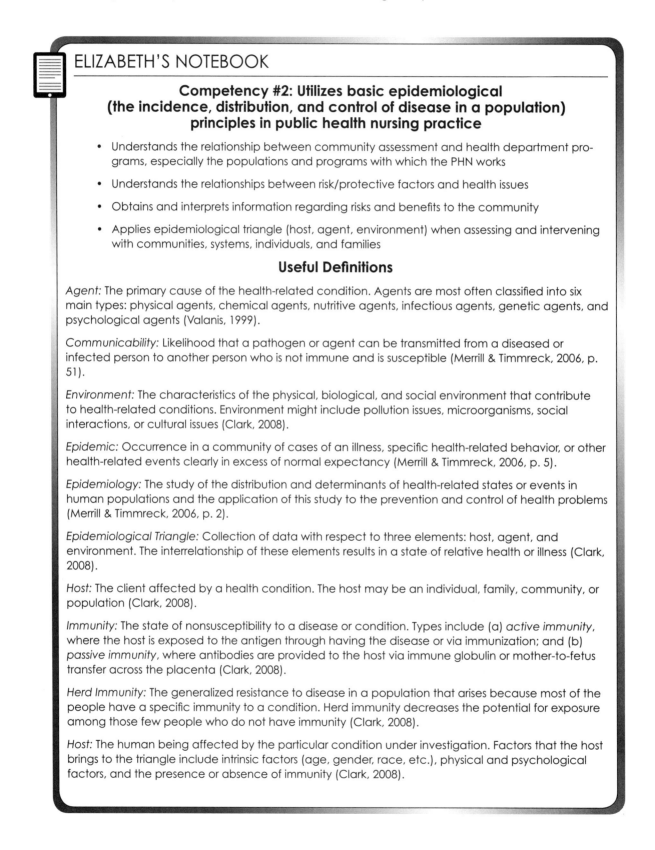

ELIZABETH'S NOTEBOOK

Competency #2: Utilizes basic epidemiological (the incidence, distribution, and control of disease in a population) principles in public health nursing practice

- Understands the relationship between community assessment and health department programs, especially the populations and programs with which the PHN works

- Understands the relationships between risk/protective factors and health issues

- Obtains and interprets information regarding risks and benefits to the community

- Applies epidemiological triangle (host, agent, environment) when assessing and intervening with communities, systems, individuals, and families

Useful Definitions

Agent: The primary cause of the health-related condition. Agents are most often classified into six main types: physical agents, chemical agents, nutritive agents, infectious agents, genetic agents, and psychological agents (Valanis, 1999).

Communicability: Likelihood that a pathogen or agent can be transmitted from a diseased or infected person to another person who is not immune and is susceptible (Merrill & Timmreck, 2006, p. 51).

Environment: The characteristics of the physical, biological, and social environment that contribute to health-related conditions. Environment might include pollution issues, microorganisms, social interactions, or cultural issues (Clark, 2008).

Epidemic: Occurrence in a community of cases of an illness, specific health-related behavior, or other health-related events clearly in excess of normal expectancy (Merrill & Timmreck, 2006, p. 5).

Epidemiology: The study of the distribution and determinants of health-related states or events in human populations and the application of this study to the prevention and control of health problems (Merrill & Timmreck, 2006, p. 2).

Epidemiological Triangle: Collection of data with respect to three elements: host, agent, and environment. The interrelationship of these elements results in a state of relative health or illness (Clark, 2008).

Host: The client affected by a health condition. The host may be an individual, family, community, or population (Clark, 2008).

Immunity: The state of nonsusceptibility to a disease or condition. Types include (a) *active immunity*, where the host is exposed to the antigen through having the disease or via immunization; and (b) *passive immunity*, where antibodies are provided to the host via immune globulin or mother-to-fetus transfer across the placenta (Clark, 2008).

Herd Immunity: The generalized resistance to disease in a population that arises because most of the people have a specific immunity to a condition. Herd immunity decreases the potential for exposure among those few people who do not have immunity (Clark, 2008).

Host: The human being affected by the particular condition under investigation. Factors that the host brings to the triangle include intrinsic factors (age, gender, race, etc.), physical and psychological factors, and the presence or absence of immunity (Clark, 2008).

Incidence: The number of individuals who develop the disease over a defined period of time (Le, 2001) or the number of new cases of a particular condition identified over a period of time (Clark, 2008).

Life Course Epidemiology: The study of long-term effects on later health or the risk of disease due to physical or social exposures during gestation, childhood, adolescence, young adulthood, and later adult life (Kuh, Ben-Shlomo, Lynch, Hallqvist, & Power, 2003, p. 778).

Prevalence: The number of existing cases of a disease or health condition within a population at some designated time (Friis & Sellers, 1999, p. 97).

Protective Factor: Health determinants that protect one from illness and/or assist in improving health (see Chapter 1).

Risk Factor: Health determinants that contribute to the potential for illness to occur or to a decrease in health or well-being (see Chapter 1).

Surveillance: The ongoing systematic collection, analysis, interpretation, and dissemination of health-related data to improve the health of populations (CDC, 2001).

Using Data to Solve Health and Disease Mysteries

Nurses often want to know why something happens or does not happen. This inquisitive nature is useful when nurses are working to prevent something from happening or to intervene before something gets worse. In some situations, if questions are not asked, credible solutions might be overlooked, and health outcomes might not be optimal. In a worst-case scenario, lives might be lost or seriously harmed if the status quo is maintained and curious questions are not asked and acted upon. At the foundation of effective population-based public health nursing is the science of epidemiology. *Epidemiology* guides the questions that PHNs ask and the steps that they take to find answers and solutions. Following is a list of questions nurses ask or should ask regularly:

- How did this occur?

- What could have prevented this outcome?

- When did the problem start (end, worsen, improve)?

- What has contributed to the change? Triggered a response?

- Why have x, y, z not improved?

- Who should be involved to contribute to the solution?

- Where are available resources to aid in addressing this situation?

- Which interventions can reduce the spread of this occurrence/disease?

- Will I be working at the individual/family, community, or systems level?

- Do I need to consider any ethical issues?

- How will I know whether the interventions are effective?

At its core, epidemiology is the study of solving mysteries—of understanding where and to what extent diseases, events, and behaviors are influencing the health of populations. Epidemiology is more than simply understanding what is going on. It also involves acting on what is understood to prevent or control problems. Similarly, a PHN should be committed not only to understanding what is contributing to a problem and the extent of the problem but also to identifying and implementing disease prevention and health promotion strategies. In fact, this use of core epidemiological pieces—namely, mathematics and data analysis—contributed to advancing the role and view of nursing in the 19th century (Earl, 2009). See the Evidence Example below to examine how Lillian Wald and Florence Nightingale used data gathering and analysis to understand and address key health problems. By doing so, they advanced the profession of nursing beyond what had, up until that time, been a fairly ill-considered occupation.

Evidence Example: Origins of Epidemiology and Nursing

Catherine Earl (2009) has written a fascinating and thorough historical article that describes the influence of epidemiology in the developing role of public health nursing. Beginning with the early 19th century, Earl presents a summary of history that reminds the reader of how far nursing and science have come in the past 200 years. Not that long ago, diseases were addressed solely within the individual, with little appreciation given for trends among the group or population. Advances in mathematical theories caused a shift, notably when Pierre Charles Alexandre Louis, a leading 19th-century physician, declared that the practice of bloodletting (often with the help of leeches) was ineffective and used statistics to support his claims. It is intriguing that, according to Earl, the use of quantitative methods was not well supported at that time and was poorly understood. This is interesting, considering that in the 21st century, quantitative analyses are core to randomized controlled trials (RCTs), which are considered the gold standard for establishing evidence.

Lillian Wald used this advance in health and science to support her work with families in New York. She advocated for nurses to live and work near and among those they were also serving. She used numbers to support her need for resources, including the number of nurses. Her successes are many, and they are in part based on her foresight and wisdom in recognizing the need for data to accomplish goals and meet the health and social needs of society. Earl summarizes well the contribution PHNs, led by Lillian Wald, made in addressing tuberculosis, because they collected and reported critical data: "Nurses' involvement in the care of TB [tuberculosis] patients in 1914 was considered a major advancement in the use of statistical methods, because nurses became involved in improving health through their role as data collectors" (p. 262).

Florence Nightingale, considered by many to be the first biostatistician and the first epidemiologist, also used data to support her efforts to address health and sanitation. In her era, it was not common for women to be educated, yet her father encouraged her to learn varied subjects, including mathematics. As a result, Nightingale had skills that enabled her to identify causes of problems and to intervene not only to heal or cure but also to prevent. As Earl states, "With an epidemiological perspective and further discussions of mortality and morbidity rates and the importance of sanitary conditions as described by Florence Nightingale, the first preventorium, a program established to save children, was designed for the prevention, not the treatment, of TB"

(p. 263). Both Lillian Wald and Florence Nightingale contributed to a significant shift from solely focusing on treatment to giving attention toward prevention, which today is also a primary focus of PHNs all over the world.

Although most PHNs are not epidemiologists, many activities that PHNs engage in parallel the work of epidemiologists. Often epidemiologists work at the systems level of a healthcare facility or state health department and are responsible for the data collection, analysis, and program development related to a particular health/medical issue. Conversely, PHNs are frequently found in the grassroots level of healthcare, working with local vulnerable populations and community partners, interpreting and promoting the recommendations, protocols, and policies that have been developed by an authoritative body. See Table 4.1 for an example list of activities that an epidemiologist often engages in and note the similarities to many public health nursing activities and interventions.

Table 4.1 Example Activities of Epidemiologists and Public Health Nurses

Epidemiologist Activities (adapted from Merrill & Timmreck, 2006, p. 3)	Public Health Nursing Activities and Interventions
Identifying risk factors for disease, injury, and death	Disease and Health Event Investigation
Describing the natural history of disease	Health Teaching
Identifying individuals and populations at greatest risk for disease	Outreach Screening Referral and Follow-Up Advocacy Case Management
Identifying where the public health problem is greatest	Surveillance Disease and Health Event Investigation
Monitoring diseases and other health-related events over time	Surveillance
Evaluating the efficacy and effectiveness of prevention and treatment programs	Evaluation is a key part of the nursing process, but it is not a specific component of the intervention wheel.
Providing information useful in health planning and decision making for establishing health programs with appropriate boundaries	Consultation Collaboration Community Organizing Policy Development and Enforcement

continues

Table 4.1   Example Activities of Epidemiologists and Public Health
Nurses   (continued)

Epidemiologist Activities (adapted from Merrill & Timmreck, 2006, p. 3)	Public Health Nursing Activities and Interventions
Assisting in carrying out public health programs	Most interventions on the Public Health Intervention Wheel
Serving as a resource	Consultation
Communicating health information	Outreach Health Teaching Social Marketing Consultation

Historically, nurses participated in epidemiologic investigations to determine the cause of a recurring problem, such as cholera outbreaks. As part of that process very early on, nurses realized that numerous risk factors often contributed to the spread of disease. This realization led to creative interventions that had multiple components to aid those already sick or affected and to prevent others from becoming sick. Quarantine (i.e., separation of an exposed individual from the rest of the community) laws are a good example of a specific effort to contain the spread of disease in the absence of other strategies. Interestingly, quarantine strategies are still used today, because some infectious viruses take time to resolve and, during set time frames, can be easily spread from person to person. Examples of such illnesses in the 21st century include pertussis, chicken pox, and the flu. When an individual is diagnosed with pertussis and other family members have been exposed, the pertussis case is strongly encouraged to stay isolated from the broader community until 5 days of antibiotic treatment have been completed. During the Sudden Acute Respiratory Syndrome (SARS) event in 2002 and 2003, quarantine of exposed individuals was key to containing the epidemic. Individuals placed under quarantine were monitored twice daily by public health workers until the SARS incubation period was completed. Although quarantines are not always enforced as they were years ago and in the SARS event, they can be effective when they are followed and when individuals and families adhere to the restrictions.

More broadly, Lillian Wald offers to us a great example of a PHN using a variety of intervention tools to address uncontrolled disease and unnecessary deaths in New York City tenements. At the individual level, she provided direct care for sick individuals in crowded apartments. At the community level, she organized community care for neighborhood children in need of a place to engage in physical activity. At the systems level, she advocated for programs that would meet the needs of many (e.g., welfare, food accessibility, child labor laws). Today's PHN needs a repertoire of intervention strategies so that when health improves, it can be maintained over time—which is sometimes hard to do. For example, if a child recovers from an illness that worsened as a result of malnourishment and lack of warmth, but the family home environment remains unchanged, the child's recovery might not be maintained. In this case, the nurse might provide a space heater as a temporary solution and connect the family to a food bank. The nurse might begin to create long-term solutions by inquiring into the reasons for the lack of heat and might help adult family members explore financial management strategies as well as possibilities for higher-paying employment or more affordable, reliable housing. Finally, the nurse might advocate for legislation that prohibits companies or landlords from turning off heat sources during cold winter months. Nurses encounter numerous possible mechanisms for influence when they face a problem that might appear to have a simple solution but often requires complex intervention approaches to keep that problem from recurring.

Understands the Relationship Between Community Assessment and Health Department Programs

Many public health agencies and community organizations use community assessments to prioritize the programs and services that they offer. Fundamental to the community assessment is the understanding of the incidence and distribution of disease in the community. The PHN often starts by reviewing the birth and death data available through the state department of health. Morbidity data can also be reviewed to determine trends in reportable diseases (such as tuberculosis or sexually transmitted infections) or case numbers of such conditions as cancers or motor vehicle fatalities or injuries. A comprehensive review of data sources generally leads and directs the community assessment process.

A variety of other strategies can be used to expand the community assessment (e.g., needs assessment via focus groups or key-informant interviews, windshield survey; see Chapter 3 for more information on community assessment). The specific approach used is based on the key questions being asked. For example, if a public health department has identified an increase in obesity in the population and plans to implement an obesity prevention program, questions might focus on identifying the groups in the community at greatest risk for obesity (e.g., age, ethnicity, neighborhood). A survey might be conducted to identify the most likely barriers to occur when the obesity prevention program is introduced. These data could then inform the steps that will be taken to optimize successful implementation of the obesity prevention program. Often, PHNs are involved in every step of this process: (a) identifying the questions that need to be asked, (b) developing the data-collection process, (c) collecting the data, (d) analyzing the data, and (e) using the data to inform future actions and program delivery.

PHNs work collaboratively in conducting assessments and using the resulting data for informing priorities and actions. Although it might be natural to focus on needs because the nurse is trying to address a problem, it is extremely valuable to take a strength- or asset-based approach toward the issue (Lind & Smith, 2008). An asset-based approach ensures that the assessment includes documentation of existing or potential strengths. In this way, the possible problem-solving strategies will ideally build on identified strengths and assets. If nurses focus only on problems, they might reach a solution that consists of outside resources rather than builds on what is available. Asset-based perspectives inherently encourage capacity building as well as self-care among individuals and families, communities, and populations (see Chapter 5 for discussion of incorporating community assets).

> *Elizabeth looked at the faxed pertussis report she had been given on 11-year-old Billy Johnson. Information included Billy's birth date, address, phone number, and laboratory results, which were positive for pertussis. Next, Elizabeth looked up Billy in the computerized state immunization registry. She saw that he had been vaccinated with five doses of DTaP vaccine, the last of which was administered at 5 years of age. Elizabeth recognized that the immunity provided by the vaccine had possibly waned.*

ACTIVITY
Reflect on the following questions:

- What has Elizabeth discovered so far?
- What are her next steps?

Understands the Relationships Between Risk/Protective Factors and Health Issues

No better classic example of understanding the relationship between a risk factor and a health issue exists than that of John Snow in mid-1800s London. For unknown reasons, many people in London began to suffer and die as a result of cholera. People were fleeing the city because of fear, and without a known cause, they had little confidence that the disease could be stopped or prevented. John Snow created a map that began to identify where the deaths from cholera were occurring across London. This now-famous map (see Figure 4.1) yielded some clues for Snow, because he managed to visualize the areas where the deaths were most heavily concentrated. He suspected a water source, so to prohibit people from accessing this source of "risk," he removed the water pump handle, as described below:

> **1854:** Physician John Snow convinces a London local council to remove the handle from a pump in Soho. A deadly cholera epidemic in the neighborhood comes to an end immediately, though perhaps serendipitously. Snow maps the outbreak to prove his point . . . and launches modern epidemiology. (Alfred, 2009, p. 1)

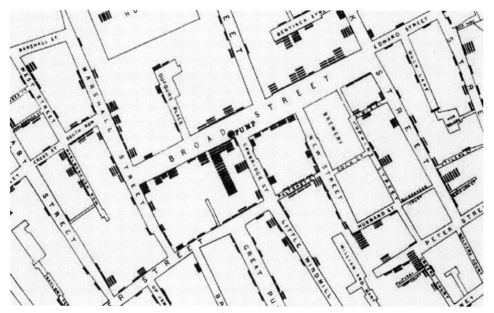

Figure 4.1
Source: Alfred, 2009

In the 21st century, PHNs continue to solve mysteries in identifying and eliminating health risks, and although conditions have improved in many parts of the world, reducing the risks from unsanitary conditions, these improvements are not universal. Consider the following observation:

> The 2010 cholera epidemic in Haiti reminds us that cholera remains a deadly disease, not all that different from the time of John Snow. While Snow debated the appropriateness of the germ theory versus the miasmatic theory for the cause of the disease, current scientists are focusing on different, but related, hypotheses. (UCLA, 2010, p. 1)

Indeed, it is true that more than a century since Snow's solved mystery, we continue to seek clearer answers and solutions regarding the risks and diseases that are present in public health settings across the globe. In the United States, PHNs face complex challenges in meeting the needs of individuals, families, communities, and populations. Nurses need to identify risk and protective factors at multiple influencing levels. For example, a nurse might be working with a child recently diagnosed with asthma. The nurse needs to identify risk factors in the family environment that might be triggers for asthma episodes. Similarly, the nurse needs to assess for protective factors in the family, such as parental commitment to preventing episodes, which is an important asset the nurse can support with education and related tools. The nurse might want to go further and explore the neighborhood environment, including the school setting, for possible risks or protections influencing the child.

It can take time to carefully and thoroughly assess risk and protective factors using a strengths-based approach. Usually, the time is well spent, because the PHN will have a very clear picture of available assets as well as deficits to address when intervening on a particular health issue. Doing this proactively is a critical part of health promotion. Conducting assessments of risk and protective factors after a health issue has become apparent is important to minimize the effect of the health problem and to encourage positive intervention results. PHNs continually reassess for risk and protective factors, because these factors can be temporal; one day a risk might exist (e.g., lack of health insurance coverage), but the following week the family might have new health insurance coverage. PHNs commit to efforts that routinely assess, intervene, evaluate, and reassess.

A PHN also stays informed about emerging diseases and pandemic threats. For example, during 2012, increased pertussis cases or outbreaks were reported in 49 states and Washington, D.C., compared with 2011. See the table below for states that had the highest reported rates of pertussis in 2012. Provisional counts from the Centers for Disease Control and Prevention (CDC) surveillance system indicate that more than 41,000 cases of pertussis were reported to the CDC during 2012. The majority of deaths continue to occur among infants younger than 3 months of age, and the incidence rate of pertussis among infants exceeds that of all other age groups. The second-highest rates of disease are observed among children ages 7 to 10 years. Rates also increase in adolescents ages 13 to 14 years.

In the case of pertussis, the PHN would recognize pertussis vaccination as a protective factor. Lack of vaccination, waning immunity from vaccination, and posing immune-compromising conditions would be risk factors.

Table 4.2   States With Incidence of Pertussis the Same or Higher Than the National Incidence During 2012 (as of January 10, 2013), Which Is 13.4/100,000 Persons

Wisconsin	104.9	Montana	44.3	Pennsylvania	14.5
Vermont	100.6	Alaska	43.3	Illinois	14.5
Minnesota *	82.9	New Mexico	35.7	Idaho	14.3
Washington	67.4	Colorado	28.9	Missouri	14.2
North Dakota	54.4	Kansas	25.5	Arizona	13.4
Iowa	53.5	Oregon	23.3	-	-
Maine	52.9	New Hampshire	16.4	-	-
Utah	47.5	New York	15.8	-	-

Source: Pertussis Outbreak Trends, Centers for Disease Control, 2013.

* Only a subset of Minnesota pertussis cases have been reported through NNDSS for 2012. These data were accessed via the Minnesota Department of Health website.

Elizabeth prepared to call Billy's parents. She placed the protocol nearby and had her report form ready. Billy's mother answered the phone, and Elizabeth introduced herself as a PHN who worked with infectious diseases. She explained how she had obtained a pertussis report on Billy and inquired whether his mother had about 15 minutes to speak with her. Billy's mother stated that she operates an in-home daycare, but most of the children had not yet arrived.

Elizabeth mentally noted this information about the daycare and then explained that the purpose of the call was to identify what could be done to prevent the spread of the disease. Elizabeth started with what she thought was the most logical question—when did this cough start? Billy's mother recalled that he started coughing on the 17th and had a paroxysmal cough without a whooping sound. He occasionally coughed so hard that he vomited. About 1 week before his cough started, he had a low-grade fever and a runny nose.

Because his cough was not getting any better, his mother brought Billy to the clinic on the 26th. Billy did not have pneumonia or any other complications of pertussis. He was given azithromycin antibiotic and was now on his third day of a 5-day course of treatment. Elizabeth jotted down a note that stated the period of infectivity started about the 10th of the month, about a week before the cough started.

Next Elizabeth asked how many other family members were in the home. Billy lived with his parents and had no siblings. Neither parent had been coughing. Elizabeth discussed with his mother the public health recommendation that other household members take a preventive course of antibiotics. She agreed to call the clinic for prescriptions.

To further assess for close contacts, Elizabeth asked questions about Billy's school. Billy told his mother "a lot of kids" were coughing in his classroom. Elizabeth stated that she would talk to the school nurse about sending a notification letter to the parents of the students in Billy's classroom, Elizabeth was careful to inform the mother that Billy would not be identified in the letter. Elizabeth explained that she would also be working with the school to identify children who sit adjacent to Billy, as they might also need preventive antibiotics.

Obtains and Interprets Information Regarding Risks and Benefits to the Community

PHNs need to have an understanding of how to find and use data. Data drive so much of what PHNs do. In fact, PHNs determine health priorities by using data to identify key problem areas or concerns. PHNs also use data to evaluate whether interventions or programs are successful in reducing the risks or health problems in a local community. Unfortunately, data are not always easy to interpret or understand; data are often presented in such formats as tables, figures or graphs, or raw numbers. They might be posed as percentages or risk ratios. Although in-depth knowledge of data, formulas, and calculations is not necessary for entry-level PHNs, they will find some awareness of how to read data and data types useful.

> **Healthy People 2020** The Healthy People 2020 website offers opportunities to explore the uses of data in public health. On the website, click "Data." From here, you can do a data search on a public health topic of interest to you. Select the health topic and then limit your search by a variety of factors, such as sex, age, race/ethnicity, and geographic location. The results are presented using the Healthy People 2020 indicators (goals/markers) and show trends over the past few years. What do you observe in the data you explore? How might these data be useful to a PHN engaged in health promotion?

Data Trend in a Graph

Often, data are presented over time by using graphs to show what is happening in a community with respect to a particular health problem or population trend. For example, a PHN might be interested in exploring trends related to tuberculosis cases in the community over the past 5 years —that is, the nurse is doing surveillance of TB in the jurisdiction (see Figure 4.2). The data in a graph form provide a snapshot of how the number of cases is increasing, maintaining, or decreasing. In the tuberculosis example, it is apparent that active TB cases are progressively increasing, whereas latent TB cases can dramatically decrease, increase, and then stabilize. This information might lead the PHN to ask questions about pulmonary versus non-pulmonary TB or population changes in the community and explore specific intervention strategies to reduce the number of active TB cases over the next few years.

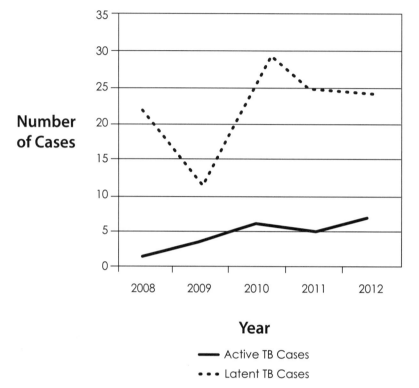

Figure 4.2. Example Trend of Active and Latent Tuberculosis Cases in a Community

Data Trend per 100,000 in a Graph

Similarly, a PHN might examine the trend of chlamydia cases over a period of 5 years. Rather than looking at the raw number of cases (as in the tuberculosis example), the PHN might prefer to examine the rate of cases, which is always based on a ratio or number of cases per 100,000 persons. The raw case number in the tuberculosis example does not give a picture of how serious the problem is, because the graph does not indicate how many people are in the community. For example, if the community population count were 100 and there were 50 cases of latent TB, the PHN would be much more concerned than if there were 50 cases in a community population of 100,000. In the chlamydia example, the rate of cases appears to be increasing, from around 90 per 100,000 in year 1 to nearly 140 per 100,000 in year 5 (see Figure 4.3). This increase is concerning by itself, but the PHN might want to compare the rate in one community with the rate in another community. Comparing rates in different communities or populations provides the PHN with perspective about the relative severity of the disease incidence or prevalence and helps determine how to prioritize efforts to prevent chlamydia's spread.

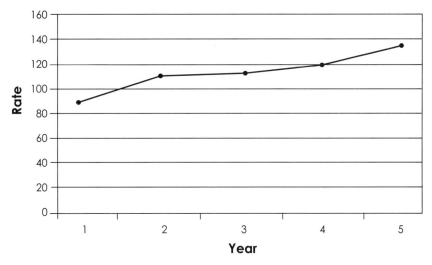

Figure 4.3. Chlamydia Example of Case Rate per 100,000 Over 5 Years

The following Evidence Example discusses using data regarding incidence rates to identify a problem and evaluate the impact of a system-wide intervention to reduce the rate of tuberculosis among inmates.

Evidence Example: Use of Epidemiological Tuberculosis Data to Inform a New York State Corrections Intervention

In a study addressing tuberculosis, data were used to inform strategies to prevent increases of tuberculosis among inmates in the New York State Corrections system (Klopf, 1998). Data indicated that the incidence of tuberculosis had increased over a 6-year period from 43 per 100,000 to 225 per 100,000, a serious problem that warranted intervention. Collaboratively, people from corrections, the local department of health, and the parole division developed a comprehensive TB control program that focused on the prevention and containment of disease. Importantly, they implemented a nurse-led case management program, using infection control nurses to carefully monitor and intervene on active and suspected TB cases. The program was truly comprehensive, including policies, development of a TB registry, surveillance, detection, and case management involving preventive and directly observed therapy among the inmates. The staff and inmates received education regarding testing, diagnoses, disease process, and treatment. It is believed that this comprehensive program contributed to the reduced incidence of TB. Six years later, the rate decreased from 225 per 100,000 to 61 per 100,000 — a 73% reduction! The data informed the need for an intervention that relied heavily on nurses. The data also demonstrated, in part, the impact of the intervention program, showing a significant reduction in the new cases of TB among New York's inmates.

Data Comparison Between State and National Sources

Comparing health and disease trends across communities can be challenging and create turmoil if it is not done in a careful manner. No community wants to appear worse than another when it comes to a health problem or condition. On the other hand, if resources are scarce, a community might want to justify acquiring greater access to available resources. Careful comparison of data within and across communities is vital to ensure that public health priorities are appropriate and that the chosen resource allocation is warranted. Comparison is useful because it can bring understanding of the severity or scope of a problem, especially if policy makers are unaware of the problem or not convinced that it requires attention.

A good example of this scenario is Lyme disease, which is contracted through exposure to ticks. The Minnesota Department of Health reports the number of Lyme disease cases since 1986, ranging from annual cases of 67 to 1,299 (see Figure 4.4). However, without being able to compare these numbers to those of another state, it is difficult to determine whether the problem is serious or relatively consistent with national trends. The PHN investigating this issue might look beyond state-level data to what is occurring nationally. Review of national data provided by the CDC would demonstrate that in 2009, Minnesota had one of the highest density areas of Lyme disease cases, second only to states along the East Coast (see Figure 4.5). The data in Figure 4.5 are from a Geographic Information System (GIS) wherein a dot is placed within the county of residence for each confirmed case of Lyme disease. GIS is an example of a mapping tool that PHNs may use for surveillance (see Innovative Data Collection below for more GIS information). These data would support efforts by PHNs to bring attention to the problem and to invest in preventive messages for Minnesotans regarding the spread of Lyme disease.

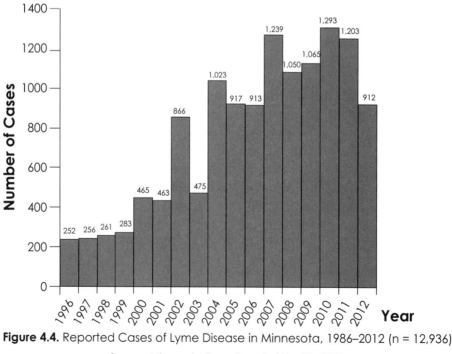

Figure 4.4. Reported Cases of Lyme Disease in Minnesota, 1986–2012 (n = 12,936)

Source: Minnesota Department of Health, 2013

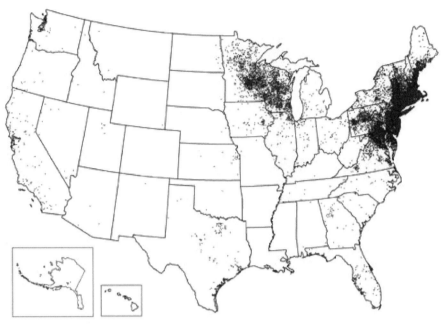

1 dot placed randomly within county of residence for each confirmed case

Figure 4.5. Reported Cases of Lyme Disease—United States, 2011
Source: Centers for Disease Control and Prevention, 2013

In this example, it is useful to point out that the data from the state and the CDC represent different years; the Minnesota data were reported through 2012, and the CDC data were from 2011. Often data are not easily and perfectly comparable between sources. An effective PHN tries to find the most comparable data possible but does point out discrepancies that exist when comparisons are made between incomparable data. Using data that are not a perfect match is not wrong, but these differences must be identified so that people can make informed decisions based on the existing data. It might not be true that people can make data say exactly what they want them to say, but it certainly is possible to inadvertently or purposefully present data in ways that might not be entirely accurate. Therefore, PHNs need to spend time practicing how to present data in meaningful, representative ways, and, equally vital, they need to have the ability to interpret and critique any data that are presented to them.

Data Comparison Between National and Global Sources

To understand the context from which a client originates, a PHN may be interested in disease incidence in other parts of the world. The earlier PHN who graphed active TB cases against latent TB cases may have found increasing numbers of families from several parts of the world now living in her community. Reviewing information from the World Health Organization (WHO) will inform her of the distribution of TB elsewhere. This information can then be applied to determine communicable disease risk related to immigration patterns into her community (see Figure 4.6). North America and Western Europe have the lowest incidence of TB, whereas Africa and Asia have the highest incidence.

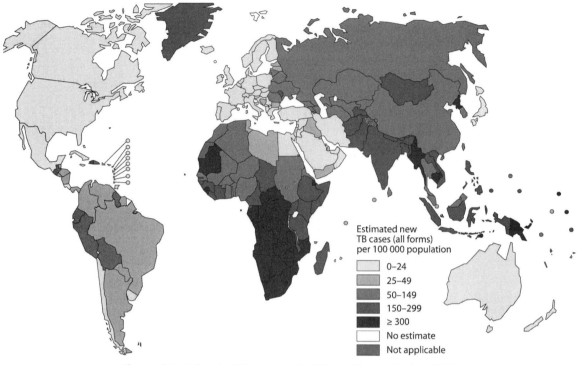

Figure 4.6. Estimated Tuberculosis (TB) Incidence Rates, 2011

Source: Global Tuberculosis Report 2012, World Health Organization

Data as Population Trends

Equally valuable are data that demonstrate population trends. These are most commonly presented in the form of a population pyramid, which at a glance provides a picture of population growth (see Figure 4.7). In this figure, it is apparent that the Hispanic population is quite young, with a large proportion of the population under age 20. In contrast, the White population appears to be more evenly distributed among the age groups. PHNs can use this information collaboratively to prioritize prevention and promotion strategies with each of these populations. For example, PHNs might examine the apparently high reproductive rate among Hispanic women and evaluate such data as birth rates and birth outcomes to determine whether an intervention to promote prenatal care is needed. Population data are important because they offer a glimpse into the big picture of how people are distributed, but the data by themselves might not be sufficient to guide intervention decisions or justify program budget priorities.

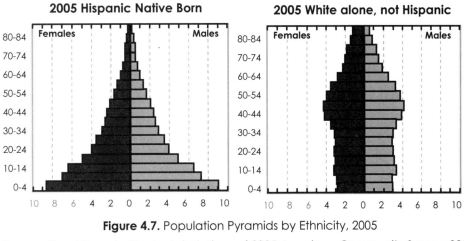

Figure 4.7. Population Pyramids by Ethnicity, 2005

Source: Pew Hispanic Center tabulations of 2005 American Community Survey, 2006

Data as Risk Ratios and Odds Ratios

Another very common tool used to examine the data regarding risks and health outcomes is a 2×2 table (see Table 4.3). This table aids in understanding how a disease is distributed in a population based on the presence or absence of a risk factor. From this table, a PHN can calculate the rate of disease in each group; the risk ratio (RR; i.e., the rate of disease for those with the risk behavior divided by the rate of disease for those without the risk behavior); and the odds ratio (OR), which is regularly used to describe the likelihood of contracting a disease for someone with the risk factor compared to someone without. In the example shown in Table 4.3, the rate of disease for the "Yes" risk behavior group is 0.75 (75/100), and the rate of disease for the "No" risk behavior group is 0.02 (2/100). Already a relationship between the risk behavior and the disease seems obvious given the raw rates (0.75 versus 0.02). Taking this a step further, you can calculate the RR (0.75/0.02 = 37.5). PHNs do not often use the RR by itself, but it is an important calculation for those who might be interested in more in-depth statistical comparisons and analysis, such as chi-square analysis. PHNs might not routinely calculate these numbers, but they often read and analyze research that includes reported rates, risk ratios, odds ratios, chi-squares, and levels of significance (i.e., $p < .001$ or $p < .05$). It is beyond the scope of this manual to completely explain how to calculate each of these, but it is useful for PHNs to have an awareness of what the numbers mean and how to appropriately interpret them.

Table 4.3 shows an example of data used to calculate odds and an OR. This ratio is useful in identifying the odds of contracting the disease, given the presence or absence of a risk factor. The formula for calculating the OR is (a/c) / (b/d) = ad/bc. Specifically, the odds of contracting the disease in the presence of the risk factor is calculated by dividing the number of people with the disease and the risk by the number of people without the disease but with the risk (i.e., 75/25), or 3. Similarly, the odds of contracting the disease but not having the risk factor can be calculated (2/98), or 0.0204. The OR is calculated by dividing the odds with the risk factor by the odds without the risk factor (3/0.0204), or 147. In this example, someone with the risk factor is 147 times more likely to contract the disease than someone without the risk factor. A PHN with this information needs to make decisions on how to act based on many factors. For example, even though the OR is so high, the disease might not be life threatening, or the risk factor might not be common. The risk factor might easily be eliminated with an intervention, or the risk factor might not be easily identified, making it difficult to intervene. PHNs need to consider numerous factors when data are interpreted and then acted upon. PHNs have an important role in helping interpret data so that they are not used inappropriately to justify action or inaction.

Table 4.3 Association Between Risk Factor and Disease

	Disease		
Risk Factor	**Yes**	**No**	**Total**
Yes	a	c	a + c
No	b	d	b + d
Total	a + b	c + d	a + b + c + d

	Disease		
Risk Factor	**Yes**	**No**	**Total**
Yes	75	25	100
No	2	98	100
Total	77	123	200

Innovative Data Collection

Data are typically collected through surveillance systems at the local, state, or national levels. Sometimes healthcare professionals provide the data, and other times, individuals are surveyed. PHNs need to be aware of the variety of tools used to collect epidemiological data, because they might participate in the data collection, interpretation, or dissemination. A GIS is an example of a tool that is growing in popularity in the field of public health (see Figure 4.8, County Health Rankings & Roadmaps, www.cnngis.org). The *County Health Rankings & Roadmaps* provide an annual check-up of the health of each county in the U.S. (County Health Rankings & Roadmaps: Health Outcomes in Minnesota, 2012). This publication shows that some places are doing very well, while others have room for improvement. Figure 4.8 shows maps that provide insights about Health Outcomes and Health Factors in Minnesota, with healthier counties depicted in lighter colors. Missouri is advancing its use of GIS to track the health of communities across the state. GIS enables the state to compile data from numerous different places into a common website that the public can explore and search to identify priority problems, strengths, and a variety of related factors. As the Missouri website explains:

> GIS has been a vital tool in promoting quality of life and health at [Department of Health and Senior Services] DHSS since 1997. GIS specializes in combining data from multiple sources and displaying that data in a geographic context. Data such as demographic information, disease prevalence, and physical environmental factors can be analyzed with GIS to reveal relationships and trends that otherwise would be very difficult to find. GIS is also a valuable management tool for policymaking and resource management. (MDHHS, 2010)

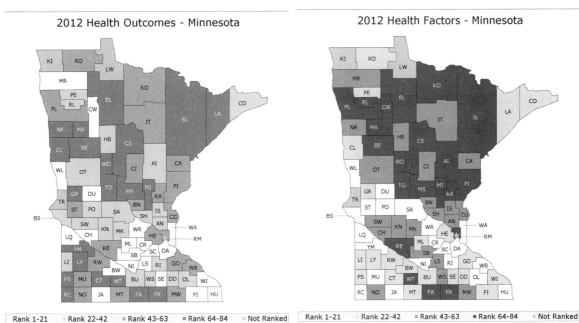

Figure 4.8. County Health Rankings and Roadmaps: Health Outcomes in Minnesota

Source: County Health Rankings & Roadmaps: Health Outcomes in Minnesota, 2012

GIS data are also being used to carefully examine community-level assets and risks related to obesity prevention. For example, GIS data can aid in understanding how communities compare in terms of access to full-scale grocery stores, corner supermarkets, gas stations, or liquor stores. Additionally, GIS data can indicate the location of parks and transpose violent crime data, which might provide insights into why youth in certain neighborhoods are reporting higher levels of physical activity than youth in other neighborhoods. In emergency situations, GIS has also played a crucial role; in Haiti in 2010, a GIS program was used within the first few hours after the earthquake to update a baseline map of Haiti. People on the ground used OpenStreetMap, a GIS crowd-sourced mapping program to modify the existing map in real time, thereby facilitating rescue efforts. The pre-earthquake terrain maps that existed were not very helpful, but the real-time maps provided valuable support to search-and-rescue teams. Technological advances make it possible for local PHNs to use GIS readily via smartphones, tablets, and laptops. GIS tools can yield data useful to a neighborhood, community, state, or country in advancing public health priorities.

Evidence Example: Screening for Neurodevelopmental Delays in Four Communities in Mexico and Cuba

Cuban and Mexican PHNs used a newly developed computerized evaluation instrument to assess and compare the prevalence of neurodevelopmental problems in three areas: language/communication, psychomotor, and hearing/vision (Guadarrama-Celaya et al., 2012). Four hundred children ages 1 to 5 years were screened using the Neuropediatric Development (NPED) screening tool in urban and suburban cities in Cuba and Mexico. Results demonstrated failures in all communities (e.g., 2.3% vision, 16.5% language) and differences by country (e.g., higher failures rate for hearing in Cuban communities). Results also demonstrated successful use of this computerized Spanish-language tool for broad community assessment of key neurodevelopmental problems among children at important stages of development. This tool could facilitate earlier identification and intervention so that long-term neurodevelopmental problems can be avoided as children develop.

Applies Epidemiological Triangle When Working With Individuals and Families, Communities, and Systems

How a PHN comes to understand a problem and its possible causes and solutions is somewhat dependent on the framework that the PHN uses. The epidemiological triangle has traditionally been used to understand disease transmission. This triangle consists of identifying a host system affected by the condition, an agent that causes the condition, and the environment that contributes to the condition. Host considerations include genetics; inherent characteristics, such as age and gender; acquired characteristics, such as immune status; and lifestyle factors. Agents are typically categorized as infectious, chemical, or physical agents. Environmental factors include anything within the host environment, such as socioeconomic factors, physical environments, and working conditions. Interactions between these three elements of the triangle are examined to determine how diseases are transmitted and how intervention strategies can be targeted to stop or prevent transmission of the health conditions. Using influenza as an example, the host would be a person who is susceptible to the flu, the agent is the influenza virus, and the environment would include factors that contribute to transmission of the virus, such as crowded housing (Clark, 2008).

This model has been adapted to consider more complex scenarios that might be contributing to disease or illness (see Figure 4.9). It is an important adaptation, because for most health problems that PHNs address, the contributing factors are complex and multifaceted. Illnesses result not merely from a simple transmission in the right time and place but also because of factors not easily controlled or resolved (e.g., poverty, inadequate housing, food shortages).

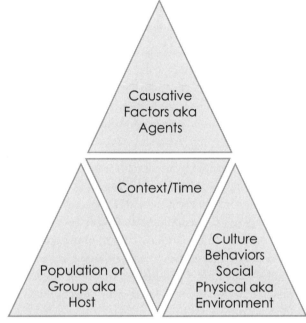

Figure 4.9. Epidemiological Triangle in the 21st Century
Source: Merrill & Timmreck, 2006, p. 15

For many in public health, complex contributing factors to poor health or well-being have been informed by such models as the web of causation. The name itself implies greater complexity than the epidemiological triangle, yet this model is also not perfect. For example, imagine a spiderweb (where the name is drawn from) and how you might use the web design to identify all the factors influencing the center of the web (i.e., the disease, such as cardiovascular disease or asthma, or the social health problem, such as teen pregnancy). After you have drawn the web, you are faced with a dilemma—specifically, which related thread to address first. How do you decide whether to prioritize a biological-related factor or a social-based factor? The web might help identify numerous potential causes, contributors, and influences, yet the model by itself does not yield readily apparent strategies or solutions. More than 10 years ago, Nancy Krieger (1997) identified these criticisms of the Web framework and proposed an ecosocial framework for developing epidemiologic theories about public health problems and possible solutions. The central question answered using an ecosocial framework is, "[W]ho and what is responsible for population patterns of health, disease, and well-being, as manifested in present, past, and changing social inequalities in health?" (Krieger, 2001a, p. 694).

A shift in thinking about traditional epidemiology models has occurred with growing recognition of the importance of social epidemiology, the field that acknowledges and seeks to address the complex combination of biological and social factors influencing health and well-being. Social epidemiology was initially defined in the 1950s but has in more recent decades grown in popularity and use among public health professionals (Krieger, 2001b). PHNs need to be aware of the trends in public health as well as the theories that guide understanding of the risk-asset-problem-intervention relationships in public health. For example, Krieger's ecosocial theory has shaped how many people now address complex public health problems. She states that the ecosocial theory is a tool that

> fosters analysis of current and changing population patterns of health, disease, and well-being in relation to each level of biological, ecological and social organization (e.g., cell, organ, organism/ individual, family, community, population, society, ecosystem) as manifested at each and every scale, whether relatively small and fast (e.g., enzyme catalysis) or relatively large and slow (e.g., infection and renewal of the pool of susceptible for a specified infectious disease). (Krieger, 2001b, p. 671)

Nursing practice should always be informed by theory. It is relatively easy in nursing practice to get caught up in the tasks one has to do and to forget, at times, to take a step back, reflect, and consider why something is being done a certain way or why certain events are occurring. Theories are always advancing, and an effective PHN strives not only to use theory but also to keep up with theoretical ideas that guide and inform practice and the care of individuals, families, communities, and populations. Epidemiology is an ideal example of the value and importance of theory as a guide for understanding and intervening on extremely complex societal health problems and conditions. The following Evidence Example is one example of a complex health problem that is best considered using an ecosocial framework.

Evidence Example: Ecosocial Framework Applied to Childhood Lead Poisoning

A study addressing childhood lead poisoning, a noninfectious disease that directly results from social environmental factors, not biological factors, used Krieger's ecosocial framework (Aschengrau & Seage, 2008). This situation is more easily understood within an ecosocial framework than through a traditional epidemiological triangle or web of causation model. Indeed, the ecosocial framework aids in the recognition of numerous contributing factors to childhood lead poisoning, including direct microlevel influences, such as substandard housing (e.g., old home that landlord has not updated to remove lead-based paint sources) and workplace exposure (e.g., Dad works with lead and wears clothing home that is contaminated and exposes the children), and indirect macrolevel influences, such as workplace policies and minimum-wage laws that limit the family's options with respect to the rent they can afford to pay. Numerous other factors can be considered in an ecosocial framework, identifying specific areas the PHN can immediately address and those that require more sustained advocacy and effort.

Another important theoretical framework in public health that PHNs should be aware of is referred to as *life course epidemiology*. Historically, as the focus of epidemiology shifted from infectious disease to chronic illness in the mid–20th century, new and expanded paradigms emerged to better recognize and understand the antecedents and causes of chronic diseases. The life course perspective views health not in stages separate from each other (infancy, early childhood, adolescence, adulthood) but as a continuum. As Krieger (2001a, p. 695) describes, "[L]ife course perspective refers to how health status at any given age, for a given birth cohort, reflects not only contemporary conditions but embodiment of prior living circumstances." A classic life course study was the research on the effects of the 1944–1945 Dutch famine that linked malnutrition with subsequent effects on human development and mental performance (Stein, Susser, Saenger, & Marolla, 1975).

Throughout the life course continuum, biological, behavioral, environmental, psychological, and social factors dynamically interact, contributing to one's health. As Matthias Richter (2010, p. 458) summarizes, "This perspective was truly helpful to contribute to a better understanding of biological, behavioural and social influences—from gestation to death—for health as well as health inequalities." The impetus of life course epidemiology was chronic disease, and, as such, the framework is grounded in a medical risk model, rather than an ecosocial model (Richter, 2010). Even so, PHNs benefit from using a life course perspective when they are designing health-promotion or disease-prevention programs, because they are encouraged to think about long-term implications and benefits. Certainly a relevant example of this is public health efforts toward obesity prevention and the myriad ways in which PHNs actively consider the life course continuum when intervening with screening, education, policy initiatives, and numerous other activities. This increased thoughtfulness about impact over time can also enhance a program's sustainability or an agency's commitment to support a long-term intervention or screening program.

In summary, public health nursing is grounded in the science of epidemiology. On numerous levels, epidemiological data help describe the scope of a problem, prioritize intervention strategies, and evaluate outcomes or trends over time. Data are presented and collected using many different formats; nurses need the skills to interpret and critique these data, regardless of how they are presented. PHNs also use epidemiological theories to inform actions and priorities for addressing public health problems. PHNs need to use and contribute to the development of theories that recognize the social complexities influencing public health problems in the 21st century.

The next area for Elizabeth to assess for close contacts was the in-home daycare. Billy's mother stated that they have a split-entry home and that the lower level is for the licensed daycare. On a normal day, she has five children who stay until 5:30 p.m. In addition, a set of 1-year-old twin girls stay until approximately 11:00 p.m. Billy's mother indicates that since Billy has been ill, he has stayed only on the upper level, away from most of the lower-level child care children. However, the situation with the twins is different: Billy eats supper with them and plays with them until bedtime. The twins have been exposed to pertussis and, according to the definition in the protocol, would be considered face-to-face contacts.

Elizabeth asks whether the twins' parents have been told about Billy's pertussis. The mother states that she has not told them because she is concerned about losing her clients and income. Elizabeth explains that the public health recommendation would be that the twins receive preventive antibiotics because of their close contact with Billy. Billy's mother agrees to notify the twins' parents by passing out to all parents a standardized notification letter from the PHN.

Ethical Considerations

As seen in the case study woven throughout this chapter, the daycare provider was concerned about a loss of income and her reputation as a provider. Many times, PHNs confront challenging situations in their practice. For example, reporting a nuisance house situation to the city building inspector might prompt the eviction of a renter or harassment from a landlord. Although they are trying to protect children living in less than desirable circumstances, PHNs' actions might have unintended consequences for entire families.

Similarly, interventions focused on reducing the exposure to lead paint in older homes might be embarrassing or financially difficult. Although the health department might offer a free home/environmental inspection for the detection of lead paint, this activity might force families to temporarily leave their homes, which some may perceive as an invasion of privacy. Moving in with relatives for a day might be embarrassing for some; for others, staying in a hotel might be beyond the family budget. Some health departments offer a free service to abate lead in a home if the family has not done so. Although this solution is helpful in covering up a lead source, the repainting services are often spotty and unsightly in appearance. The benefits of reducing lead exposure to children must be weighed against the other consequences for the family. See Table 4.4 for ethical perspectives and applications relevant to epidemiological principles in public health nursing.

Table 4.4   Ethical Action in Using Epidemiological Principles in Public Health Nursing

Ethical Perspective	Application
Rule Ethics (principles)	• PHNs should use epidemiology to assess and develop interventions that promote beneficence. • PHNs can support the autonomy of those they are working with, even when uncomfortable changes are needed to minimize the spread of disease.
Virtue Ethics (character)	• PHNs need to demonstrate respect for individuals, families, and communities when suggesting promotion or prevention strategies; this can be challenging but necessary, especially when some might refuse to adhere to the actions being recommended. • PHNs should be persistent in understanding the complexity of factors contributing to a problem so that potential solutions are comprehensive and yield lasting changes.

Feminist Ethics (reducing oppression)

- PHNs can advocate for system-level changes that promote the well-being of those who often feel they have no voice (e.g., tenants who are unable to ask a landlord to maintain heat levels during the winter).
- PHNs should explore societal changes that can improve the underlying environment for people, such as increasing the minimum-wage law so that families have additional resources to sustain and promote health.

 ## Key Points

- Epidemiology is an important foundation to the work of PHNs.
- There is a growing shift from traditional epidemiological models toward more complex models that consider social influences on health, such as a social epidemiological model.
- Epidemiological data, including prevalence and incidence data, help set national and local public health priorities.
- PHNs can and should use epidemiological data to advocate for health promotion priorities in their areas of influence.

Learning Example for Effective Use of Epidemiological Principles in Public Health Nursing Practice

The following learning example builds on the epidemiological concepts presented in the chapter and offers a real-life situation in which a PHN used data to address an important public health concern.

Somewhere County Learning Example: Using Population-Based Data

The following infectious disease data were obtained by the local PHN: 24 cases of amebiasis, 169 cases of chlamydia, 4 cases of dengue fever, and 18 cases of Kawasaki disease. A quick review made it clear that chlamydia was the most concerning infectious disease issue, based on the actual number of cases. Using the U.S. Census website, the PHN obtained the estimated population for her jurisdiction (124,768). Calculate the rate of chlamydia for this population. (Check the table that follows to ensure that you obtained the correct answer.)

Next she gathered more data to determine the trend of cases over 5 years in the jurisdiction. Compute the rate per 100,000 population and fill in the chart below.

Year	Number of Chlamydia Cases	Population	Rate per 100,000 Population
1	111	123,119	
2	136	123,402	
3	138	123,895	
4	148	124,002	
5	169	124,768	135

The incidence of chlamydia was definitely increasing, but the PHN wanted a larger context or comparison, so she computed the rate per 100,000 for neighboring jurisdictions.

Year 5	Rate per 100,000 Population
The nurse's area	135
Area to the south	123
Area to the west	143
Adjacent metro area	483

The PHN created this comparison table for each of the preceding 4 years. She discovered that overall, the rate of chlamydia was similar in her area to that of other adjacent areas, except the metro area, where there was greater ethnic diversity, lower insurance rates, and more campus college settings (all possible explanatory factors for the different rates).

She then examined additional factors that were contributing to the snapshot of her jurisdiction. The following is her summary of the chlamydia cases that occurred in Year 5 in her jurisdiction:

- 70% female

- 47% from Happyville, 21% from Somewherecity, and 21% from Wheresitville

- 61% Caucasian (including 1% Hispanic) and 8.3% African-American

- Co-infection rate with gonorrhea – 3.8%

- No co-infection with syphilis

- Heterosexual spread

- Top five diagnostic sites included sites outside the jurisdiction. No cases reported from Wheresitville Clinic.

- Age distribution:
    - Ages 15–19: 24.2%
    - Ages 20–24: 37.7%
    - Ages 25–29: 21.5%

Based on this summary of the PHN's analysis and comparison:

1. Which next steps do you think she should take in addressing the problem of chlamydia in her community?

2. Whom might she target for health education or screening activities?

Develop a plan of action she might implement with the goal of reducing the transmission of chlamydia in her community.

 Reflective Practice

Investigating outbreak possibilities can be challenging, but it can also present opportunities to practice great intercommunication skills. Elizabeth handled a situation that could have been extremely difficult in a professional, thoughtful manner. She asked the right questions and managed to express concern rather than judgment. By building a good relationship right away, Elizabeth received honest responses from the child care provider, and together they determined who had been exposed and an appropriate course of action.

1. What do you imagine will be some follow-up steps that Elizabeth will take in this situation?

   _____

   _____

2. How can Elizabeth be a resource for the child care provider if her clients grow angry when they are informed about the possible exposure?

   _____

   _____

3. Who might be additional partners to Elizabeth within the health department as she follows this case through until it is resolved?

   _____

   _____

4. How might Elizabeth address an ethical issue, such as whether some of the exposed refuse preventive treatment?

_____

_____

5. How will Elizabeth know whether this case investigation has been successful? What will be important for Elizabeth to document?

_____

_____

6. How will the numbers that Elizabeth has collected as part of this investigation be useful to others at her local health department? At the state level? At the national level?

_____

_____

7. How might Elizabeth use each of the Cornerstones of Public Health Nursing (see Chapter 1) in this case investigation?

_____

_____

 Application of Evidence

1. What are some ways you can use the ecosocial framework to examine contributing and influencing factors on complex public health problems in the United States in the 21st century, such as obesity or adolescent pregnancy?

2. Examine the different types of data presented in this chapter (e.g., odds ratios, rates) and identify some of the pros and cons associated with the use of each of them.

3. As a PHN working in a community, identify three to five sources of state- or federal-level data you would want to use in demonstrating how your community issues compare to others.

 Think, Explore, Do

1. Look through your local newspaper (or a national online news source) and identify all the articles that describe problems a PHN might be involved in addressing. How will the tools of epidemiology assist in identifying ways to intervene on the problems?

2. Develop an ecosocial model that portrays contributing factors to the problem of childhood obesity.

3. Explore the mobile applications available for a smartphone or tablet. Specifically, identify GIS applications and how these could be used for public health nursing epidemiological purposes (e.g., ArcGIS by Esri). The CDC has an application game in which you try to prevent an outbreak (Solve the Outbreak) or you can attempt to spread a virus through the popular application Plague Inc.

4. Read *The Ghost Map: The Story of London's Most Terrifying Epidemic—and How it Changed Science, Cities, and the Modern World* by Steven Johnson (2006; New York: Riverhead Books) or *Flu: The Story of the Great Influenza Pandemic of 1918 and the Search for the Virus That Caused It* by Gina Kolata (2001; New York: Touchstone) and reflect on whether PHNs should be concerned about these types of pandemic threats resulting in an outbreak in the United States. Which changes (positive or negative) contribute to your opinions (e.g., global travel in 21st century, communication capabilities via text, IM, etc.)?

5. Read about the United States Agency for International Development (USAID) Emerging Pandemic Threat program. Reflect on the benefits of interdisciplinary efforts (animal, human, and environmental health professionals) working together to prevent outbreaks locally and globally.

6. Visit the CDC website and search for two of the three short videos (see titles below). Consider the epidemiologic activities of a PHN in addressing these public health concerns:

   - The Obesity Epidemic

   - Healthy Swimming Is No Accident

   - Global Disease Detectives

References

Alfred, R. (2009). *Sept. 8, 1854: Pump shutdown stops London cholera outbreak.* Retrieved from http://www.wired.com/thisdayintech/2009/09/0908london-cholera-pump

Aschengrau, A., & Seage, G. R. (2008). *Essentials of epidemiology in public health, 2nd ed.* Sudbury, MA: Jones and Bartlett.

Centers for Disease Control and Prevention (CDC). (2001). Updated guidelines for evaluating public health surveillance systems: Recommendations from the Guidelines Working Group. *MMWR, 50*(RR13), 1–35. Retrieved from http://www.cdc.gov/mmwr/preview/mmwrhtml/rr5013a1.htm

Centers for Disease Control and Prevention (CDC). (2013). *Pertussis outbreak trends.* Retrieved from http://www.cdc.gov/pertussis/outbreaks/trends.html

Centers for Disease Control and Prevention (CDC). (2013). *Reported cases of Lyme disease—United States, 2011.* Retrieved from http://www.cdc.gov/lyme/stats/maps/map2011.html

Clark, M. (2008). *Community health nursing: Advocacy for population health, 5th ed.* Upper Saddle River, NJ: Pearson Education.

County Health Rankings and Roadmaps: Health Outcomes in Minnesota. (2012). University of Wisconsin Population Health Institute. Retrieved from http://www.countyhealthrankings.org/app/minnesota/2012/rankings/outcomes/overall

Earl, C. (2009). Medical history and epidemiology: Their contribution to the development of public health nursing. *Nursing Outlook, 57*(5), 257–265.

Friis, R. H., & Sellers, T. A. (1999). *Epidemiology for public health practice, 2nd ed.* Gaithersburg, MD: Aspen.

Guadarrama-Celaya, F., Otero-Ojeda, G. A., Pliego-Rivero, F. B., Porcayo-Mercado, M., Ricardo-Garcell, J., & Perez-Abalo, M. C. (2012). Screening of neurodevelopmental delays in four communities of Mexico and Cuba. *Public Health Nursing, 29*(2), 105–115.

Klopf, L. (1998). Tuberculosis control in the New York State Department of Correctional Services: A case management approach. *American Journal of Infection Control, 26*(5), 534–538.

Krieger, N. (1997). Epidemiology and the web of causation: Has anyone seen the spider? *Social Science and Medicine, 39*(7), 887–903.

Krieger, N. (2001a). A glossary for social epidemiology. *Journal of Epidemiology and Community Health, 55*(10), 693–700.

Krieger, N. (2001b). Theories for social epidemiology in the 21st century: An ecosocial perspective. *International Journal of Epidemiology, 30*(4), 668–677.

Kuh, D., Ben-Shlomo, Y., Lynch, J., Hallqvist, J., & Power, C. (2003). Life course epidemiology. *Journal of Epidemiology and Community Health, 57*(10), 778–783.

Le, C. T. (2001). *Health and numbers: A problem-based introduction to biostatistics, 2nd ed.* New York, NY: Wiley-Liss.

Lind, C., & Smith, D. (2008). Analyzing the state of community health nursing: Advancing from deficit to strengths-based practice using appreciative inquiry. *Advances in Nursing Science, 31*(1), 28–41.

Merrill, R. M., & Timmreck, T. C. (2006). *Introduction to epidemiology, 4th ed.* Sudbury, MA: Jones and Bartlett.

Minnesota Department of Health (MDH). (2013). *Reported cases of Lyme disease in Minnesota by year, 1986–2012.* Retrieved from http://www.health.state.mn.us/divs/idepc/diseases/lyme/casesyear.html

Missouri Department of Health and Senior Services (MDHSS). (2010). *Geographic Information Systems (GIS) and maps.* Retrieved from http://www.dhss.mo.gov/GIS/

Pew Hispanic Center. (2006). *Population pyramids by ethnicity, 2005.* Cited in Hakimzadeh, S. (2006). 41.9 million and counting: A statistical view of Hispanics at mid-decade. Retrieved from http://pewresearch.org/pubs/251/419-million-and-counting

Richter, M. (2010). It does take two to tango! On the need for theory in research on the social determinants of health. *International Journal of Public Health, 55,* 457–458.

Stein, Z., Susser, M., Saenger, G., & Marolla, F. (1975). *Famine and human development: The Dutch hunger winter of 1944–45.* New York, NY: Oxford University Press.

University of California, Los Angeles (UCLA). (2010). *John Snow.* Retrieved from http://www.ph.ucla.edu/epi/snow.html

Valanis, B. (1999). *Epidemiology in health care, 3rd ed.* Stamford, CT: Appleton and Lange.

World Health Organization (WHO). (2012). *World: Estimated tuberculosis (TB) incidence rates, 2011 (as of 5 Nov 2012).* Retrieved from http://reliefweb.int/map/world/world-estimated-tuberculosis-tb-incidence-rates2011-5-nov-2012

COMPETENCY #3
Utilizes Collaboration to Achieve Public Health Goals

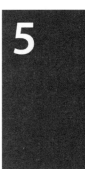

5

Marjorie A. Schaffer
with Joyce Bredesen, Carol L. Hargate, and Rose M. Jost

Jake is a public health nursing student who has 10 years of experience in the acute care setting as an associate degree nurse. His expertise has been in the area of cardiac care, working in the Coronary Care Unit at a local hospital. Jake has returned to school to complete a baccalaureate degree in nursing. The community surrounding the university that Jake attends has identified a need to address healthcare access for the homeless population. A local church approached the university to work with it to develop a clinic for the homeless by using resources in the community and students for the delivery of care for this underserved population. Jake's preceptor, Linda, a public health nurse (PHN), is representing the local public health department at planning meetings. Jake will have the opportunity to learn how professionals, community members, and organizations collaborate to contribute to the development of a community clinic that serves a vulnerable population. Jake has many questions, such as: Who would he collaborate with to contribute to this goal? Whom should be invited to be partners in the collaboration? How does such a diverse group work together? What is the PHN's responsibility in collaborative work?

Before Jake attends the first planning meeting with Linda, he picks up his notebook to review the population-based public health nursing competency list and concentrates on Competency #3, which focuses on collaborative practice.

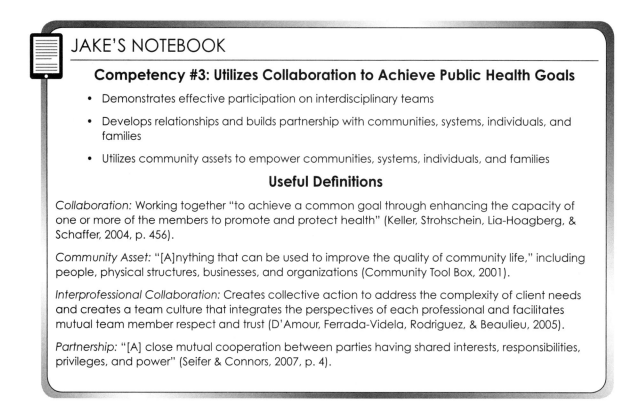

Accomplishing More by Working Together

PHNs work with many individuals and community organizations. Collaboration can be between two or more individuals or between organizations. PHNs collaborate with representatives of the population, other professionals, and organizations to contribute to healthcare planning and promote health (ANA, 2013; Chaudry, Polivka, & Kennedy, 2000). An important skill for PHNs is learning how to develop the collaborative community partnerships to bring about community and systems change for improving health (Fawcett, Francisco, Paine-Andrews, & Schultz, 2000; Franklin, Exline, & Stringer, 2002).

Building capacity for partnership and engaging community members is an important focus for PHNs. In a study of public health nursing practice, PHNs said their goal was to make a difference in the lives of their patients by focusing on "doing with" rather than on "doing for" (Aston, Meagher-Stewart, Edwards, & Young, 2009). They wanted to empower their patients to take responsibility and ownership for health decisions. The PHNs identified several strategies for empowering their patients: Begin with the patient's perspective, tune into the readiness of the patient, assess holistically (refer to Public Health Nursing Competency #10 in Chapter 12), and build rapport with the patient.

The study also suggested strategies to encourage community member participation in health programs and initiatives. The PHNs involved community members in decision-making groups, focused on community assets, and gave positive feedback and encouragement by affirming what was working well. The PHNs involved people who normally might not have the opportunity to participate in decision-making groups, such as youth living in poverty and mothers who were isolated. At every group meeting, the PHNs asked, "So who is missing and who needs to be here?" PHNs often initiate the process of uniting people around a problem they all care about. PHNs encourage group ownership and often look for community members to take the lead in problem solving. PHNs can assist with the group process, but ideally community members should control the flow and process toward finding and implementing solutions. Collaboration works best when everyone has the opportunity to share thoughts and ideas. One PHN in the study used the word *catalyst* to describe an approach that draws the voices and participation of community members. This means that someone needs to initiate the collaborative process, which then continues to develop with the input of the people who contribute their perspectives and skills to the collaboration.

The PHNs in the study also talked about how important it was to connect community members and groups to existing social networks, which could include neighborhood groups; community organizations, such as churches; or programs that provide food. The PHNs talked about building these connections as "creating participatory infrastructure." This means the PHNs linked people and community organizations that were working on similar goals but had not yet worked together. PHNs created infrastructure by "building partnerships among clients, establishing self-help groups, advocating for clients by connecting them to other agencies, and linking together agencies to provide the best possible service for clients" (Aston et al., 2009, p. 30). One PHN talked about finding "the movers and shakers" in the community by reaching out to community groups, such as men's or women's groups, church groups, and community health boards. These strategies encourage the collective voice of community members and foster citizen participation. PHNs can also bring their expertise in health promotion to existing collaborative groups that are already established in communities.

Interprofessional collaboration (IPC) is central to improving health outcomes in public health nursing practice. Interprofessional collaborative practice is both community- and population-oriented and patient- and family-centered. Teamwork and team-based care involve engaging other health professionals, specific to the care environment, to participate in client-centered problem solving. George Thibault (2012) has identified four domains of interprofessional practice:

1. Teamwork and team-based practice, which means engaging other professionals in shared problem solving

2. Interprofessional communication practices, which refers to active participation in timely, sensitive, and instructive sharing/feedback

3. Roles and responsibilities for collaborative practice, which refers to communicating one's role and responsibilities to patients/families, community groups, and other professionals

4. Values/ethics for interprofessional practice, which means acting with honesty and integrity in all relationships and modeling respect, confidentiality, and dignity for clients and team members

The "professional" part of IPC refers to individuals who have specific knowledge and skills that they can use to contribute to community well-being. Interprofessional education occurs when professions "learn about, from, and with each other to enable effective collaboration and improve health outcomes"

(WHO, 2010). Grant and Finnocchio (1995) have identified barriers to effective IPC and strategies to overcome them (see Table 5.1).

Table 5.1   Interprofessional Collaboration (IPC): Common Barriers and Strategies for Overcoming Them

Barriers	Overcoming Barriers
Team Level	**Team Level**
• Lack of a clearly stated, shared, and measureable purpose	• Reach agreement on unifying philosophy focused on the primary care of the client/ community.
• Lack of education/training in IPC	
• Ambiguity in member roles and leadership	• Develop a commitment to the unifying philosophy and common collaborative goals.
• Difference in levels of authority, power, and expertise	
• Difficulty engaging the community	• Increase knowledge about other professions and their roles.
• Traditions/professional cultures, particularly professions with a history of hierarchy	• Work to establish a method for negotiation and renegotiation of goals and roles over time.
• Conflict around individual relationship to client as a team member	• Establish a mechanism for resolving conflicts between team members.
Individual Level	• Commit to consistently working to overcome barriers.
• Divided loyalties between team focus and own discipline	
• Varied responsibilities and job titles	**Individual Level**
• Gender-, race-, or class-based bias	• Respect the skills and knowledge of others.
• Presence of a defensive attitude	• Demonstrate positive attitudes about own profession.
• Reluctance to accept ideas from team members from other professions	• Work to cultivate trust between members.
• Absence of trust in the collaborative process	• Be prepared to share responsibility for client/community care.

Source: Grant, 1995

Collaboration Example

PHNs collaborate with individuals and families, community groups, and systems. A local church hosts a Wellness Center to serve the needs of persons living in the community who have health needs and difficulty accessing healthcare. Many clients need dental care, so PHNs collaborate at all levels of practice and across professions to respond to this need.

Individual level: When clients at the Wellness Center complain of toothaches, PHNs refer them to low-cost dental care and arrange transportation to the community site where dental care is provided.

Community level: PHNs collect information on agencies and organizations that provide low-cost dental care and create a handout or pamphlet to communicate that information to potential clients and other community locations where persons in need can learn about resources. In addition, PHNs could provide social marketing to local schools about resources for dental care.

Systems level: PHNs advocate for policy change to include dental care in health programs that serve individuals and families without employer-provided insurance.

Best Practices for Collaboration

Collaboration is important because with the input of several stakeholders (individuals and organizations), the pooling of expertise can lead to expanded ideas and strategies for improving population health outcomes. Collaboration might also lead to community organizing or coalition building that mobilizes a community to promote health (Findley et al., 2003). The creativity and synergy that can result from collaboration provide energy and a sense of purpose in reaching a common goal (Gamm, 1998). Together with community partners and other professionals, PHNs strive to identify mutual goals for the collaboration and expected outcomes (see Table 5.2 for a summary of best practices for effective collaborative action).

Table 5.2 Best Practices for Collaboration

- Effective leadership
- Commitment of the participants
- Shared values and a sense of purpose
- Mutual respect for team members
- Linkages between groups and individuals
- Identification of strategies and resources to achieve the goals, a structure to support the collaborative work
- Internal systems to support the structure (for example, communication mechanisms, a place to meet, time available in assigned workload)

Collaboration With Other Professionals and Communities

Depending on their practice setting, PHNs work with a variety of other professionals, groups, and organizations. For example, a PHN working in a school collaborates with teachers, families, students, school administration, primary care providers, other health and special education professionals, social workers, and groups that address such health needs as chronic illness and mental health services. The following are possible partners in public health nursing networks:

- Schools
- Child care programs and providers
- Primary care providers (physicians, nurse practitioners, physician assistants)
- Clinical nurse specialists
- Dental care providers (dentists, dental hygienists, dental assistants)
- Traditional/Native healers
- Clergy
- Psychologists
- Mental health centers
- Speech therapists
- Physical therapists
- Occupational therapists
- Audiologists
- Nutritionists
- Extension agents
- Early childhood development programs
- Businesses
- Social services
- Colleges and universities
- Special education
- Housing programs
- Battered women's shelters
- Services for children with special needs
- Financial assistance
- Food shelves
- Jobs and training services
- Transportation services
- Literacy programs
- English as a second language learner programs
- Women, Infants, and Children (WIC)
- Services for vision and hearing impaired
- Legal aid
- Ombudsmen
- Meals on Wheels
- Energy assistance
- Community service organizations (Rotary, Lions)
- City council
- Community residents
- Complementary/alternative therapy programs
- Head Start
- Community action programs
- Alcoholics Anonymous
- Chemical dependency programs
- Home care agencies
- Law enforcement
- Congregate dining
- Homeless shelters
- Environmental health programs
- Vulnerable adult programs
- Child protection and welfare programs
- Planned Parenthood
- Volunteers
- Artists
- Musicians

Evidence Examples of Interprofessional Collaboration

As you read through these examples of IPC, think about your community and how you could collaborate with other professionals to improve the health of the population.

Evidence Example: A Collaborative Approach to Fall Prevention

The Geriatric Emergency Management-Falls Intervention Team (GEM-FIT) project was a nurse-led research initiative developed to improve fall prevention in the elderly (Merrett, Thomas, Stephens, Moghabghab, & Gruneir, 2011). IPC included PHNs and occupational therapists who evaluated participants before and after fall-prevention interventions. The project outcome was a modest improvement in participant outcomes and a decline in modifiable risks.

Evidence Example: Collaborating for Information Literacy

Nurse educators and health science librarians collaborated to provide workshops for nurses practicing in community settings (Miller, Jones, Graves, & Sievert, 2010). In this initiative, effective collaboration involved mutual understanding of discipline-specific information, known as silos, as shared cooperation to achieve teaching and learning goals. One workshop example is the presentation on management of lice in the school setting to school nurses. As a collaborative effort, the nurse educator presented evidence-based practice guidelines, and the librarian presented methods for finding and using credible information sources. Both presenters discussed implications for practice. Effective collaboration increased nurses' information literacy skills, leading to improved health outcomes.

Evidence Example: A Collaborative Response to Postpartum Depression

A collaborative mental health initiative was established between a community-based mental health program and public health centers (Wood, Middleton, & Leonard, 2010). Because early screening for postpartum depression (PPD) is crucial to timely interventions for the mother, infant, and family, PHNs served as consultation liaisons and had the opportunity to screen for PPD (secondary prevention) during home visits to new mothers. The collaborative partnership on screening led to referrals for interventions for mothers at risk. Several positive outcomes resulted: Women with PPD had quicker access to psychiatric services and more seamless entry into the mental health system, and PHNs' confidence in collaboration and communication with primary care providers was enhanced.

As a PHN, you are going to work with many people who have different educational backgrounds, different experiences, and different philosophies of life from your own and from each other. As a result, you are going to encounter many different perspectives about which issues are most important and what should be done to address specific health concerns. You need to become familiar with some common differences to avoid making assumptions about the viewpoints of community partners and members of the community. Sometimes tension and conflict occur as collaborators work through different perspectives and ideas about how to respond to a problem. However, in most cases, the result of the collaboration is more effective than what one individual or one professional group could accomplish. Conflict that can be worked through has the potential to lead to effective collaboration and positive change.

As you begin your practice, ask questions of persons with different educational preparation and roles about what they think about a situation. Many will be pleased that you ask about their perspectives. Differences can be as basic as using different terminology for similar work, practices, or interventions. What you call an *assessment* might be called something different in another profession. Take enough time to communicate and make sure that all collaborators are on the same page. Time limitations and a sense of urgency in responding to a public health problem can sometimes create barriers to collaboration. However, time spent getting to know one another can prevent tension and conflict, which would likely take more time to resolve at a later point or result in the collaboration's failure.

To collaborate effectively with people representing different organizations, an understanding of group dynamics is useful. A framework for understanding how a collaborative group develops its relationships and interaction patterns for working on a common public health goal is Bruce Tuckman's (1965) stages of normative group development (Table 5.3): forming, storming, norming, and performing. After the forming phase, most groups will move through a storming phase. Conflict-management skills can be helpful in the storming phase to identify participant interests and positions, create new options through brainstorming, and negotiate a plan for moving forward (Bazarman, 2005). After moving through the norming phase into the performing phase, the group aims to work together collaboratively to achieve an agreed-upon goal. A healthy functioning group creates energy that moves the group toward goal accomplishment.

Table 5.3   Normative Group Development

Forming	Storming	Norming	Performing
• Members work to understand one another. • The group determines its boundaries and focus. • Group leaders emerge.	• Conflict emerges. • Some members may be resistant to following group direction. • People express concern about the right way to do things.	• Trust develops. • Members identify as a group. • The group experiences cohesion in choosing a goal.	• The group focuses on accomplishing tasks. • Members establish rules for working together.

The first planning meeting Jake attended included 32 people (the pastor, the assistant pastor, a police liaison, two social workers, four nurses from various clinical backgrounds, two alternative healers, two chiropractors, two community members, two people from the church's board of directors, a director from a local clinic, a block nurse coordinator, three homeless persons, two faculty from the university Jake is attending, two staff members from the surrounding homeless shelters, an insurance representative, a local physician, a musician, and two other nursing students). The group met early in the evening to accommodate the participants' different schedules. It took most of the first meeting to introduce everyone and to allow each person to share an opinion of what the wellness clinic's vision would be.

Jake was shocked to realize that for such a large group to come to a consensus about a vision, at least six meetings would be needed. He realized the group members needed time to talk so that they could determine their goals and how they were going to work together. During the initial meeting, the police liaison, who was also a social worker and a member of the church, emerged as the natural leader of the project. His skills and experiences had prepared him for a leadership role. He also had experience working with the homeless population in the neighborhood. After the meeting, Jake asked his preceptor, Linda, several questions. He wondered how a group of people with such a variety of backgrounds and experiences could create one plan. What would the group do if everyone had different ideas about how to develop the clinic? Which services did the clinic need to provide to meet the needs of the homeless population?

As the meetings progressed, some community members dropped out of the group, feeling frustrated as they perceived that their ideas were not being considered. As Jake continued to work on the planning team, he realized that conflict-management skills and leadership skills were essential to work with such a large group. Jake marveled at the police liaison's ability to calm the waters and return focus to the group's vision to serve the homeless population through this community outreach project. Decision making involved negotiation and compromise among the group members.

New members would sometimes come to one meeting and then be gone at the next. This spotty attendance meant that at each meeting, new members needed to be introduced and time was needed to explain the vision and review the group's planning phase. After about 10 meetings, a core group of community members had been identified through their commitment and attendance at meetings. Jake observed that this smaller group more easily came to a consensus about the project's vision and purpose and that the members began to trust each other and understand their roles in the group.

Each group member was focused on the delivery of services to assist the homeless. Each member brought unique gifts and contributions to the table. Jake was excited to be a part of this collaborative endeavor. He was asked to develop a flyer that would promote and advertise the wellness clinic, which would be open on Wednesday evenings.

 ACTIVITY

Identify the forming, storming, norming, and performing stages in the preceding scenario.

Building Partnerships With Communities, Systems, Individuals, and Families

Effectively collaborating and developing partnerships require equality among the partners (Kenny, 2002). Equality in collaborative relationships is promoted through listening, being respectful, appreciating differences, and developing trust. To encourage effective collaborative relationships with communities, professionals need to give up control, set aside the "rightness" of their views of healthcare, and trust the process of community participation (Clatworthy, 1999; Lindsey, Sheilds, & Stajduhar, 1999). Collaborative relationships work best if they are nonhierarchical in nature. Power to influence the collaboration is based on knowledge or expertise rather than on role or function (Henneman, Lee, & Cohen, 1995). Ineffective relationships result from power inequities (Foss, Bonaiuto, Johnson, & Moreland, 2003). To reduce power inequities, you need to pay attention to how the partnership is structured, who controls resources, and the amount of time participants are expected to commit to partnership work.

Guidelines for effective partnerships (Seifer & Connors, 2007) include the following:

- Partnerships involve mutual relationships that are based in trust, respect, authenticity, and commitment.

- Partnerships recognize and build on strengths and assets of individuals and communities.

- Partners strive to communicate clearly and openly and establish a process for decision making and conflict resolution.

- Partnerships involve balancing power and sharing resources.

Healthy People The Healthy People 2020 website offers suggestions useful for collaboration and building partnerships. On the website, click "Get Involved" and "Stay Connected." Explore the featured partnership. How might PHNs use Healthy People 2020 goals and resources as they collaborate with professionals and communities? Which strategies can PHNs use to stay updated on Healthy People 2020 resources and initiatives?

Jake realized that the tone of the meetings had changed to a collaborative relationship of listening to each other, respecting differences, and valuing each other's input in the process—traits representative of an effective partnership. The members who were homeless were key partners and helpful in identifying needs and offering suggestions for delivery of services. Jake felt the strength of the bond of the collaborative partnership team in a shared vision. Jake observed that the team members were sharing resources and ideas with the group and striving for positive outcomes for the wellness clinic.

When Jake's preceptor, Linda, asked him which characteristics and skills he thought were needed for partnerships to be effective in planning such a challenging project, he answered that being committed, tactful, and persistent was important. He commented that it was really hard when people dropped out of the planning group in the early stage. However, the people who stayed with the project proved themselves to be committed and persistent. Jake also said that he thought it was very important to have people in the group who had some influence in the community.

Using Community Assets to Empower Communities, Systems, Individuals, and Families

PHNs identify assets that exist within a community. In addition, they strengthen these community assets through collaborating with others to identify community resources. To increase the inclusion of community assets when planning interventions, PHNs can use specific strategies, such as asset mapping and community-based participatory research.

How Can PHNs Use Community Assets in Planning Interventions?

To be effective collaborators, PHNs must recognize and emphasize community assets in planning interventions to promote public health. Community groups and organizations, such as churches, social service agencies, and neighborhoods, can identify assets within the community that provide building blocks for public health initiatives. Partnerships with social organizations, such as a neighborhood community center, can build community capacity to achieve public health core functions: assessment, policy development, and assurance (Kang, 1995). See Table 5.4 for an example of how using community assets can contribute to efforts to reduce youth violence. An intervention that builds on a foundation of community assets is sometimes referred to as a *strengths-based intervention*, which means that an intervention is selected and/or enhanced because it is already a resource or strength that exists within the community.

Table 5.4 Building Community Capacity for Responding to Youth Violence

Core Function	Community Asset	PHN Action
Capacity for Assessment	Parents, schools, and police department can provide data about youth violence in the community.	Recruit key community members to form an advisory group, which can help interpret assessment findings.
Capacity for Policy Development	Community advisory committee has knowledge of key resources and possible solutions for creating effective programs and policies to reduce youth violence.	Collaborate with others on advisory committee to identify recommendations for an evidence-based policy and/or program to reduce youth violence; communicate advisory group recommendations to decision makers (might be governmental or nonprofit organizations).
Capacity for Assurance	Lay helpers and persons from the community can effectively deliver health messages; such organizations as churches, schools, and neighborhood centers can provide resources for supporting a policy or developing a program.	Provide tools and evidence-based strategy ideas for community members who select the strategy that best meets the needs and characteristics of both the community environment and the population targeted for the program or policy change.

Source: Kang, 1995

Tools for Strengthening Communities

Asset Mapping

Karen Goldman and Kathleen Schmalz (2005) contrast a needs-based assessment approach with an asset-based assessment approach. Looking for needs results in looking for what is wrong with the community and determining how "to fix" the problems, while looking for assets results in building on community strengths and mobilizing resources within the community to promote community health (see Table 5.5).

Table 5.5   Needs Assessment vs. Asset Mapping

Needs Assessment	Asset Mapping
• Community need is based on deficiency or problem.	• Community assets include people, places, businesses, and organizations that can be mobilized for improvement.
• Looks at what is wrong with the community and how to fix it.	• Focuses on positive aspects (strengths).
• Leads community to seek assistance rather than in-house skills and change agents.	• Leads community to look within for solutions and resources to solve problems.
• Discourages community members.	

Source: Goldman & Schmalz, 2005

Assessing community assets means listening carefully to the voices of community members through interviews, meetings, focus groups, and asset-based inventories. Strengths of individuals, community groups, and community organizations are identified in an asset-based inventory. Strategies to conduct an inventory may also include conducting a walking or windshield survey in which community strengths are noted and using maps to document assets with a Geographic Information System (GIS).

Asset mapping can benefit the community in several ways. This approach empowers people to think more positively and encourages them to discover their abilities to contribute to their own health. They also learn to listen and value the contributions of others. Asset mapping is an inclusive process, which results in highlighting information and resources that can be used to mobilize individual and community assets (Fuller, Guy, & Pletsch, 2002; Kretzmann & McKnight, 1993; Morgan & Ziglio, 2007).

John Kretzmann and John McKnight (1993) have identified five categories of community assets: physical, individual, associations, institutions, and economic. Luther Snow (2004) and John Hammerlinck (2013) propose asset-mapping questions, which can be adapted to help community groups explore their assets (see Table 5.6).

Table 5.6   Questions for Community Groups to Promote Thinking About Assets

Asset Category	Questions
Physical	What are two or three physical assets in your community (neighborhood, buildings, parks, space, land, natural resources)?
Individual	What are your talents, experience, perspectives, and skills? What do you care about? What do you know about? Whom do you know?
Associations	What is your participation in formal or informal voluntary groups, networks, and organizations of individuals who gather to do or enjoy something they cannot do alone? Which groups are you part of? Which groups do you know about?
Institutions	Which institutions (such organizations as businesses, nonprofit agencies, government, and schools) are located in your community? What do these organizations contribute to your community?
Economic	What is something you spend money on? What is something you make or do that people would pay you for? Where do you invest your money? What are unique economic assets in your community?

Source: Hammerlinck, 2013; Snow, 2004

Once the community group has identified its assets, the next step is to review and consider how these assets can be tapped. In a group exercise, group members can list assets on pieces of paper or sticky notes and talk about how they are connected and can be used to improve the health and well-being of the community (Snow, 2004).

 Evidence Examples for Asset Mapping

Promoting healthy eating behaviors. Gayle Timmerman (2007) explores barriers experienced by women who were underserved and attempted to adopt healthy eating behaviors. Collaboration occurred by involving women in focus groups to understand women's experience with ways to improve nutrition. Key aspects of the collaboration included establishing a personal connection with the women, emphasizing respect, facilitating reciprocity, and providing feedback (Crist & Escandon-Dominguez, 2003). Timmerman explains that using an asset-based approach (as opposed to the traditional needs-based approach) led to identifying community resources that could help sustain changes in behavior. Additional important components included having a shared vision and purpose for recommended changes in health strategies and employing workers from the community. The African-American participants in the focus groups suggested that churches should be a central place for health promotion activities, because churches were viewed as trustworthy and convenient for participants to access (*individual and community levels*). Possible partners for nutrition interventions included local grocery stores, restaurants, schools, farmer's markets, food banks, and public transportation to increase access to nutritious affordable food (*community and systems levels*) (Timmerman, 2007).

Partnership to decrease childhood obesity. An initiative to address childhood obesity used asset mapping to identify individual and community strengths in the targeted population, a public school district in upstate New York. The goal was to reduce television viewing time. Partners in the initiative included child care staff, school and college staff and faculty, primary healthcare staff, local businesses, social and faith-based organizations, the local library, and students from all educational levels. Partners networked to involve others in the community; community groups offered 40 different afterschool and weekend activities in 11 public locations for preschool children and their families in a sponsored "TV turn-off week." Community groups collaborated on a variety of family activities, such as sports, lessons, music, dancing, and arts and crafts. Outcomes based on feedback from questionnaires and partner debriefing sessions indicated that more parents enrolled their children in programs that encouraged physical activity (*individual level/family level*), the library decided to continue to offer storytelling hours (*community level*), and child care providers changed their policies for viewing media (*systems level*) (Baker et al., 2007).

PHNs can make the best use of community resources by selecting evidence-based public health interventions. Community-based participatory research (CBPR) is a research strategy in which PHNs can partner with community members and organizations to investigate interventions that will be most effective with at-risk population groups. CBPR requires establishing a trusting relationship with community partners and engaging in collaboration between researchers and community members as equals (Israel, Eng, Schulz, & Parker, 2005; Savage et al., 2006; Schaffer, 2009). The expertise of community members enriches and adds authenticity to research findings. CBPR methods help overcome some of the challenges of conducting research with at-risk populations and are more likely to result in meaningful data that lead to effective strategies for improving health status in the community. PHNs can use a CBPR approach to build evidence for their practice in communities.

Evidence Examples for Community-Based Participatory Research (CBPR)

Improving maternal and infant health in an African-American community. Nurse researchers, a parish nurse, an African-American nurse, and community stakeholders interested in infant health joined community residents to collaboratively complete their research plan and develop recruitment strategies. Community partners provided essential information about the neighborhoods and enhanced the interpretation of the data in ways that would not have been known by the researchers if they had worked independently. For example, a participant complained about "black bars" in the neighborhood; the community partners explained that black bars were actually black wrought-iron fences that were placed between buildings to provide barriers to criminal activity (Savage et al., 2006).

PhotoVoice as a CBPR method for influencing social change. PhotoVoice offers participants visual evidence through photographs to help identify problems and influence potential solutions

(Goodhart et al., 2006; Wang, Morrel-Samuels, Hutchinson, Bell, & Pestronk, 2004). For a doctor of nursing practice (DNP) project that featured the voices of families who were experiencing homelessness, Joyce Bredesen (2012) provided cameras to families and individuals who were currently homeless. The participants were instructed to take pictures of things that affected their health in their daily lives. Through a series of three meetings, participants were encouraged to discuss their photographs and describe the personal meaning of each image they photographed (see Figure 5.1 for a photo example). Bredesen then compared the realities of those experiencing homelessness with the recommendations of the national guideline *Adapting Your Practice: General Recommendations for the Care of Homeless Patients* (Bonin et al., 2010). The results of the comparison as well as the pictures and stories of the participants were shared at a community forum attended by local leaders, policy makers, healthcare providers, representatives of the homeless population, and community members. The information from the forum was shared with local healthcare and service providers within the community. The outcomes of the project included empowerment of the participants, increased awareness of healthcare needs of homeless families within the community, and promotion of dialogue among local leaders, policy makers, and community members that potentially will lead to improvements in the delivery of services to the homeless.

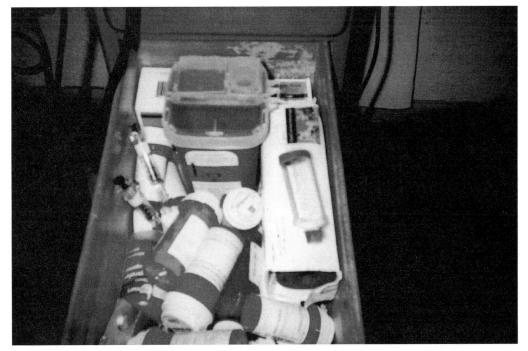

Figure 5.1.   "These are all the meds that are combined with my daughter's that we have. It's a lot to keep up with, when to take them, how many to take, what to take with them. It's really difficult, you know, but it's a part of my health and a part of her health. All these meds went in my bag with me everywhere. This fills up my backpack."

Source: Bredesen, 2013

Jake realized the importance of knowing community assets and working with other professionals. The pastor knew the neighborhood and community well and had space and people resources for serving the meal on Wednesday evenings to the homeless. The social worker had experience with chemical dependency patients and the skills needed to address drug-abuse issues or concerns among the homeless. Another nurse was a mental health specialist who knew about useful referrals for homeless people. The police liaison knew many people who were homeless and was very well respected in the community. The insurance representative could help find resources to increase people's access to healthcare by identifying funding options and programs. The PHN knew about social service resources and possible sources of healthcare funding. Even Jake, as a student nurse, brought his gifts of delivery of care by doing blood pressure screenings, health teaching, and foot care at the wellness clinic. The programs planned at the wellness clinic were services the collaborative community members could offer or find others to come in and provide.

Jake was present the first night the wellness clinic opened. As he sat down to share a meal with some of the individuals who visited the wellness clinic, he realized the value in this statement: "It takes a community to take care of its own." The strengths of each collaborative partner were needed to develop the wellness clinic.

Ethical Application

When PHNs collaborate with other professionals, community members, and community organizations, ethical concerns often center on selecting interventions that promote social justice for vulnerable populations that have fewer resources for improving their health. However, as PHNs work to promote a healthier life for community members, they must also consider how community members are going to view and experience the interventions they develop. In addition, collaboration often requires courage to work with others who have different views and persistence to keep working together even when disagreements and tension about the right way to proceed exist. All voices need to be heard in the decision-making process. In collaboration, an emphasis on community assets leads to inclusion, diversity, empowerment, and advocacy (see Table 5.7 for the application of ethical perspectives to collaboration).

Table 5.7   Ethical Action in Collaboration

Ethical Perspective	Application
Rule Ethics (principles)	• The goal is beneficence or promoting good (improvement in health status) for the community and community members.
	• Encourage autonomy of community members by ensuring that their perspectives contribute to determining interventions to improve health.
Virtue Ethics (character)	• Be courageous in working with those with different views and perspectives.
	• Be persistent in working through disagreements and tension in collaboration with others.

Feminist Ethics (reducing oppression)	<ul><li>Encourage including the voices of all stakeholders in the collaboration.</li><li>Respect everyone.</li><li>Strive for equality in the provision of programs and services.</li><li>Emphasize community strengths.</li><li>Advocate for individuals and community groups who have less power.</li></ul>

When Jake first started the community health course, he believed that, although important, the delivery of services to persons who were homeless was someone else's concern, not his. He also wondered why individuals who were homeless were included in the planning group. In the early meetings, he observed that the participants who represented the homeless population were very quiet, so many other members of the group were talking about what they thought homeless people wanted. In the third meeting, the police liaison who had emerged as the group's leader asked the members who represented the homeless population to offer their opinions on some of the ideas that had been expressed. He explained that they were "experts" on what it meant to be homeless and would therefore have good ideas about which services and resources would best help meet their health needs. The police liaison also did not back away from conflict but continued to emphasize the common goal of the group.

After being a part of the project and actually spending time with individuals who were homeless, Jake now understood why it was important to include persons who have experienced homelessness in planning the clinic. The planning group empowered the group members who were homeless to participate as equal partners and take a leadership role in creating solutions.

As Jake provided foot care for a middle-aged man one evening, the man shared his story of how he worked for a big company, lost his job as the company downsized, coped by drinking, lost his house and his family, and finally lost his sense of self-respect. As Jake reflected on this story, he reflected that each of us could find ourselves in a similar situation. Through collaboration, Jake realized that a community can use its strengths and resources to make a difference.

Key Points

- PHNs collaborate with many partners, including other nurses, health professionals, lay workers, community members, healthcare and community organizations, businesses, and government organizations.

- Effective partnerships share a common goal and require respect for and equality among partners.

- Partnership development requires trust between partners and a commitment to spend the time needed to develop that trust.

- When building IPC relationships, pay attention to the following: teamwork, communication practices, roles and responsibilities, and values.

- Collaborative partnerships for promoting the health of the public should integrate community assets that contribute to the identification of intervention strategies and design interventions in collaboration with community members. Tools for identifying community assets include asset mapping and CBPR.

Learning Examples for Effective Collaboration Strategies

You can find abundant examples in the literature of learning opportunities for collaborating with others to improve population health. The following examples illustrate collaboration with other nurses, professionals, community members, or organizations. As you read through these examples, think about your community and how you could collaborate with other health professionals, people, and organizations to improve the health of the population.

Infection Control and Emergency Preparedness Toolkit for the Faith Community

- Collaborators included six health departments, parish nurses, a county emergency preparedness coordinator, public health nursing consultant, and nurse educators in Wisconsin.

- A toolkit included resources for faith communities: fact sheets, posters, bulletin announcements, resources for children and church nurseries, recommendations for faith-based emergencies, and pandemic planning and emergency preparedness instructions for individuals and families.

- A follow-up survey revealed an increase in awareness about infection control and an increase in the number of resources that faith communities determined they would use to prevent the transmission of infection (Reilly et al., 2011).

Worksite Health Promotion

- The Office of Health Promotion and Wellness at the University of Alabama and a college of nursing collaborated to encourage employees to engage in healthy behaviors.

- The health and wellness program provided health assessment, screening, and health advising meetings and facilitated identifying and monitoring individual health goals.

- IPC included participation from health professionals, undergraduate nursing students, and graduate students in nursing, dietetics, psychology, and kinesiology (Carter, Kelly, Montgomery, & Cheshire, 2013).

Project Hope: A Partnership Between a City and a School of Nursing

- Pairs of nursing students in an RN-BSN program in Denver, Colorado, conducted outreach with an outreach worker in downtown parks and a mall. They carried backpacks with supplies for assessment and wound care and gloves, hats, socks, and water to give to homeless individuals.

- Nursing students also provided assessment and health-related education in a downtown shelter for homeless individuals and families.

- Assessment, health teaching, and referrals were the most frequently provided interventions (Pennington, Coast, & Kroh, 2010).

 ## Reflective Practice

Developing a clinic for the homeless is a complex project that involves many stakeholders and community organizations. Before partners begin to collaborate, reflecting on the goals of the collaborative project is essential. When partners are gathered together, they need to reach consensus on a shared goal. Now that you have learned about collaboration and the knowledge and skills needed to collaborate effectively, consider the following questions:

1. What does Jake need to consider about effective partnerships before collaborating on developing a clinic for the homeless?

   _____

   _____

2. Consider the barriers to IPC and strategies for overcoming them, as shown in Table 5.1. For the scenario about the clinic for the homeless, what do you see as possible barriers the team might encounter? What can they do to effectively manage those barriers?

    _____

    _____

3. What information about the population and community organizations will be needed for planning? What is an effective way to gather the information?

    _____

    _____

4. What would be important to include on the agenda for the first planning meeting?

    _____

    _____

5. How can the group explore individual and community assets that can be mobilized?

    _____

    _____

6. Which additional questions will you need to ask to partner effectively to develop a clinic for the homeless population?

    _____

    _____

7. Refer to the Cornerstones of Public Health Nursing in Chapter 1. Which of the Cornerstones are consistent with and support the development of a clinic for individuals and families who are homeless?

    _____

    _____

After you have worked through these questions, develop an outline of possible partners and collaborative strategies. Propose relevant Public Health Intervention Wheel interventions and the level of each intervention that may be part of the plan.

Application of Evidence

1. Which responses would you expect from the planning group based on Tuckman's phases of group development?

2. Which partnership guidelines would you apply to increase the likelihood of partnership success?

3. How could you use asset mapping or CBPR to achieve partnership goals?

Think, Explore, Do

1. Which previous experiences have you had with collaboration or working in a partnership to promote health (student work groups or task forces)? What do you think went well, and what did not go well? Which factors contributed to the partnership's success (or lack thereof)?

2. How have you been included or excluded as a collaborator in contributing to improving your own health?

3. Which types of responses from others help you feel respected and included?

4. Which assets in the community where you live do you think promote population health?

5. Which organizations in the community or state could provide additional resources to promote the health of the homeless population in the scenario?

6. Which actions do you think are essential for developing an effective partnership?

7. What can you do to promote equality when power differences exist among partners?

8. What can you do to promote buy-in for committing to the partnership among community members and organizations?

9. What can you do to "learn about, from, and with" as you collaborate with professionals from other disciplines in public health nursing practice?

References

American Nurses Association. (2013). *Scope and standards of public health nursing practice.* Silver Spring, MD: Nursebooks.org.

Aston, M., Meagher-Stewart, D., Edwards, N., & Young, L. M. (2009). Public health nurses' primary health care practice: Strategies for fostering citizen participation. *Journal of Community Health Nursing, 26,* 24–34.

Baker, I. R., Dennison, B. A., Boyer, P. S., Sellers, K. F., Russo, T. J., & Sherwood, N. A. (2007). An asset-based community initiative to reduce television viewing in New York state. *Preventive Medicine, 44*(5), 437–441.

Bazarman, M. H. (Ed.). (2005). *Negotiating, decision making and conflict management.* Cheltenam, UK: Edward Elgar Publishing United.

Bonin, E., Brehove, T., Kline, S., Misgen, M., Post, P., Strehlow, A. J., & Yungman, J. (2010). *Adapting your practice: General recommendations for the care of homeless patients.* Nashville, TN: Health Care for the Homeless Clinicians' Network, National Health Care for the Homeless Council, Inc.

Bredesen, J. A. (2012). *A comparison of recommended practice guidelines for health care of the homeless and the current health status of homeless families in St. Paul, Minnesota, as assessed through the use of PhotoVoice methodology.* Doctor of Nursing Practice Project.

Carter, M. R., Kelly, R. K., Montgomery, M., & Cheshire, M. (2013). An innovative approach to health promotion experiences in community health nursing: A university collaborative partnership. *Journal of Nursing Education, 52*(2), 108–111. doi:10.3928/01484834-20130121-04

Chaudry, R. V., Polivka, B. J., & Kennedy, C. W. (2000). Public health nursing director's perceptions regarding interagency collaboration with community mental health agencies. *Public Health Nursing, 17*(2), 75–84.

Clatworthy, W. (1999). Community care: Collaborative working. *Journal of Community Nursing, 13*(4), 4.

Community Tool Box. (2001). Identifying community assets and resources. Retrieved from http://ctb.ku.edu/en/tablecontents/sub_section_main_1043.aspx

Crist, J. D., & Escandon-Dominguez, S. (2003). Identifying and recruiting Mexican American partners and sustaining community partnerships. *Journal of Transcultural Nursing, 14*(3), 266–271.

D'Amour, D., Ferrada-Videla, M., Rodriguez, L., & Beaulieu, M. (2005). The conceptual basis for interprofessional collaboration: Core concepts and theoretical frameworks. *Journal of Interprofessional Care, Suppl. 1,* 116–131.

Fawcett, S. B., Francisco, V. T., Paine-Andrews, A., & Schultz, J. A. (2000). A model memorandum of collaboration: A proposal. *Public Health Reports, 155*(2–3), 174–190.

Findley, S. A., Irigoyen, M., See, D., Sanchez, M., Chen, S., Sternfels, P., & Caesar, A. (2003). Community-provider partnerships reduce immunization disparities: Field report from northern Manhattan. *American Journal of Public Health, 93*(7), 1041–1044.

Foss, G. F., Bonaiuto, M. M., Johnson, Z. S., & Moreland, D. M. (2003). Using Polivka's model to create a service-learning partnership. *Journal of School Health, 73*(8), 305–310.

Franklin, L., Exline, J., & Stringer, K. (2002). Using coalition and community-based partnerships to improve immunization rates in Mississippi: A case study. *Texas Journal of Rural Health, 20*(3), 31–37.

Fuller, T., Guy, D., & Pletsch, C. (2002). Canadian Rural Partnership asset mapping: A handbook. Canadian Rural Partnership: Canada. Retrieved from http://www.planningtoolexchange.org/browse/results/asset%20mapping%20handbook

Gamm, L. D. (1998). Advancing community health through community health partnerships. *Journal of Healthcare Management, 43*(1), 51–67.

Goldman, K. D., & Schmalz, K. J. (2005). "Accentuate the positive!" Using an asset-mapping tool as part of a community-health needs assessment. *Health Promotion Practice, 6,* 125–128.

Goodhart, W., Hsu, J., Baek, J. H., Coleman, A. L., Maresca, F. M., & Miller, M. B. (2006). A view through a different lens: PhotoVoice as a tool for student advocacy. *Journal of American College Health, 55*(1), 53–56.

Grant, R. W., & Finnocchio, L. J. (1995). *Interdisciplinary collaborative teams in primary care: A model curriculum and resource guide.* San Francisco, CA: Pew Health Professions Commission.

Henneman, E. A., Lee, J. L., & Cohen, J. I. (1995). Collaboration: A concept analysis. *Journal of Advanced Nursing, 21*(1), 103–109.

Israel, B. A., Eng, E., Schulz, A. J., & Parker, E. A. (Eds.). (2005). *Methods for community-based participatory research for health.* San Francisco, CA: Jossey-Bass.

Kang, R. (1995). Building community capacity for health promotion: A challenge for public health nurses. *Public Health Nursing, 12*(5), 312–318.

Keller, L. O., Strohschein, S., Lia-Hoagberg, B., & Schaffer, M. A. (2004). Population-based public health interventions: Practice-based and evidence supported. Part 1. *Public Health Nursing, 21*(5), 453–468.

Kenny, G. (2002). Children's nursing and interprofessional collaboration: Challenges and opportunities. *Journal of Clinical Nursing, 11*(3), 306–313.

Kretzmann, J. P., & McKnight, J. (1993). *Building communities from the inside out: A path toward finding and mobilizing a community's assets.* Chicago, IL: ACTA Publications.

Lindsey, E., Sheilds, L., & Stajduhar, K. (1999). Creating effective nursing partnerships: Relating community development to participatory action research. *Journal of Advanced Nursing, 29*(1), 1238–1245.

Merrett, A., Thomas, P., Stephens, R. M., Moghabghab, R., & Gruneir, M. (2011). A collaborative approach to fall prevention. *Canadian Nurse, 107*(8), 24–29.

Miller, L. C., Jones, B. B., Graves, R. S., & Sievert, M. C. (2010). Merging silos: Collaborating for information literacy. *Journal of Continuing Education in Nursing, 41*(6), 267–272.

Morgan, A., & Ziglio, E. (2007). Revitalizing the evidence base for public health: Assets model. *Promotion & Education, Suppl. 2,* 17–22.

Pennington, K., Coast, M. J., & Kroh, M. (2010). Health care for the homeless: A partnership between a city and school of nursing. *Journal of Nursing Education, 49*(12), 700–703. doi:10.3928/01484834-20100930-02

Reilly, J. R., Hovarter, R., Mrochek, T., Mittelstadt-Lock, K., Schmitz, S., Nett, S., . . . Behm, L. (2011). Spread the word, not the germs: A toolkit for faith communities. *Journal of Christian Nursing, 28*(4), 205–211. doi:16.1097/CNJ.06013c31822afc7f

Savage, C. L., Xu, Y., Lee, R., Rose, B. L., Kappesser, M., & Anthony, J. S. (2006). A case study in the use of community-based participatory research in public health nursing. *Public Health Nursing, 23*(5), 472–478.

Schaffer, M. A. (2009). A virtue ethics guide to best practices for community-based participatory research. *Progress in Community Health Partnerships: Research, Education, and Action, 3*(1), 83–90. Retrieved from http://muse.jhu.edu/login?auth=0&type=summary&url=/journals/progress_in_community_health_partnerships_research_education_and_action/v003/3.1.schaffer.pdf

Seifer, S. D., & Connors, K. (Eds). (2007). Faculty toolkit for service-learning in higher education. Community-Campus Partnership for Health, Learn and Serve America's National Service-Learning Clearinghouse. Retrieved from http://www.servicelearning.org/filemanager/download/HE_toolkit_with_worksheets.pdf

Snow, L. K. (2004). *The power of asset mapping.* Herndon, VA: Alban Institute.

Thibault, G. E. (2012). Core competencies for inter-professional collaborative practice. Institute of Medicine Global Forum on Innovation in Health Professional Education. Retrieved from http://iom.edu/~/media/Files/Activity%20Files/Global/InnovationHealthProfEducation/2012-MAR-08/Thibault_Core-Competencies-for-Inter-Professional-Collaborative-Practice.pdf

Timmerman, G. M. (2007). Addressing barriers to health promotion in underserved women. *Family & Community Health, Supplement, 30*(15), S34–S42.

Tuckman, B. W. (1965). Development sequences in small groups. *Psychology Bulletin, 63*(6), 384–399.

Wang, C. C., Morrel-Samuels, S., Hutchison, P. M., Bell, L., & Pestronk, R. M. (2004). Flint PhotoVoice: Community building among youths, adults, and policymakers. *American Journal of Public Health, 94*(6), 911–913.

Wood, A., Middleton, S. G., Leonard, D. (2010). "When it's more than the blues": A collaborative response to postpartum depression. *Public Health Nursing, 27*(3), 248–254.

World Health Organization. (2010). Framework for action on interprofessional education and collaborative practice. Retrieved from http://whqlibdoc.who.int/hq/2010/WHO_HRH_HPN_10.3_eng.pdf

COMPETENCY #4
Works Within the Responsibility and Authority of the Governmental Public Health System

Marjorie A. Schaffer

with Bonnie Brueshoff and Raney Linck

Dan was recently employed as a public health nurse (PHN) by a county health department. After 2 months on the job, he was asked to staff a clinic to respond to the vaccination needs for the H1N1 pandemic influenza virus. The county health department had received a limited supply of vaccine, so the state health department directed that the vaccine first be given to children ages 9 and under. To reach a large number of children and maximize available staff, the public health director (acting as incident commander) made the decision to offer two mass clinics at health department sites.

Dan had never worked for the government. Through the orientation process, he began to wonder whether he would ever understand how the different levels of government worked together. He referred to his orientation materials for Population-Based Public Health Nursing Competency #4, which focuses on working with governmental systems. He commented to his supervisor, Carol, "This competency has so many parts. How will I ever understand what all these terms mean for the work I am doing?"

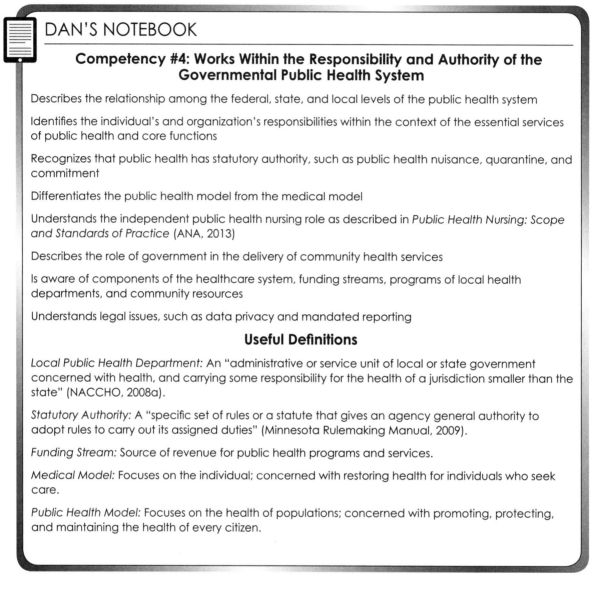

DAN'S NOTEBOOK

Competency #4: Works Within the Responsibility and Authority of the Governmental Public Health System

Describes the relationship among the federal, state, and local levels of the public health system

Identifies the individual's and organization's responsibilities within the context of the essential services of public health and core functions

Recognizes that public health has statutory authority, such as public health nuisance, quarantine, and commitment

Differentiates the public health model from the medical model

Understands the independent public health nursing role as described in *Public Health Nursing: Scope and Standards of Practice* (ANA, 2013)

Describes the role of government in the delivery of community health services

Is aware of components of the healthcare system, funding streams, programs of local health departments, and community resources

Understands legal issues, such as data privacy and mandated reporting

Useful Definitions

Local Public Health Department: An "administrative or service unit of local or state government concerned with health, and carrying some responsibility for the health of a jurisdiction smaller than the state" (NACCHO, 2008a).

Statutory Authority: A "specific set of rules or a statute that gives an agency general authority to adopt rules to carry out its assigned duties" (Minnesota Rulemaking Manual, 2009).

Funding Stream: Source of revenue for public health programs and services.

Medical Model: Focuses on the individual; concerned with restoring health for individuals who seek care.

Public Health Model: Focuses on the health of populations; concerned with promoting, protecting, and maintaining the health of every citizen.

Taking Responsibility for Improving Population Health

You can find PHNs working in all levels of government; in urban, suburban, and rural settings; and in a variety of community agencies and organizations. Federal, state, and local governments all provide essential resources for contributing to the public's health. This chapter discusses how levels of government work together to promote public health and how PHNs work with the government to deliver population-based public health services.

How Are the Federal, State, and Local Levels of Public Health Connected?

At the *federal* level, the U.S. Department of Health and Human Services (DHHS) oversees many other agencies that focus on the health and well-being of U.S. citizens. One of these agencies is the Centers for Disease Control and Prevention (CDC). The CDC keeps track of disease outbreaks and health statistics and protects the health and quality of life for U.S. populations. The CDC website is a good source for statistics and other information you need for public health interventions. For example, a PHN could use the CDC website to find updated statistics on state and national obesity trends and evidence-based strategies for obesity prevention.

Other examples of agencies that come under the DHHS umbrella are those that oversee Medicare and Medicaid Services; research and healthcare quality; substance abuse and mental health services; and the safety of food, cosmetics, medications, biological products, and medical devices. For example, a PHN could access information on food-safety alerts. Past examples include the contamination of ground beef (salmonella, typhimurium) and salad bars (norovirus).

State health departments often work with both the federal and local levels of government. State health departments regulate facilities and organizations that influence health as well as health professionals, including nurses. State functions include financing and administering programs (Stanhope & Lancaster, 2008) and offering technical assistance to local health departments for program development and services (MDH, 2009a). The organization and functions of state healthcare departments can differ greatly among the states. Regardless of the organizational structure, a strong partnership between state and local health departments is essential.

Local public health departments display considerable variability in the populations they serve and how they accomplish their work. A 2010 report identified the following characteristics of local health departments (NACCHO, 2011):

- About 63% of local health departments served populations with fewer than 50,000 persons, while 6% served populations of 500,000 or more.

- There was great variability in annual expenditures, dependent on population size, ranging from a median of $512,000 for departments serving fewer than 25,000 persons to a median of $58.5 million for those serving populations of one million or more.

- Jurisdiction types varied from county, to combined city-county, to local boards of health.

The report (NACCHO, 2011) also revealed that nursing staff decreased from 19.8% of local health department staff in the 2008 report to 17.4% in 2010. Local health departments (96%) employed 1 to 65 nurses, depending on the size of the population served.

The skills and expertise of PHNs are valued and needed to effectively deliver public health services. See Table 6.1 for an example of how the three levels of government worked together during a flu pandemic.

Table 6.1   Example: Three Levels of Government Working Together

2009–2010 H1N1 Flu Pandemic: Dakota County's Response

Background
- On April 27, 2009, the CDC declared a public health emergency.

- On June 11, 2009, the World Health Organization (WHO) determined that scientific evidence was sufficient to declare the H1N1 virus as the first global pandemic of the 21st century.

- The Dakota County Public Health Department collaborated with the Minnesota Department of Health and other health agencies to implement the pandemic flu response plans that had been previously developed.

Governmental Actions
- **Federal**—The CDC ordered H1N1 vaccine from manufacturers and identified priority groups for vaccine (initially pregnant women and children).

- **State**—The Minnesota Health Department directed local health departments.

- **Local**—The Dakota County Public Health Department coordinated plans with community organizations and worked with health clinics and providers in the county to redistribute vaccine doses.

Dakota County Response
- The county opened a Department Operations Center (DOC) to monitor the situation, coordinate response efforts, and provide updates to community stakeholders (schools, clinics, hospitals, long-term care facilities, police, fire, and emergency response units).

- When manufacturing problems delayed vaccine delivery, the local health department identified priority risk groups as caregivers of infants, pregnant women, healthcare workers, and first responders.

- Vaccinations were provided at scheduled immunization clinics, H1N1 appointment and walk-in clinics, and four mass vaccination clinics.

- A telephone and appointment system offering recorded messages in English and Spanish was established to respond to the surge of phone calls.

- Expanded groups became eligible to receive the vaccine as vaccine supplies increased.

- The Dakota County Public Health Department distributed 12,494 doses of vaccine by March 31, 2010.

- Minnesota ranked eighth in the nation for the percentage of residents who had received the H1N1 vaccine.

- Minnesota ranked first in the nation for vaccination of people ages 25 to 64 who had medical conditions placing them at a higher risk for H1N1 flu-related complications.

Source: 2009 H1N1 Flu Pandemic: Dakota County's Response (2010)

In 2011, a national voluntary accreditation program for local, state, territorial, and tribal leaders was established (CDC, 2013c). The Public Health Accreditation Board (PHAB) oversees the accreditation process and measures the accomplishment of the three core functions of public health (assessment, assurance, policy development) and the 10 essential public health services.

How Do the Essential Public Health Services and Core Functions Guide the Public Health Department and Your Work as a Public Health Nurse?

You first learned about the essential public health services and core functions in Chapter 1. The following section shows how PHNs accomplish the work that is outlined in the essential services and core functions and contribute to the well-being of populations. In a survey of 57 PHNs working in local and state governments and representing 28 states, they identified the amount of time they spent providing each of the essential services. The percentage of time spent on each essential service ranged from 7% to 14% (Keller & Litt, 2008). See Figure 6.1.

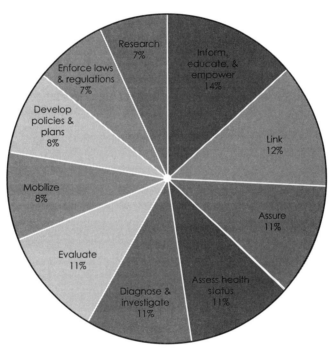

Figure 6.1. Percentage of PHNs' Time Dedicated to Essential Services (*n* = 57)

Dan remembered seeing the Public Health Core Functions in his orientation manual—assessment, policy development, and assurance. He said to Carol, "Let's see if I understand how this works. For the H1N1 flu clinic, I can see assessment happening when we are identifying how many children in the targeted age group live in our county. For policy development, we are following the directives given by CDC and the state department of health for vaccine administration. I can see how we are working with and through others to ensure that as many children as possible have access to the vaccine. Assurance happens when we make sure the vaccine is accessible to the population groups that need to be vaccinated and that the vaccine has been administered to them. Our health department redirected vaccine supplies to many area medical clinics so they could provide vaccinations."

Carol affirmed Dan's analysis of how the core functions were represented in the vaccine availability and distribution by the health department. Dan then said, "I am not sure about all those essential services. Do they all happen with our H1N1 response?"

Carol answered, "Let's analyze how each of the essential services happens when our health department responds to the H1N1 pandemic. Let's develop a handout to put into the orientation manual to help everyone understand how we are providing the essential services." See Table 6.2 for the handout that Dan and Carol developed.

Table 6.2   Essential Services in H1N1 Flu Clinic

Essential Service	Application Example
1. Monitor Health	Monitored county-specific data on school closures, hospitalization, and fatalities
2. Diagnose and Investigate	Communicated with school nurses about H1N1 flu symptoms and reporting requirements
3. Inform, Educate, and Empower	Worked with local media outlets to advertise H1N1 flu clinics and communicated educational information about protective measures, such as hand hygiene and "cover your cough"
4. Mobilize Community Partnerships	Worked with Medical Reserve Corps volunteers to assist in mass clinics
5. Develop Policies	Adopted policies from CDC and state department of health on priority setting of who should first receive the vaccine
6. Enforce Laws	Activated Emergency Response Plan following the CDC declaration of a public health emergency
7. Link to/Provide Care	Referred population to state flu telephone line to be assessed for influenza-like symptoms; local health department engaged local pharmacies to participate as dispensing sites for antiviral medications
8. Assure Competent Workforce	Provided training for staff prior to and day of mass clinics to ensure competence for roles and responsibilities

| 9. Evaluate | Held "hotwash" after each clinic (people in command positions identified what worked well and what needed improvement); completed formal "after action report" (AAR) |
| 10. System Management and Research | CDC provided information about system effectiveness in reaching population for administration of H1N1 flu vaccine |

Working toward public health accreditation provides local public health departments with the opportunity to document their capacity to deliver the 10 essential services. The accreditation process gives the assurance of which public health services should be provided to community residents (CDC, 2013c).

How Do Public Health Nurses Use Statutory Authority?

Statutory authority refers to the rules or statutes (laws) through which the government gives authority to agencies to carry out specific duties. In the public health arena, PHNs are responsible for following public health laws that have been enacted to protect and promote the health of communities (NACCHO, 2010). Public health laws might be federal, state, or local, but many public health laws are carried out at the local level. Laws concerned with public health include public health nuisance; quarantine; mandated reporting of communicable disease; mandated reporting of suspected abuse and neglect of children, the disabled, and the elderly; and commitment. See examples of local public health laws in Table 6.3.

Table 6.3   Local Public Health Law Examples

Type of Law	Key Features	Example
Public health nuisances	Conditions that threaten the health of the public, including garbage accumulation, sewage, noise, junked cars, abandoned swimming pools, rodent infestation, and faulty electrical wiring or plumbing	Top three complaints were mold, garbage houses, and accumulation of rubbish or junk (MDH, 2011)
Quarantine	Provides for isolating individuals and/ or groups to prevent the spread of communicable disease; restricts activities or travel of an otherwise healthy person with possible exposure to a communicable disease to prevent disease transmission	Can be used to reduce the effects of bioterrorism or pandemic events, such as the spread of avian influenza

Table 6.3   Local Public Health Law Examples   (continued)

Type of Law	Key Features	Example
Mandated reporting of communicable disease	Mandates reporting of communicable diseases so that surveillance of the occurrence of the disease can be monitored	During the H1N1 epidemic during the fall of 2009, surveillance of incidence of H1N1 cases helped determine the number of flu clinics that needed to be offered and provided data for determining whether schools needed to be closed.
Civil commitment	Protects mentally ill individuals from being dangerous to themselves or others; process of obtaining a court order to obtain treatment for mental illness when individuals are unable or unwilling to seek treatment voluntarily and need protection from harming themselves or others due to illness	PHNs collaborate with family members, other health professionals, community agencies, and the government in the civil commitment process.
Mandated reporting of child abuse	Professionals in relevant disciplines who have a reason to believe a child is being neglected or abused are obligated to report the information to the local welfare agency.	PHNs are engaged in the healing arts and are mandated reporters for child abuse and neglect.

Sources: Minnesota Department of Health, 2005a; Minnesota Department of Health, 2005b; Minnesota Department of Health State Community Health Services Advisory Committee, 1992; Minnesota Statutes, 2005, Section 144.419; National Alliance on Mental Illness, 2006; Office of the Reviser of Statutes, 2012

A website that compiles information and resources about public health law at all levels of government is the Network for Public Health Law. It identifies primary legal issues and offers technical assistance for a variety of topics.

What Is the Difference Between the Public Health Model and the Medical Model?

As you think about how government organizations guide and deliver public health services and the responsibilities of the government and PHNs for improving the health status of individuals and populations, consider how PHNs use a public health model in contrast to a medical model. One difference is that the public health model focuses on populations, whereas the medical model focuses on individuals. Another difference is the public health focus on prevention of disease as opposed to the medical model focus on treatment of disease. In the public health model, healthcare is viewed as a right, whereas in the medical model, healthcare is a service. PHNs can use the public health model (see Table 6.4) to help frame their practice as prevention-oriented and population-based. You must consider how the public health model differs from the traditional medical model when planning interventions to improve health status among populations to ensure that interventions are consistent with the mission of public health.

Table 6.4 Differences Between the Public Health and Medical Models

Public Health Model	Medical Model
Mission is to promote, protect, and maintain the health of every citizen.	Mission is to restore health to those who seek care (i.e., treatment and cure).
Focus is on the primary health needs of communities and populations.	Focus is on the primary health needs of individuals.
Health is seen as a birthright of every citizen.	Healthcare is seen as a service to be sought.
Goal is client/family and population self-sufficiency.	Goal is providing quality service to meet immediate medical care needs.
Focus is on prevention.	Focus is on treatment.
It seeks to protect the public's health before problems arise.	It seeks to meet the needs of patients who present for care of an existing problem.
It reaches out to identify individuals, families, and populations with service needs (case-finding).	It addresses the needs of patients who present for care.
Focus is on populations, the community, and the family.	Focus is on the individual.
It provides services that others cannot or will not provide.	It generally provides services that are reimbursable.
It seeks social change to improve the health status of populations.	It seeks change to improve status of an individual.
It provides services primarily in community settings.	It provides services primarily in healthcare facilities.
It provides services in the home that are holistic in nature; might provide services for medically necessary needs or refer those individuals with medically necessary needs to a home care agency.	It provides home care services for medically necessary needs related to disease and disability.

Some services might be provided in both public health and medical settings, but their approaches to healthcare differ. For example, childhood screening is provided in public health programs to improve the well-being of the population of children in the community. From the perspective of the medical model, an individual child is screened on routine visits in a clinic to evaluate that child's health status. For childhood obesity prevention, consider how a PHN could provide interventions that are consistent with the public health model (see Table 6.5).

Table 6.5 Public Health Model vs. Medical Model for Childhood Obesity Prevention

Public Health Model Example	Medical Model Example
• Framed as a disease that affects a population	• Framed as a physical problem for individual child
• Results from individual vulnerability and environmental factors	• Treatment of the individual through clinic services
• Interventions are targeted toward changing environmental factors (e.g., guidelines for nutritious day care and school lunches and snacks).	• Focus is on behavioral changes and personal responsibility.

Source: Schwartz & Brownell, 2007

The PHN who provides interventions for childhood obesity prevention within a framework of the public health model could consult with school administration and teachers on the implications of policies and guidelines for nutrition for school children (systems level), use social marketing to communicate the benefits of healthy eating (community level), and provide health teaching to groups of school children on fun ways to eat better (individual level). A public health approach often involves a greater number of interventions with a holistic and environmental approach to promoting well-being.

After the flurry of responses to the flu pandemic had subsided, Dan reflected on how his work differed from that of his previous position as a nurse for a pediatric clinic. Dan commented to his supervisor, Carol, "I never realized how the government is responsible for public health. I now think about people who need the flu vaccine not as individuals, but as populations. We prioritized which populations should receive the vaccine first—those who had the greatest need for protection from complications of influenza. We also made sure that the vaccine was available to everyone, regardless of whether they could pay for the vaccine. In the clinic, we followed a medical model that approached clients as individuals."

Carol added, "Yes, the public health model is oriented to finding people who need health services rather than always waiting for persons to identify their needs. In addition, public health is oriented toward changing health and social systems to create environments that encourage improvement in health status. By reaching out to those populations most in need of the flu vaccination, we have actually created an environment that will help keep people healthy in the communities served by our agency."

How Do the Scope and Standards of Public Health Nursing Guide the Public Health Nurse in Independent Practice?

The American Nurses Association (ANA) published an updated version of *Public Health Nursing: Scope and Standards of Practice* in 2013. This publication explains the professional role expectations for PHNs. It has two sections—standards of practice and standards of professional performance. The standards of practice detail how the nursing process is applied in public health nursing (see Figure 2.1 in Chapter 2). Table 6.6 analyzes how each of these role expectations occurred in the implementation of an H1N1 flu clinic.

Table 6.6 Standards of Professional Performance—Application to H1N1 Flu Clinic in Dakota County, Minnesota

Standard	Example
Ethics	Decided and adhered to prioritization plan for which groups received the vaccine first
Education	Provided education on roles, responsibilities, and incident command structure for staff working in the H1N1 mass clinics
Evidence-Based Practice and Research	Accessed information from the CDC for vaccine safety and adverse reactions
Quality of Practice	Contracted with Minnesota Visiting Nurse Agency (MVNA) to provide vaccinations, which received the *Mark of Excellence Award*, the Minnesota Department of Health flu-shot provider award
Communication	Discussed the formula to use for distributing a limited supply of vaccine within the region during the early phase of the pandemic
Leadership	Activated DOC to coordinate the response and work with local organizations
Collaboration	Worked with another county to share utilization of Medical Reserve Corps for staffing clinics
Professional Practice Evaluation	Completed After Action/Improvement Plan that follows guidelines from the Homeland Security Exercise and Evaluation Program
Resource Utilization	Worked with local city police department for security and assistance with traffic during mass clinics

continues

Table 6.6 Standards of Professional Performance—Application to H1N1 Flu Clinic in Dakota County, Minnesota (continued)

Standard	Example
Environmental Health	Promoted practices that reduced exposure to those most at risk within the community
Advocacy	Provided outreach throughout the county to promote and encourage vaccination and communicate flu clinic schedules

How Is the Government Involved in the Delivery of Community Health Services?

Often, governmental organizations collaborate with private and nonprofit organizations to deliver community health services. How do the core functions of assessment, policy development, and/or assurance take place in the following evidence examples?

Evidence Example: Action Plan for Asthma Management

A university collaborated with county PHNs and Head Start teachers and managers to conduct a needs assessment and develop an action plan for asthma management. In a community participatory action approach, focus groups with Head Start staff resulted in identification of challenges in asthma management—occurrences of asthma that were undiagnosed and not reported, coordination of plans with parents, issues with medication administration, and variability in the plans (Garwick, Seppelt, & Riesgraf, 2010). Recommendations were made for PHN leadership in developing an action plan that focused on early screening of asthma, evidence-based policy development, teaching Head Start staff about asthma management, and coordination of asthma care.

Evidence Example: Mock Vaccination Exercise

A county health department collaborated with a Medical Reserve Corps Unit (volunteers of trained medical and community health personnel) in St. Louis County in Missouri (Curtis, 2010). A mock vaccination exercise took place at a local high school to provide training for the members of the reserve unit and nursing students. The mock screening instructed the participants in the correct and efficient administration of vaccines to more than 5,000 individuals at five vaccine clinics.

Evidence Example: The Business Case for Breastfeeding

The Health Resources and Services Administration's Maternal and Child Health Bureau (which resides within the DHHS) provides a resource toolkit on its website titled *The Business Case for Breastfeeding* (Health Resources and Services Administration, 2013). The website provides guidelines for privacy to express milk, flexible hours, education, and support and extols the benefits of breastfeeding for health and work productivity.

What Should the Public Health Nurse Know About the Healthcare System?

PHNs need to have specialized skills and knowledge to effectively meet the expectations for their role, including knowing how public health is funded, having the skills necessary to function in specific public health programs, and understanding the referral process for connecting people with community resources. Funding of public health affects the ability of state and local health departments to provide adequate public health services. In your work as a PHN, you might be called on to contribute to planning and writing grant applications for funds for specific public health programs. In larger health departments, you might become more specialized with skills and knowledge for a specific public health program, such as follow-up for clients with tuberculosis or family-planning clinics. In rural health departments, your skill set and knowledge may have to be broader, because you might work in a variety of programs and settings. Also, you would be expected to have knowledge about the many resources that are available to individuals, families, and communities and the referral process needed to receive services from those resources.

Funding Streams

Funding for local public health comes from a mix of local, state, and federal funds, fees, and reimbursements, and it varies across states. In a 2011 state example of funding streams, the local tax levy accounted for 30% of local health department expenditures (MDH, 2012). Other sources of funding included reimbursements and fees for services, reimbursements from Medicare and Medicaid, and state general funds that provided a local public health block grant. Evidence shows that funding is linked with both public health department performance and population health outcomes (MDH, 2012). Because of the multiple sources of funding for public health, budgets are complex and vary each fiscal year. Funding sources are often focused on responding to current crises, such as the federal funding that was made available for the H1N1 pandemic response. Public health funding is dependent on a flourishing economy; a downturn in the economy means that public health resources might be more limited.

Another example of funding streams is the provision of home visits to high-risk families, which involves a mix of public and private funding. One family home-visiting program provided by a visiting nurse agency typically focuses on pregnant and parenting families and children with illnesses who live in a large metropolitan area. PHNs staff the program at 7.5 FTEs (full-time equivalent). Funding sources for the home visits from PHNs include third-party reimbursement from Medicaid and insurance companies (55%), funds from the city local government (43%), and special project funds (2%). For this program, much of the reimbursement from insurance comes through state public programs that contract with the insurance company to deliver healthcare services for a specified population. Special projects focus on a specific service that is provided, such as a one-time assessment of pregnant women or an asthma grant, which focused on low-income children who had been diagnosed with asthma. All visits provided by the PHNs must have an identified payment source (either public or private). Families frequently move between public and private sources, many times related to the fact the families served are often on the edge of homelessness and are very mobile (C. Lanigan, personal communication, 2013).

Programs of Local Public Health Departments

Although variation exists among programs that local public health departments provide, some public health services are provided more frequently, such as immunizations and surveillance and epidemiology for communicable/infectious diseases. In addition, population-focused home-visiting programs can be offered that target specific vulnerable or high-risk populations, such as parenting adolescents.

Local health departments have numerous responsibilities and activities; percentages of the occurrence of specific activities in local health departments are listed below (NACCHO, 2011, p. 52):

- Adult immunization provision (92%)
- Communicable/infectious disease surveillance (92%)
- Child immunization provision (92%)
- Tuberculosis screening (85%)
- Food service establishment inspection (78%)
- Environmental health surveillance (77%)
- Food-safety education (76%)
- Tuberculosis treatment (75%)
- Schools/daycare center inspection (74%)
- Population-based nutrition services (71%)

The *National Association of County and City Health Officials* (NACCHO) report showed that emergency preparedness has become an important responsibility of public health, with 65% of health departments including designated emergency preparedness staff. Local health departments provided screenings for a number of diseases and conditions in addition to tuberculosis, including high blood pressure, blood lead, diabetes, cancer, and cardiovascular conditions. Maternal and child health (MCH) services included Women, Infants, and Children (WIC) services, MCH home visits, family-planning services, well-child clinics, and prenatal care. Additional health services that may be provided by local health departments are oral health, home healthcare, primary care, and mental health and substance abuse services.

Increasingly, local health departments are employing informatics specialists, given the growth in the use of information technology (IT). The NACCHO (2010) report identified the following uses of IT in local health departments (p. 75):

- Have electronic health records (EHRs) or plan to implement EHRs (34%)
- Use Facebook (28%)
- Use Twitter (13%)
- Have electronic immunization registries (75%)
- Use an electronic syndromic surveillance system (56%)
- Use an electronic surveillance system to detect influenza-like illness (89%)

How Does the Affordable Care Act Contribute to Access to Care and Influence Healthcare Delivery?

PHNs work with populations that will have increased access to healthcare through the Affordable Care Act (ACA), passed by Congress in March 2010. Although political controversy surrounded the passage of the act, the law is increasing access to healthcare for Americans who previously lacked healthcare coverage. The ACA is the biggest change in American healthcare policy since the establishment of Medicare and Medicaid in 1965. The intent of the ACA is to increase access to healthcare and control escalating healthcare costs. One of the strategies is to provide more preventive care, which is aimed at reducing the use of hospital emergency departments (EDs) by persons who lack healthcare coverage. The ACA does not cover persons who are not American citizens (see Table 6.7 for some of the key provisions of the ACA).

Table 6.7   Key Provisions of the Affordable Care Act

Insurance Reform
• More people covered through Medicaid expansion, insurance exchanges, no denial of insurance because of preexisting conditions, coverage of young adults on parents' plans until age 26, and penalties for Americans who do not purchase insurance
• More benefits and protections through preventives services provided by insurance at no cost to enrollees, a minimum set of benefits, no lifetime or annual limits, and rate restrictions on higher rates based on gender or health status
• Lower costs for consumers and government through insurance exchange subsidies; prescription drug rebates for Medicare enrollees; and other restrictions on rates, payments, and how insurance companies spend premium dollars

Health System Reform
• Improved quality and efficiency through new structures, such as accountable care organizations, medical homes, quality measures, and incentive payments based on quality measures
• Stronger workforce infrastructure through community and school-based health center funding, increased payments for Medicare and Medicaid providers, loan repayments, and public health workforce development
• A greater focus on public health and prevention through new funding and grants for prevention efforts, public health education campaigns, community health needs assessments, and nutrition labeling

Source: American Public Health Association, 2012

As part of the ACA, the National Prevention Strategy: America's Plan for Better Health and Wellness (HealthCare.gov, 2013b) includes four major strategies:

- Building healthy and safe community environments
- Expanding quality preventive services in clinical and community settings

- Empowering people to make healthy choices
- Eliminating health disparities

The seven priority areas are (1) tobacco-free living, (2) preventing drug abuse and excessive alcohol use, (3) healthy eating, (4), active living, (5) injury and violence-free living, (6) reproductive and sexual health, and (7) mental health and emotional well-being. The National Prevention Strategy identifies evidence-based recommendations for reducing the incidence of preventable death and major illness.

Because service delivery is changing, new initiatives are also restructuring the healthcare system, including the following:

- **Health insurance exchange:** Provided by state or federal government; virtual marketplaces where individuals, families, and small businesses can comparison shop for health coverage; useful for those with no access to employer-based insurance coverage and who do not qualify for Medicaid or Medicare; subsidies available for low-income individuals and families

- **Accountable Care Organization (ACO):** A group of healthcare providers who provide coordinated care, chronic disease management to improve the quality of patient care and health outcome, resulting in reduced costs (HealthCare.gov, 2013a)

- **Healthcare or Medical Home:** Provides coordination of healthcare; "primary care providers, families and patients work in partnership to improve health outcomes and quality of life for individuals with chronic health conditions and disabilities" (MDH, 2013)

In addition, new IT infrastructures are being planned to improve the sharing of data through interoperable EHRs. In 2009, the Health Information Technology for Economic and Clinical Health (HITECH) Act identified EHR meaningful use as a critical national goal (CDC, 2012). HITECH has identified four areas in public health to be improved by moving from current processes (such as paper forms or telephone calls) to secure electronic reporting directly from the EHR:

- **Syndromic Surveillance (SS):** Improving public health monitoring in real time through digital submission of pertinent health data from hospital and clinic EHRs to public health agencies for analysis and planning. Current SS examples include monitoring for injury trends, such as bicycle accident–related injuries; tracking the burden of disaster-related conditions in hospitals following a natural disaster, such as a tornado; and tracking the severity of asthma and upper respiratory tract infections during allergy season (International Society for Disease Surveillance, 2012).

- **Immunization Information Systems (IIS):** Creating a centralized repository of all immunization data with two-way electronic record exchanges that include sending and receiving immunization histories for individuals and related demographic information as well as observations about an immunization event, such as reactions or eligibility for a funding program (Savage, 2011).

- **Electronic Laboratory Reporting (ELR):** State and local laws require the reporting of particular lab results to public health agencies regarding communicable diseases, such as anthrax, botulism, smallpox, and more. Through reporting, these agencies can act quickly to control the spread of the disease, such as vaccinating or treating close contacts of a patient, identifying contaminated foods, or uncovering industrial practices that cause toxic exposures (Georgia Department of

Public Health, n.d.). The goal is to improve timeliness and thoroughness of reporting as well as to reduce the number of manual data-entry errors (CDC, 2013a),

- **Cancer Registry:** Population-based cancer surveillance is essential for coordination of care, activities, and resource allocation to decrease the mortality and morbidity of this disease, which is the second-leading cause of death in the United States (CDC, 2013b).

EHR meaningful use is being planned in a three-stage rollout, with the public health initiatives being emphasized in Stages 2 and 3, beginning in 2014 and 2016, respectively. An exciting sign of things to come is the Beacon Community Program, which provided federal grants to 17 diverse communities from Maine to Hawaii so they could innovate and test new health IT approaches to improve public health (Rein, 2012). Although great progress has been made, there are still many issues left to resolve regarding the cost and feasibility of managing such large amounts of data at the state and local agency levels.

Community Resources

Local health departments cannot carry out their mission without community partnerships and resources. PHNs build cooperative partnerships with community agencies, organizations, other professionals, and community groups to respond to community health concerns. Many nonprofit organizations are vital partners that assist in working on and achieving public health goals. *Nonprofit organizations* provide services that contribute to the well-being of persons, communities, or society and do not aim to make a profit. They might be funded by grants or donations and sometimes receive funds from governmental organizations. For example, the MVNA was an invaluable partner in providing the nurse staff capacity for mass clinics in response to the H1N1 pandemic. In many communities, the visiting nurse agency is a primary provider of community health services.

 Evidence Example: American Lung Association Open Airways for Schools

For children with asthma, the American Lung Association is a nonprofit organization that provides important information to schools, nurses, and parents about responding to asthma. The American Lung Association website offers classroom kits that include a curriculum guide, posters, activities, and handouts (American Lung Association, 2010). The curriculum, available in English and Spanish, offers an interactive teaching approach that helps children and parents learn about self-management of asthma. Columbia University conducted a study of the program's effectiveness with a diverse group of 239 children from 12 elementary schools in New York City. Results showed that the school children who finished the program managed their asthma more effectively, had improved school performance, and had fewer episodes of asthma. Parents were also more involved in helping their children manage their asthma, and the school environment increased its support for children with asthma.

Dan noted that nurses from the Medical Reserve Corps were volunteering to help staff some of the flu clinics. He asked one of the nurses, Grace, how she became involved in the Medical Reserve Corps. Grace commented, "I have a regular job at the hospital in my community, but when I heard about the Medical Reserve Corps, I decided I wanted to help my community if a disaster occurred. I am a volunteer. I found out about this organization when some of my friends went to New Orleans to help with health needs after Hurricane Katrina."

Dan later spoke with his supervisor, Carol, about the Medical Reserve Corps (MDH, 2008; NAC-CHO, 2008b). Carol said, "Since Hurricane Katrina, many healthcare workers in our state have signed up to be in the program, and now it includes more than 7,000 volunteers. This program strengthens the public health response, which we call public health infrastructure, when a disaster occurs. Local coordinators oversee the program and provide training and support so that volunteers are ready to respond to the disaster. Our health commissioner can mobilize volunteers when they are needed."

Dan responded, "The Medical Reserve Corps is a great community resource. I am going to tell my friends from my last job at the hospital about this wonderful volunteer opportunity."

Healthy People 2020 On the Healthy People 2020 website, go to 2020 Topics and Objectives, A–Z, and under "P" click "Preparedness." "Preparedness involves Government agencies, nongovernmental organizations, the private sector, communities, and individuals working together to improve the Nation's ability to prevent, prepare for, respond to, and recover from a major health incident" (Healthy People, 2013). What are some ways that PHNs can use the information in this section to contribute to accomplishing the goal of "improve[ing] the Nation's ability to prevent, prepare for, respond to, and recover from a major health incident" (Healthy People, 2013)? Think about actions that will address the needs of individuals, families, and communities during a major health incident. Which levels of government will be involved in PHN responses?

Which Legal Issues Are Important for Public Health Nurses to Understand?

The examples below include federal and state legal issues that are important for PHNs to understand.

Data Privacy

The federal government administers the Health Insurance Portability and Accountability Act (HIPAA) of 1996. PHNs are accountable for ensuring HIPAA's data-privacy aspect. You are certainly familiar with this law from day one of your clinical experiences or working in a healthcare setting. In some states, laws specify that information important for ensuring public health can be disclosed. For example, Minnesota's Data Sharing Law allows the sharing of immunization data with schools and child care providers without parental permission (MDH, 2003b). In addition, healthcare providers can share information about communicable diseases with the state health department without patients' permission (MDH, 2003a).

Mandated Reporting

All states have laws that protect abused children and require certain professionals, including nurses, to report suspected child abuse. Many states also offer civil immunity for people who make reports and/or penalties if suspected child abuse is not reported (Pozgar, 2005). Although the first case of child abuse was addressed under a law that prevented cruelty to animals in the 1870s, it was not until the 1960s and 1970s that all states had mandatory reporting laws (Encyclopedia of Everyday Law, 2010). Marie Land and Lesley Barclay (2008) have explored Australian nurses' perceptions about how they protected children and the barriers they experienced. Nurses were concerned they would have to appear in court and were also concerned about their personal safety if they reported abuse. Authors of the study recommended that nurses needed education about their legal responsibilities for child protection and suggested that changes in organizational structure and culture were necessary to promote interdisciplinary collaboration and the sharing of health information between professionals.

School-Entry Laws

PHNs who practice in school settings are involved in the enforcement of school-entry laws, which mandate evidence of vaccination for specific communicable diseases or a legal exemption signed by a parent. School-entry laws have been in existence since the 1960s and have led to increased vaccination rates and decreased rates of childhood communicable diseases (Horlich, Shaw, Gorji, & Fishbein, 2008). Some parents might object to compulsory vaccinations for their children, believing that the government is taking away their authority.

Ethical Application

One of the ethical problems involved in implementing flu-vaccine clinics is prioritizing which populations should receive the vaccine first. This decision sometimes creates an ethical problem when the benefits for the many (the population group) are deemed to be more important than the needs or interests of one person. Another ethical problem that PHNs might encounter regarding immunizations for children is that some parents are concerned that immunizations can cause their children harm (for example, the worry about the measles vaccination causing autism). An important role for PHNs is to be knowledgeable about evidence on the effects of immunizations to communicate to parents (see Table 6.8 for the application of ethical perspectives to immunization).

Table 6.8   Ethical Action in Providing Immunizations to Children

Ethical Perspective	Application
Rule Ethics (principles)	• Promote justice by providing access to immunizations for families with children, which is consistent with school-entry laws. • Prevent harm to the children by promoting immunization for this population. • Use evidence about immunization's effectiveness and debunk misinformation to provide education about immunization's benefits.
Virtue Ethics (character)	• Respect individual parental rights to refuse immunization for their children per the law, which allows parental exemption based on religious or other values.
Feminist Ethics (reducing oppression)	• Be aware of using authority in a manner that oppresses parents. • Encourage parents' voices and perspectives in making decisions about what to do.

 Key Points

- All levels of government (local, state, and federal) have responsibility for promoting public health and often work together.

- Ten essential services and three core functions of public health determine the goals of public health departments.

- PHNs who are employed by governmental agencies are responsible for upholding specific laws that protect the public health.

- The public health model focuses on populations and prevention in contrast to the medical model, which focuses on individuals and provides healthcare services in response to illness and injury.

- Funding for public health comes from public and private sources and determines the programs and services that local public health departments can provide.

- Local public health departments work with nonprofit organizations to improve the health status of populations.

- The Affordable Care Act (ACA) increases access to healthcare for more Americans.

Learning Examples for Working With Governmental Systems

Following are four learning examples. Useful websites from governmental organizations that provide additional information and strategies can help you generate evidence-based approaches to the public health concern. See Chapter 6 Resources, Appendix B, for website URLs.

Emergency Preparedness

(Carter, Kaiser, O'Hare, & Callister, 2006)

- Participate as a volunteer in a mock pandemic or biological terrorism event; reflect through writing or in a clinical conference discussion about the effectiveness of the governmental response to the event.

- In a clinical group, review the emergency response plan of a selected agency in the community. Evaluate the plan and summarize what the group has learned. Evaluate or develop a risk communication plan.

- Study a natural disaster (hurricane, tornado, or flood) and review the literature about the governmental response (Carter et al., 2006).

Review the CDC National Emergency Preparedness websites:

- Preparation and Planning
- Natural Disasters and Severe Weather

Updating Immunization Records

- Update immunization data on student health records at a charter school by accessing the immunization database on the state health department website.

- Review data privacy and requirements for immunizations for school children.

Implementing Nutrition Policy for School Children

- Review the following governmental guidelines and educational strategies for promoting healthy eating:

  - U.S. Department of Health and Human Services. (2013). Dietary guidelines for Americans.

  - Centers for Disease Control and Prevention. (2008). Make a difference at your school: Key strategies to prevent obesity.

  - Centers for Disease Control and Prevention. (2013). Competitive foods in school.

- U.S. Department of Agriculture, Food and Nutrition Service. (2013). Nutrition education.

- U.S. Department of Agriculture, Food and Nutrition Service. (2013). Nutrition standards for school meals.

- Robert Wood Johnson Foundation. (2009). Improving child nutrition policy: Insights from national USDA study of school food environments.

- Discuss how each of the three levels of government would be involved in implementing nutrition policy for school children.

- Identify interventions from the Public Health Intervention Wheel that you find represented by suggested strategies.

Reducing Youth Access to Tobacco

- Review the following resources and information about strategies for reducing youth access to tobacco:

  - Centers for Disease Control and Prevention. (2013). Youth tobacco prevention.

  - Minnesota Department of Health. (2013). Youth tobacco reports.

  - Minnesota Department of Health. (2013). Youth tobacco prevention.

- Identify PHN interventions for reducing youth access to tobacco.

- Identify governmental and community resources for reducing youth access to tobacco.

 # Reflective Practice

Governmental organizations develop and enforce regulations and laws to prevent disease and promote the health of populations. They also provide the resources needed to improve the public health. These resources include staff members with expert knowledge and funds to support public health programs and services. As a PHN working for a governmental organization, it is both a responsibility and honor to contribute to improved population health through one's expert knowledge and skills. Consider the public health response to a flood occurring in a community and answer the reflective practice questions that follow.

In 2009, the Minnesota Department of Health (MDH) opened its DOC in response to flooding of the Red River (MDH, 2009b). The MDH coordinated communication, activities of MDH employees in several counties, and volunteers to help local agencies and healthcare facilities. In addition, the MDH responded to resource requests. Social media tools facilitated communication; FirstLink (a call center), Twitter, Facebook, a blog that provided access to news releases and alerts, and mapping for showing evacuation areas all facilitated preparing for and responding to the flood emergency.

Review the following resources on guidelines for responding to a flood disaster (web links are provided in Chapter 6 Resources, Appendix B):

- Minnesota Department of Health. (2010). Information and guidelines for healthcare facilities and providers in the event of spring flooding or other natural disasters.

- Minnesota Department of Health. (2010). Floods: Protecting your health.

- Minnesota Department of Health. (2010). Floods: Caring for yourself.

Then answer the following questions:

- What are the responsibilities of the local, state, and federal levels of government in responding to major flooding in a community?

  _____

  _____

- How could community resources be involved in responding to the consequences of the flood in the community (disease prevention and health promotion)?

  _____

  _____

- How does a PHN use expert skills and knowledge to respond to a flood disaster?

  _____

  _____

- How are PHN actions in response to a flood disaster consistent with the Cornerstones of Public Health Nursing? (See Chapter 1.)

  _____

  _____

 ## Application of Evidence

1. Which essential services would be most relevant in responding to the natural disaster of flooding in a community?

2. Give a practice example that illustrates each of the three core functions for responding to a flood in a community.

3. Refer to Table 6.6, which identifies the ANA Standards of Professional Performance for Public Health Nursing. How do the following standards apply to the example of a flooding disaster: education, collaboration, resource utilization, leadership, and advocacy?

4. For the same flooding scenario, which public health laws and legal issues do PHNs need to keep in mind when responding to a flood disaster?

Think, Explore, Do

1. Choose a public health concern applicable to a population group. Analyze how the three levels of government are involved in responding to the public health concern.

2. Locate the annual report for the local health department (city or county) in which you have your clinical experience or where you live. (Annual reports are usually available on health department websites.) Find the financial report and identify revenue and expenses for provided services. Analyze the sources of public and private funding streams for public health in the county or city.

3. Discuss the mandate for reporting suspected child abuse, which is a responsibility of the professional nurse. Which public health interventions would the PHN use in working with a family in which child abuse might be occurring? How could community resources contribute to the prevention of child abuse?

4. Make a list of public health programs and services provided by the local health department in which you work or have your clinical experience. Analyze how the programs and services are consistent with the public health model. (See Table 6.4 for how the public health model contrasts with the medical model.)

5. How can you prepare yourself to be ready for the challenge when a disaster happens in your community? How can nurses and community organizations collaborate with the government to deliver healthcare during emergencies and disasters?

6. Read about the following U.S. governmental health services to learn their purpose, how they are organized, services that are provided, and who is eligible for and receives services:

   - U.S. Department of Veterans Affairs
   - DHHS Indian Health Services
   - U.S. Public Health Services
   - Military Health System

7. Explore the HealthCare.gov website:

   - Listen to some of the featured videos.
   - Click on *Prevention, Wellness, and Comparing Providers* in the toolbar.
   - Explore the webpage. Watch some of the short videos.

8. Explore the Beacon Community Program website:

   - Read inspiring stories from diverse communities that received federal grants to implement innovative new uses of health IT to improve public health.

References

2009 H1N1 Flu Pandemic: Dakota County's response. (2010 May). Dakota County Public Health Department.

American Lung Association. (2010). About OAS. Retrieved from http://www.lungusa.org/lung-disease/asthma/in-schools/open-airways/about-oas.html

American Nurses Association. (2013). *Public health nursing: Scope and standards of practice.* Silver Spring, MD: Author.

American Public Health Association. (2012). *Affordable Care Act Overview.* Retrieved from http://www.apha.org/advocacy/Health+Reform/ACAbasics/default.htm

Carter, K. F., Kaiser, K. L., O'Hare, P. A., & Callister, L. C. (2006). Use of PHN competencies and ACHNE essentials to develop teaching-learning strategies for generalist C/PHN curricula. *Public Health Nursing, 23*(2), 146–160.

Centers for Disease Control and Prevention. (2012). *Meaningful use introduction.* Retrieved from http://www.cdc.gov/EHRmeaningfuluse/introduction.html

Centers for Disease Control and Prevention. (2013a). *Electronic lab reporting.* Retrieved from http://www.cdc.gov/EHRmeaningfuluse/elr.html

Centers for Disease Control and Prevention. (2013b). *National Program of Cancer Registries: Meaningful use of electronic health records.* Retrieved from http://www.cdc.gov/cancer/npcr/meaningful_use.htm

Centers for Disease Control and Prevention (2013c). *National voluntary accreditation for public health departments.* Retrieved from: http://www.cdc.gov/stltpublichealth/hop/pdfs/NVAPH_Factsheet.pdf

Curtis, M. P. (2010). Community collaboration in a community H1N1 vaccination program. *Journal of Community Health Nursing, 27,* 121–125.

Encyclopedia of Everyday Law: Child Abuse/Child Safety/Child Discipline. (2010). Retrieved from http://www.enotes.com/everyday-law-encyclopedia/child-abuse-child-safety-discipline#history

Garwick, A. W., Seppelt, A., & Riesgraf, M. (2010). Addressing asthma management challenges in a multisite, urban Head Start Program. *Public Health Nursing, 27*(4), 329–336.

Georgia Department of Public Health. (n.d.). "Meaningful use" submissions of reportable laboratory results. Retrieved from http://www.health.state.ga.us/programs/meaningfuluse/labresults.asp

Health Resources and Services Administration. (2013). The business case for breastfeeding. Retrieved from http://mchb.hrsa.gov/pregnancyandbeyond/breastfeeding

HealthCare.gov. (2013a). *Glossary: Accountable care organizations.* Retrieved from http://www.healthcare.gov/glossary/a/accountable.html

HealthCare.gov. (2013b). *National Prevention Strategy: America's Plan for Better Health and Wellness.* Retrieved from http://www.healthcare.gov/news/factsheets/2011/06/prevention06162011a.html

Healthy People. (2013). *Preparedness.* Retrieved from http://www.healthypeople.gov/2020/topicsobjectives2020/overview.aspx?topicid=34

Horlich, G., Shaw, F. E., Gorji, M., & Fishbein, D. B. (2008). Delivering new vaccines to adolescents: The role of school-entry laws. *Pediatrics, 121,* S79–S84.

International Society for Disease Surveillance. (2012, November). *Electronic syndromic surveillance using hospital inpatient and ambulatory clinical care electronic health record data: Recommendations from the ISDS meaningful use workgroup.* Retrieved from http://www.syndromic.org/storage/ISDS_2012-MUse-Recommendations.pdf

Keller, L. O., & Litt, E. A. (2008). *Report on public health nurse to population ratio.* Association of State and Territorial Directors of Nursing (ASTDN).

Land, M., & Barclay, L. (2008). Nurses' contribution to child protection. *Neonatal, Paediatric and Child Health Nursing, 11*(10), 18–24.

Minnesota Department of Health. (2003a). *Communicable disease reporting and HIPAA. Immunization sharing and HIPAA.* Retrieved from http://www.health.state.mn.us/divs/idepc/dtopics/reportable/rule/hipaacomm.html

Minnesota Department of Health. (2003b). *Immunization sharing and HIPAA.* Retrieved from http://www.health.state.mn.us/divs/idepc/immunize/hippadata.html

Minnesota Department of Health. (2005a). *Isolation and quarantine procedures.* Retrieved from http://www.health.state.mn.us/divs/opa/isolation05.pdf

Minnesota Department of Health. (2005b). *Communicable disease rule, Chapter 4605.* Retrieved from http://www.health.state.mn.us/divs/idepc/dtopics/reportable/rule/rule.html

Minnesota Department of Health. (2008). *Minnesota responds Medical Reserve Corps volunteer protections.* Minnesota Department of Health fact sheet. Retrieved from http://www.health.state.mn.us/divs/opa/mrcfs08.pdf

Minnesota Department of Health. (2009a). *Local Public Health Act Overview.* Retrieved from http://www.health.state.mn.us/divs/cfh/lph/docs/lphoverview_factsheet.pdf

Minnesota Department of Health. (2009b). *Ready to respond: MDH Preparedness Newsletter.* Retrieved from http://www.health.state.mn.us/oep/news/09july.pdf

Minnesota Department of Health. (2011). *Local public health act overview.* Retrieved from http://www.health.state.mn.us/divs/cfh/lph/docs/lphoverview_factsheet.pdf

Minnesota Department of Health. (2012). *Financing local public health services in Minnesota: Trends in local tax levy expenditures.* Retrieved from http://www.health.state.mn.us/divs/cfh/ophp/system/ran/docs/1210ran_lhdfinancing.pdf

Minnesota Department of Health. (2013). *Health care homes.* Retrieved from http://www.health.state.mn.us/healthreform/homes/index.html

Minnesota Department of Health State Community Health Services Advisory Committee. (1992). *Controlling public health nuisances: A guide for community health boards.* Retrieved from http://www.health.state.mn.us/divs/eh/local/chsboardguide.pdf

Minnesota Rulemaking Manual. (2009). *Chapter 3—Rule Development.* Retrieved from http://www.health.state.mn.us/rules/manual/chapters.html

Minnesota Statutes. (2005). *Section 144.419. Isolation and quarantine of persons.* Retrieved from http://www.revisor.leg.state.mn.us/data/revisor/statutes/2005/144/419.html

National Alliance on Mental Illness. (2006). *Understanding the civil commitment process.* Retrieved from http://www.namihelps.org/assets/PDFs/civilcommitmentSinglePg102108.pdf

National Association of County and City Health Officials (NACCHO). (2008a). *Fast facts: 2008 national profile of local health departments.* Retrieved from http://www.naccho.org/topics/infrastructure/profile/resources/2008report/upload/profilebrochure2009-10-17_COMBINED_post-to-web.pdf

National Association of County and City Health Officials (NACCHO). (2008b). *Medical Reserve Corps.* Retrieved from http://www.naccho.org/topics/emergency/MRC/index.cfm

National Association of County and City Health Officials (NACCHO). (2010). *Public health law.* Retrieved from http://www.naccho.org/topics/infrastructure/PHLaw/index.cfm

National Association of County and City Health Officials (NACCHO). (2011). *2010 national profile of local health departments.* Retrieved from http://www.naccho.org/topics/infrastructure/profile/resources/2010report/upload/2010_Profile_main_report-web.pdf

Office of the Reviser of Statutes. (2012). *2012 Minnesota Statutes. 626.556 Reporting of maltreatment of minors.* Retrieved from http://www.revisor.mn.gov/statutes/?id=626.556

Pozgar, G. D. (2005). *Legal and ethical issues for health professionals.* Sudbury, MA: Jones and Bartlett.

Rein, A. (2012, June 3). *Beacon policy brief 1.0: The Beacon Community Program: Three pillars of pursuit.* Academy Health and the Office of the National Coordinator for Health Information. Retrieved from http://www.healthit.gov/sites/default/files/beacon-brief-061912.pdf

Savage, R. (2011, September 15). *HL7 Version 2.5.1: Implementation guide for immunization messaging, release 1.3.* Centers for Disease Control and Prevention and American Immunization Registry Association. Retrieved from fhttp://www.cdc.gov/vaccines/programs/iis/technical-guidance/downloads/hl7guide-2011-08.pdf

Schwartz, M. B., & Brownell, K. D. (2007). Actions necessary to prevent childhood obesity: Creating the climate for change. *Journal of Law, Medicine & Ethics, 31*(1), 78–89.

Stanhope, M., & Lancaster, J. (2008). *Public health nursing: Population-centered health care in the community.* St. Louis, MO: Mosby Elsevier.

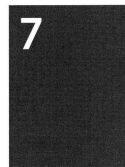

COMPETENCY #5
Practices Public Health Nursing Within the Auspices of the Nurse Practice Act

Marjorie A. Schaffer
with Carol Flaten

Jennifer, a public health nurse (PHN), has worked for the Weaver County Health Department for 10 years. Jennifer's first nursing position after completing her bachelor of science in nursing (BSN) and passing nursing boards was on a medical-surgical unit in a large metropolitan hospital. Since her public health experience in nursing school, she had been anxious to find a PHN position. In her search for a PHN position, Jennifer focused on three states in the Midwestern part of the United States that interested her. Within several months, she found a position at a small local health department in the town of Aurora, the county seat of Weaver County.

Aurora is surrounded by an agricultural community. Corn, soybeans, and sugar beets are the major crops. Cattle are also raised in this area. The town of Aurora has a population of 15,000. German immigrants settled Aurora in the 1850s. Today, Aurora is a multicultural community. The racial makeup is 91% Caucasian, 2% African-American, 2% Hispanic or Latino, 1% Native American, 1% Asian, 1% Pacific Islander, and 1% other. The median income is $30,000.

Weaver County has a significant population of migrant workers from Mexico who provide a large portion of the workforce for many farms in the area and also provide the labor for a poultry-processing company located on the northern edge of the county. This processing company opened 10 years ago. The town has needed to learn to adapt to a new cultural group.

Sarah, a public health nursing student, has been assigned to work with Jennifer to complete her public health nursing field experience. She is excited to start this experience. Sarah is completing her undergraduate BSN degree at a university about 45 miles from Weaver County. She is familiar with Weaver County only through the media reports regarding the difficult racial issues in the county over the past years. Sarah grew up in an urban area, where a variety of cultures and races were represented. She is Korean and was adopted into an American family as an infant. Sarah is eager to learn not only about the role of the PHN but also how the community environment affects the work of the Weaver County Public Health Department and its PHNs.

As Sarah has been reflecting on her public health nursing class, she remembers the three core functions of public health—assessment, policy development, and assurance. Along with this underlying framework, Sarah also knows the importance of the Cornerstones of Public Health Nursing. She is particularly interested in learning about how independent nursing practice is carried out and how PHNs use the Public Health Intervention Wheel in Weaver County. Sarah will spend 5 weeks with Jennifer, learning as much as possible about public health nursing.

SARAH'S NOTEBOOK

Competency #5: Practices Within the Auspices of the Nurse Practice Act

Understands the scope of nursing practice (independent nursing functions and delegated medical functions)

Establishes appropriate professional boundaries

Maintains confidentiality

Demonstrates ethical, legal, and professional accountability

Delegates and supervises other personnel

Understands the role of a PHN as described under public health nursing registration

Useful Definitions

Confidentiality: Nondisclosure of health information that is considered to be private.

Delegation: "The transfer of responsibility for the performance of a task from one individual to another while retaining accountability for the outcome" (ANA, 2010, p. 64).

Independent Practice: Professional decision-making guided by professional standards of the profession; scope of practice that includes independent functions might also be defined legally.

Nurse Practice Act: State statute that describes the practice of nursing; describes scope of professional nursing practice.

Professional Boundaries: Limits that allow for safe connections and situations in professional interactions with clients; in the professional relationship, expert knowledge is assumed on the part of the professional, and the relationship is directed at meeting the needs of the client, but not the needs of the professional (Gallop, 1998; Jacobson, 2002).

Public Health Nursing Registration: Requirements for practicing public health nursing, which are not universal across all states.

Supervision: Directing, guiding, and influencing the outcome of an individual's performance of a task (ANA, 2012).

Understanding Public Health Nursing Roles Ethically, Legally, and Professionally

This chapter discusses the Nurse Practice Act and how state legislation guides independent practice in public health nursing. Every state has its own Nurse Practice Act that lays out legal specifications for definitions, titles, licensing, and other parameters for the practice of nursing. Because much of public health nursing involves independent decision-making on the part of nurses and in collaboration with others, PHNs need to be aware of how the Nurse Practice Act for their states guide their professional role and define professional accountability.

Each state has a board of nursing that develops guidelines through rules and regulations that go through a public review before they are enacted. The board of nursing also sets standards for prelicensure nursing education and clinical learning experiences and reviews complaints of misconduct and follows up with any needed disciplinary action. Although Nurse Practice Acts vary somewhat among states, they all include the following components (Russell, 2012, p. 37):

- Definitions

- Authority, power, and composition of the board of nursing

- Educational program standards

- Types of titles and licenses

- Protection of titles

- Requirements for licensure

- Grounds for disciplinary action, other violations, and possible remedies

 Evidence Example: Core Elements of U.S. Nurse Practice Acts

Jarrin (2010) conducted an analysis of the core elements of Nurse Practice Acts in the United States for all 50 states and the District of Columbia. The researcher used qualitative analysis software to identify the major themes and frequency of occurrence in the Nurse Practice Acts (Table 7.1).

Table 7.1   Nurse Practice Act Themes

Theme	Percentage of occurrence
Care in the context of nursing	98%
Nursing process	88%
Supervision or delegation of nursing	82%
Executing the medical regimen	73%
Health maintenance and prevention	65%
Teaching nursing	65%

Source: Jarrin, 2010, p. 170

When PHNs practice independently, they make decisions based on their own expert knowledge and skills, professional standards, and the best evidence that guides nursing practice. Independent practice in public health settings differs from the experience of nurses in hospitals and other structured settings, in which medical orders are required for many nursing tasks. On some occasions in public health settings, a physician's order is needed for reimbursement from insurance, Medicare, or Medicaid for provided services. Also, a physician's order, although not legally required, might be necessary to make a referral for public health nursing services to obtain reimbursement. PHNs might refer to other members of the interdisciplinary team, such as a lactation consultant or a physical therapist, but again, a physician's order might be required for authorization of payment.

What Is the Scope of Public Health Nursing Practice?

Chapter 1 explains that the scope of practice refers to the boundaries of safe and ethical practice. The Public Health Intervention Wheel describes what PHNs do and further explains activities that fall within the scope of public health nursing practice. In public health nursing, PHNs often collaborate with staff from different disciplines. It is important to clarify job descriptions and professional roles so that representatives from each discipline make the best use of their specific expertise as they work together on reaching a common goal.

A study on the work of PHNs (Keller & Litt, 2008) demonstrated the breadth and consistency of public health nursing practice. The researchers used an online survey to complete a task analysis of 60 PHNs who represented 28 states. Many of the tasks identified were consistent with the interventions from the Public Health Intervention Wheel and represented the scope of public health nursing practice (see Table 7.2 to find out which interventions PHNs in the study used most often).

Table 7.2   Task Analysis of PHN Interventions

Frequency	Task/Intervention
100%	Emergency preparedness
100%	Health teaching to individuals and families
100%	Receive and make referrals
93%	Immunization clinics
88%	Health promotion/prevention programs in the community
88%	Case management
87%	Facilitate vulnerable individuals' access to services
87%	Work with groups related to public health issues
83%	Home visits
82%	Health teaching to groups
81%	Vulnerable children and/or adults
78%	Investigate disease and other health threats

78%	Health screening
73%	Educational classes, meetings, workshops for providers
70%	Advocate for increased healthcare availability and access
60%	Community organizing activities
47%	Lead groups related to public health issues

Source: Keller & Litt, 2008

This table shows that 88% of the PHNs in the sample used the intervention of Case Management. PHNs will have future opportunities to function as care coordinators (Case Management on the Intervention Wheel). Healthcare reform initiatives emphasize care coordination as a strategy to improve the quality of care and reduce costs (Robinson, 2010). PHNs' expertise and knowledge of community resources and advocacy are important in the skill set of empowering family participation in care coordination. Functioning in this role is consistent with recommendations in the Institute of Medicine's report on the future of nursing: "[N]urses should practice to the full extent of their education and training" and "nurses should be full partners, with physicians and other healthcare professionals, in redesigning healthcare in the United States" (Institute of Medicine, 2010, pp. 2–3).

Evidence Example: Hepatitis B Prevention in Case Management for Pregnant Women

In Hennepin County, Minnesota, the Perinatal Hepatitis B PHN serves a growing population of refugees and immigrants. The program provides case management, contact investigation of household members, monitoring of immunizations and titers for exposed infants, and education to address cultural myths about Hepatitis B for pregnant women who are antigen-positive. The PHN collaborates with the medical provider, social worker, mental health worker, and family members at clinic visits and, through case management, makes any needed referrals. Program effectiveness is measured by improved outcomes in vaccine and serology completion for infants (from 92% to 100%), increases in the number of women referred to liver specialists for follow-up, and increases in the number of referrals of sexual partners and household members for follow-up (Przybilla, Johnson, & Hooker, 2009).

Evidence Example: Case Management of Children in Foster Care

PHNs in California collaborated with foster caregivers and social workers to help children in foster care obtain needed health services. The PHNs assisted with interpretation of healthcare reports, development of health plans, referrals for care, and evaluation of placements in meeting healthcare needs. To be effective in working in the multidisciplinary model, the PHNs needed skills and knowledge that included flexibility, clear communication, the ability to prioritize, and an understanding of health and social services at the county and state levels. PHNs provided all 17 interventions from the Public Health Intervention Wheel in their case management of foster care children (Schneiderman, 2003, 2006).

In Schneiderman's (2003) study of 12 nurses working in the child welfare system and the school district, school nurses most often used the interventions of Screening, Health Teaching, and Surveillance, whereas the child welfare nurses more often used the interventions of Consultation, Referral and Follow-up, Surveillance, and Case Management. Schneiderman suggested that the collaborative work of PHNs within the child welfare system could be enhanced by developing clear job descriptions, having a structure that identifies the workflow for PHNs, and providing education for other professionals on the competencies, skills, and knowledge of professional nurses.

Evidence Example: The Independent Practice of Public Health Nurses

Researchers conducted a study with 23 focus groups in six Canadian geographic regions to identify organizational attributes that contributed to a successful experience in providing public health nursing interventions. Focus groups were held with 156 PHNs and were divided into staff PHNs and PHNs who were in management or policy making. These groups were also divided by place of practice—urban or rural/remote. Analysis of focus group data revealed that organizational leadership needed to support public health nursing practice autonomy, which is consistent with independent practice. Staff PHNs wanted nursing management to trust their ability to work independently. Although they wanted clear guidelines and specified roles for their work, they also wanted flexibility in deciding with their clients the best approach to use, because different ways of reaching the same goal exist. The focus group data revealed the importance of defining roles in terms of "what" needs to be accomplished rather than focusing on "how" an outcome should be accomplished. The study also noted that "champions" are needed at the organizational level to increase public awareness of the work of PHNs (Underwood et al., 2009).

PHNs may also work in or receive referrals from Nurse-Managed Health Clinics (NMHCs), which have interprofessional teams that include nurse practitioners, physicians, and social workers. NMHCs often provide health services encompassing primary care, health promotion, and disease prevention to persons with limited access to healthcare (American Association of Colleges of Nursing, 2013). The focus is on integrating preventive care and wellness approaches into primary care. Outcomes show a reduction in hospitalization and use of the emergency department (ED) for patients who receive services from NMHCs (Coddington & Sands, 2008; National Nursing Centers Consortium, 2011). In addition, NMHCs provide high-quality healthcare based on a favorable comparison with national benchmarks; they also have high levels of patient satisfaction (Barkauskas, Pohl, Tanner, Onifade, & Pilon, 2011).

Evidence Example: Nurse-Managed Health Clinics (NMHCs)

North Metro Pediatrics is a community-based NMHC that provides affordable pediatric care to a suburban pediatric population on a sliding-fee scale and a flexible payment system. Services provided include immunizations; physicals for sports, camps, and schools; chronic disease management; and prevention education. In addition, a marriage and family therapist provides mental health services, a university mobile dental clinic provides preventative oral health services, and case management is available for children with stable complex medical conditions. The clinic collaborates with other healthcare programs and community resources to promote family well-being (Bredow, personal communication, 2013).

Sarah's first day of her public health nursing clinical experience with Jennifer began right away on Monday morning (see Table 7.3 for Jennifer's schedule). Sarah met Jennifer at the Public Health Office at 7:30 a.m. She had met Jennifer briefly a week earlier, but this would be the first time that Sarah would have the opportunity to observe nursing through the eyes of a PHN. Sarah was on time and ready to enter the building at 7:28 a.m., but the door was locked! Sarah worried. This never happened at the hospital. She tried to open the door several times. It did not budge. She checked her calendar to be sure she had the correct day and time. She did. Within a minute, Jennifer drove up. They were off to their first visit.

Sarah rode with Jennifer. Jennifer had three home visits scheduled for the morning, followed by two home visits in the afternoon. At the end of the day, Jennifer had a planning meeting for a health fair. Jennifer briefly described the three morning home visits, which were to families whom she knew from previous visits: (1) a 93-year-old woman with congestive heart failure who lived alone, (2) a toddler with an elevated lead level whose parents had emigrated from Mexico last year, and (3) a 17-year-old with a 3-month-old girl. After the morning visits, Jennifer planned to return to the office for a short time to make any follow-up phone calls and review plans for the afternoon home visits. The last hour of the day, they would meet with the new director of an alternative learning center in the school district who had identified a need among her students for a health fair that focused on healthy foods.

Table 7.3   Jennifer's Schedule

Day/Time	Monday	Tuesday	Wednesday	Thursday	Friday
8am–9am	Home visit: Hanson	Staff Meeting	Immunization Clinic	Women Infants and Children Clinic	Alternative Learning Center Health Fair
9am–10am	Home visit: Vu	Diversity Coalition Meeting	Immunization Clinic	Women Infants and Children Clinic	Alternative Learning Center Health Fair
10am–11am	Home visit: Loften	Diversity Coalition: Collect county data for grant application	Inventory and order supplies for Immunization Clinic	Women Infants and Children Clinic	Alternative Learning Center Health Fair

continues

Table 7.3   Jennifer's Schedule   (continued)

Day/Time	Monday	Tuesday	Wednesday	Thursday	Friday
11am–12pm	Office: Follow up on calls, new referrals, plan for Health Fair	Office: Phone Triage	Meet with Program Manager to determine funding for Asthma Coalition	Women Infants and Children Clinic	Office: Phone Triage
12pm–1pm	Lunch	Lunch	Lunch	Lunch	Lunch
1pm–2pm	New Referral	Home visit: Ahmed	Prep for Foot Clinic at Community Center	Office: Follow up on phone calls and referrals, pack up supplies for Health Fair	Write report for Alternative Learning Center Health Fair
2pm–3pm	New Referral	Home visit: Johnson	Foot Clinic	Home visit: Wallis	Immunization Clinic
3pm–4pm	Meet with Director of Alternative Learning Center to plan for Health Fair	Home visit: Freeman	Foot Clinic	Home visit: Froeland	Immunization Clinic

Expanded Description of Activities

Alternative Learning Center Health Fair: The alternative learning center is part of the public school system. It offers middle and high school curricula for students who benefit from smaller class sizes and alternative methods of course content delivery. Many of the teachers at the school felt a need to provide "healthy lifestyle habits" information to the students. The school nurse contacted the public health office to collaborate with the PHNs to design a morning "Health Fair." The focus will be on including healthy snacks and exercise in your day, with demonstration stations on how to make a snack, followed by an opportunity for the students to make and eat their own snacks.

Asthma Coalition: One of the school nurses in Aurora noticed that more and more children with asthma were coming to her office every year. She mentioned this concern to a local physician, who had also noticed an increase in pediatric patients needing asthma-related care. The school nurse contacted the public health department to find out whether it was aware of an increase in asthma rates in the county or state. The timing of that call was good—the public health nursing director had just learned of funds that were available for starting a coalition related to asthma in children. The state and county statistics were showing an increase in asthma cases over the past 5 years. Out of these conversations, a coalition was formed. Currently one of the PHNs is the chairperson of this coalition, which meets monthly to identify ways to increase public and provider awareness of methods to manage asthma. This coalition includes school nurses, nurse practitioners, physicians, PHNs, coaches, and parents of children with asthma.

Diversity Coalition: This is a group of community partners (educators, healthcare providers, local business owners) who are interested in supporting the various groups represented in Aurora. The overall goal of this group is to make Aurora a welcoming community for everyone. One of the elementary school teachers in town initiated this group, as he was observing segmentation of racial groups that led to tension not only in the elementary school but also in the community at large.

Foot Care Clinic: Twice a month, the PHNs hold a clinic to provide foot care for senior citizens at the community senior center. The PHNs worked with a podiatrist in the community and the public health medical director to develop a foot-clinic protocol and referral system. Because an identified need existed in the community to provide basic skin and nail care and assessment for elderly citizens, this has been a very popular clinic. Two PHNs staff it.

Immunization Clinic: Each week, the public health office holds an immunization clinic where people can receive low-cost vaccinations for children or adults in their families. The clinic is held at the local health department, which is centrally located. It is a walk-in clinic, so no appointments are required. Each PHN takes a turn staffing the clinic. One PHN oversees the clinic by ordering vaccines, following current protocols for administration, and informing the PHNs of updated information.

Phone Triage: The PHNs all take turns on "phone triage." During this time, the PHN works on documentation or projects at his or her desk and answers calls that come to the agency that require a PHN to assess and provide feedback. Calls can range from parents needing to know which immunizations their children need and low-cost places to get those vaccinations to a landlord worried about bedbugs in a vacated apartment unit.

WIC Clinic: Women, Infants, and Children (WIC) is a federally funded food program administered by states and counties that provides screening, nutrition counseling, and health referrals for pregnant and breastfeeding women and their children from birth to 5 years of age. In Aurora, PHNs and nutritionists from the health and human services department staff this clinic twice a month at the public health nursing office. Jennifer's role is to provide height and weight checks for the children and review their immunization status.

Sarah's assignment for the day was to observe Jennifer's communication and actions. Sarah planned to take notes about her observations and communication between the PHN and client. See Sarah's notes.

SARAH'S NOTEBOOK

Activity	Sarah's observations
Visit 1: Lily Hanson, a 93-year-old woman with congestive heart failure. Lives alone.	Arrived at a four-plex apartment building. The yard and building were maintained well, with big shade trees, grass, and flower beds surrounding the building. Lily's apartment was on the first floor (no steps). Jennifer knocked on the door and opened it slightly; Lily called to Jennifer to come in. Lily was sitting at the dining room table and using her portable oxygen, neatly dressed, with her pill bottles lined up. The apartment was well-kept, with many photos on the walls.
	A fan was running quietly in the corner of the living room. Jennifer completed a heart and lung assessment and asked Lily about her activity level. Lily reported that even in the hot, humid weather, if she stayed indoors with the fans running, she felt comfortable. Jennifer filled Lily's pillbox for the week. Jennifer also asked Lily about alternate plans if her apartment became too hot for her to tolerate. Lily reported that she had had a window air conditioner, but it broke, and she did not have enough money to buy a new one. Jennifer suggested that Lily call the County Senior Support Network (SSN). The SSN has funds for elders in need of basic housing supplies. In this heat wave, Jennifer has learned that SSN will provide air conditioners.
	Jennifer talked to Lily so naturally. Jennifer explained that she had known Lily for 3 years. The first year she came to visit, Lily was not friendly at all. She thought Jennifer was visiting to get information that would cause her to go to a long-term care facility. After that first year and many short conversations, Lily accepted that Jennifer was trying to help her maintain her independence so that she could continue to live in her apartment. Jennifer hypothesized that her persistence and nonjudgmental attitude helped Lily realize she was there to support her.
Visit 2: Toddler with an elevated lead level whose parents emigrated from Mexico last year	Drove to an older part of town with many single-family homes. Much of the paint had worn off or was peeling. In most of the yards, the grass was worn away, and there were many children's toys. Jennifer rang the doorbell, knocked, and called in the front window, but there was no response. There was no response to a phone call either. Jennifer explained that sometimes families might not be home even though an appointment had been made for the visit. Persons living in poverty experience more frequent crises and with fewer resources might live from day to day, with less emphasis on future planning.

Visit 3: First-time 17-year-old mom, Ann, who has a 3-month-old girl	Stopped at an old apartment building that had broken glass on the front steps. Entry security system was working. Ann responded cheerfully to Jennifer. Ann lived on the third floor. No elevator. Smelled musty. Ann had the door open for us. It was 90 degrees out at 10 a.m. Ann had the shades pulled to keep the sun out, but there were no air conditioners or fans in the efficiency apartment. Jennifer focused this visit on baby Kayla's development. She used the Ages and Stages Questionnaire that has questions specific to development expected for the age of the child. I noticed Jennifer also gave some suggestions to Ann about what she could expect to happen in Kayla's development over the next few months.
Office (and lunch)	Jennifer checked for messages and had a message from the Garcia family—They will not be home today. Completed some charting. Checked for new referrals. Made calls to these families.
New Referral: Active case of tuberculosis (TB)	Met Mr. Adams at his house. Mr. Adams was diagnosed with TB (tuberculosis) about 4 months ago. He likely acquired TB working overseas in a disaster relief effort. He recently moved to Aurora to be near his aging parents. Jennifer will be providing Directly Observed Therapy (DOT) for Mr. Adams. In DOT, Jennifer will observe Mr. Adams to make sure he takes his medication correctly. When too many people take their TB medication inconsistently, the TB bacteria can become resistant to medication. In comparison to Jennifer's interaction with Lily earlier today, this was a very formal meeting. Jennifer asked questions to get the intake information. She also inquired about Mr. Adams's preferences for DOT. After the discussion and a brief health history, Jennifer observed Mr. Adams taking the medication and left.
New Referral: Postpartum visit	We met Amy Chan. She is 2 weeks postpartum. Her baby boy is doing well. However, Amy is anxious and nervous about her son, as her first child died of Sudden Infant Death Syndrome (SIDS) 3 years ago. Jennifer provided positive feedback regarding the care that Amy was providing for her son. Short messages and positive feedback seemed to help Amy. Jennifer suggested a support group for Amy.
Met with Director of alternative learning center	Jennifer met with the director, two of the teachers, and the school health aid. The director is very concerned about the nutritional status of the students. Many of the students drink sodas and eat chips for snacks at school and often skip lunch. Jennifer suggests planning a health fair that will focus on healthy snacks and provide samples.

Sarah spoke with Jennifer after the first day of her clinical experience. Sarah commented, "I don't know how I will ever become independent in my decision-making about what to do."

Jennifer suggested, "Let's review the day. Then we can analyze what we did today and which independent public health nursing interventions were accomplished. Also, I will have you look at my schedule for the rest of the week. You can begin to think about which interventions you would consider to be independent practice and how you might collaborate with others. We can discuss the skills and knowledge a PHN needs for these interventions."

ACTIVITY

Review Jennifer's schedule for the week (Table 7.3) and answer the following questions:

Which public health interventions from the Public Health Intervention Wheel did Jennifer use?

Which interventions were independent, and which were delegated functions?

What skills and knowledge enabled Jennifer to practice independently?

How did Jennifer collaborate with other individuals, groups, professionals, or organizations?

Healthy People 2020 On the Healthy People 2020 website, go to 2020 Topics and Objectives, A–Z, and under "M" click "Maternal, Infant, and Child Health." Read about factors that affect pregnancy and childbirth. Review determinants of health for mothers and infants. Scroll down to the box on the left side of the web page and click "Social Determinants of Health." Refer to the 17-year-old mother described in Sarah's journal. Which social determinants of health are important to consider and address for this young mother? Return to the "Maternal, Infant, and Child Health" page and click "Interventions and Resources." Find one intervention among the suggestions that the PHN could use to address the needs of this young family.

How to Establish Professional Boundaries in Public Health Nursing

On Tuesday, Jennifer has a visit scheduled with one of her favorite clients, Mindy, who is 16 and lives with her mother. Mindy has a 6-month-old baby girl. Mindy's former boyfriend, the baby's father, had been physically abusive to Mindy during her pregnancy. Mindy has developmental delays and struggles with school and fitting in. Mindy was referred to public health nursing after her first prenatal clinic visit when she was 6 months' pregnant. Mindy and Jennifer have developed a good relationship. Mindy has worked hard to follow through with good parenting practices and has been receptive to Jennifer. Jennifer checked her Facebook account last night and saw that Mindy had added her as a friend. Jennifer feels torn between the professional, therapeutic, and supportive roles she provides for Mindy.

Understanding professional boundaries is essential for all nurses. PHNs practice in environments that are sometimes more challenging for maintaining professional boundaries, such as in homes, schools, and other community settings that have different norms of behavior in contrast to the hospital setting. In the hospital setting, professional and client roles are more clearly defined. In community and home settings, relationships and the norms of interaction need to be differentiated from more casual social relationships. Sometimes students and PHNs find it difficult to keep from moving into a social friendship with the client as the relationship progresses over time. PHNs must clarify their role and the purpose of the relationship with clients to maintain professional boundaries.

Gloria Jacobson (2002) identified potential areas for boundary violation that need clarification about the nursing role. Confusion about the nurse's role can occur in situations of gift-giving or offering money. Although PHNs do not wear uniforms, they need to choose professional-appearing attire that is comfortable. Individuals from some cultures might frown on clothing that they consider too revealing and might be reluctant to believe what the PHN is saying is important if the PHN is not professionally dressed. PHNs need to be alert for any situation or conversations that might result in self-disclosure. PHNs need to ask themselves whether what they are doing is what a nurse would typically do. PHNs can use touch as a comfort measure but need to consider the meaning of any physical contact to the nurse and client. Touch and eye contact are not considered accepted practices in some cultures.

On some occasions, physical assessment is required, and although it is a norm for adults and children to remove clothes for physical exams in the hospital and clinic settings, removing clothes is not a norm in a community setting. If infants and children require a physical examination, the PHN should ask the parent or the child, if old enough, to remove the child's clothes.

Evidence Example: Defining Boundaries in Public Health Nursing

Five PHNs in a qualitative study described the challenge of defining boundaries as they worked with clients. They described situations of being persuaded to do something and then feeling regret that they had not said "no." The authors of the study suggested that one's professional ethical responsibility does not mean doing what another demands. Closer relationships that develop over a long-term time period with clients can lead to a sense of duty, which can result in overinvolvement and possible development of a friendship, which is a potential professional boundary violation. "Each nurse has to make decisions that are not only based on quality standards, but also on their professional intuition and personal involvement" (Clancy & Svensson, 2007, p. 163).

Maintaining professional boundaries does not mean being detached from clients. At the same time, the PHN does not fulfill the role of being a friend to a client. In a qualitative study of the ethical problems that 22 PHNs experienced in Canada, those who practiced in rural areas found it more difficult to separate their personal and professional lives to keep client confidentiality (Oberle & Tenove, 2000). In a study on maintaining personal and professional boundaries, McGarry (2003) identifies concerns about the PHN giving too much emotionally and spending too much time, which could lead to negative consequences for both the nurse and the client. The client might become too attached, the nurse might become too vulnerable, and the boundaries might become blurred. PHNs might experience a challenge in finding a balance between creating a participative, trusting relationship with the client while maintaining a separate professional identity.

ACTIVITY

When is it helpful to share something personal about yourself with a client? When is it not helpful?

What are some "red flags" indicating that you might not be maintaining professional boundaries with clients?

Is it a boundary violation to attend a patient's baby shower? A funeral for a client? Why or why not?

How do you think Jennifer should handle Mindy's Facebook request?

How Do Public Health Nurses Establish and Maintain Confidentiality?

Confidentiality in public health nursing often goes hand in hand with professional boundaries. Maintaining professional boundaries requires that PHNs keep health information private. PHNs must consider with whom they speak about clients and the confidentiality of their documentation processes. The Health Insurance Portability and Accountability Act (HIPAA), which specifies how health information may be communicated, is discussed in Chapter 6. Respecting patient confidentiality is a professional and legal duty (Griffith, 2007). However, PHNs must also balance this duty against the need to disclose information to protect someone from harm, such as in situations of suicide ideation. When vulnerable adults or children are involved, the duty to protect outweighs the duty to keep health information in confidence. Competing interests can exist—disclosure can be justified for the public good, an individual's protection, or the prevention or detection of a crime (Griffith, 2007).

> *Jennifer was well known at one of the apartment buildings in Aurora where many elderly adults lived. Jennifer had made many visits to residents in this complex over the years. The residents, although not related, had become like family to each other and welcomed Jennifer. They had an informal system of checking on each other daily and helping each other with trips to the grocery store or pharmacy. Often as Jennifer exited a client's apartment after a visit, several residents would stop Jennifer to ask how her client was doing. The neighbors were genuinely concerned and wanted to be helpful in any way possible.*

Question: How should Jennifer respond to the residents' questions about the clients she has visited?

Evidence Example: Maintaining Boundaries and Confidentiality in Working With Families with Intimate Partner Violence

Evanson (2006) investigates the role of PHNs who conducted home visits with families who had experienced intimate partner violence. The PHNs who worked in rural settings had more challenges in keeping confidentiality, helping women find resources, getting their own support, and keeping professional and personal boundaries. Although all the PHNs viewed setting boundaries as an essential part of their work with families who were experiencing intimate partner violence, Evanson concludes that the boundaries between personal and professional lives for rural PHNs are less clear than those for nonrural nurses. The rural PHNs had learned to be flexible with boundaries because they were highly visible in the community and often knew their clients personally through attending the same church, having children who were friends, or knowing mutual acquaintances. Personal ties were perceived as being a barrier to disclosure of the interpersonal violence. Rural PHNs needed to be vigilant about maintaining confidentiality and at times needed to withhold the truth from others within a client's family or community. Evanson recommends that rural agencies provide support opportunities through staff meetings and case conferences to help nurses who work with families experiencing intimate partner violence cope with the emotional labor of their jobs.

What Do Ethical, Legal, and Professional Accountability Mean in Public Health Nursing?

Ethical and professional standards and legal guidelines drive accountability in public health nursing practice. *Public Health Nursing: Scope and Standards of Practice* (ANA, 2013) specifies areas of accountability for PHNs (see Chapter 1). PHNs have more accountability to populations in comparison to nurses in other practice settings. The PHN is accountable for improving population health. *Legal* accountability is discussed in Chapter 6; this chapter focuses to a greater extent on PHNs' *ethical* accountability.

PHNs consider individuals, families, and communities as their clients. PHNs might experience ethical problems when they have to consider the impact or benefits and burdens of their decisions on multiple clients, population groups, and communities (Racher, 2007). Culturally diverse societies and communities might have moral standards different from each other's and from those of the PHNs, which could lead to conflicts between the PHNs and clients. Ethnic diversity in the community requires a complex ethical framework that includes the complementary approaches of rule ethics, virtue ethics, and feminist ethics (Racher, 2007; Volbrecht, 2002).

Rule ethics uses a framework of guiding principles for decision-making (Racher, 2007). Examples of rules or principles include autonomy, beneficence (promoting good), nonmaleficence (preventing harm), justice, loyalty, truth-telling, and respect (Aiken, 2004; Beauchamp & Childress, 1979; Purtilo, 2005; Scoville Walker, 2004). Rule ethics is based on a biomedical model of decision-making.

In contrast, *virtues ethics* is based on good character (Racher, 2007). One's actions are evaluated in the context of one's community. Examples of nursing virtues include compassion, honesty, courage, justice, self-confidence, resilience, practical reasoning, and integrity (Volbrecht, 2002).

Feminist ethics focuses on building relationships and reducing oppression in society (Volbrecht, 2002). Key values in a feminist ethics approach are inclusion, diversity, participation, empowerment, social justice, advocacy, and interdependence (Racher, 2007). Table 7.4 provides additional explanations about these three ethical approaches.

Table 7.4 Ethical Framework for Public Health Nursing Practice

Rule Ethics
- Rule ethics defines rules or principles that are based on perceptions of fairness.
- Ethical principles are standards of conduct that guide behavior and specify moral duties and obligations (Racher, 2007).
- Community rights might be given priority over individual rights in some situations.
- Resources are given based on need and thus might be distributed unequally (distributive justice).
- Those who have been unfairly burdened or harmed are compensated (compensatory justice).

Virtue Ethics
- Virtue ethics identifies characteristics of the individual (moral agent) and that person's intentions and behaviors.
- An individual is responsible for developing good character and good community (Volbrecht, 2002).
- This type of ethics provides the foundation for professional ethics, which specifies professional values and virtues.

Feminist Ethics
- A core ideal is achieving social justice; feminist ethics applies social justice and distributive justice to social structures and context.
- This ethical approach focuses on characteristics of relationships, strengthens relationships and connectedness, eliminates oppression, and realigns power imbalances.
- Feminist ethics is committed to restructuring relationships, social practices, and institutions so that people can live freer and fuller lives (Volbrecht, 2002).

Public health ethics is driven by social justice. The aim is to create a flourishing community for all rather than satisfying individual self-interests. A bioethics perspective focuses more on autonomy and individual rights (Easely & Allen, 2007). Ethical challenges in public health nursing can result from the conflict between protecting the community and respecting individual autonomy. For example, individuals might be required to take medication to treat tuberculosis (even when they would prefer to choose otherwise) to protect others' health. Protecting individual rights to privacy might conflict with the need to share information to benefit the public's health, such as in the case of reporting cases of communicable diseases to the health department so that disease incidence can be monitored (Racher, 2007).

In the study by Clancy and Svensson (2007), PHNs expressed that they thought they had a greater sense of responsibility than hospital nurses, because the PHNs primarily worked on their own. They expressed that they felt alone with their worries and their uncertainties about what to do. Ethical decision-making does not occur in a vacuum. Resolutions will be better with input from other experts in the field. PHNs need to seek out collegial and organizational support for their decision-making to ensure ethical, legal, and professional accountability.

Evidence Example: Ethical Problems in Public Health Nursing

A qualitative study of 22 PHNs in Canada (11 in rural settings and 11 in urban settings) revealed five categories of ethical problems they experienced in their work: (1) relationships with healthcare professionals; (2) systems issues, such as distribution of resources and consequences of policies; (3) character of relationships with clients; (4) respect for persons; and (5) putting self at risk, which involved value conflicts or potential physical danger. Most of the ethical problems the PHNs identified focused on relationships: "Decision making in public health might be equated with a juggling act in which the nurse tries to keep many balls in the air simultaneously, always in the interests of doing 'good' for the client. Difficulties arise in defining 'good' and determining whose good should be promoted. Moreover, good must also be defined in the long term, not just the immediate present" (Oberle & Tenove, 2000, p. 436). The authors recommend that PHNs have opportunities for dialogue with administrative leaders, that dialogue be multidisciplinary, and that public health nursing leaders provide support and mentorship for ethical decision-making.

What Should I Know About Delegation and Supervision in Public Health Nursing?

PHNs practice within their professional scope and standards of practice as well as within the guidelines of state Nurse Practice Acts, which define the legal parameters of nursing practice. Delegation is based on requirements addressed in each state's Nurse Practice Act. PHNs may be in the role of accepting delegated activities, such as carrying out provider orders for administering immunizations or monitoring respiratory status. PHNs may be in the role of delegating specific functions to unlicensed assistive personnel (UAP) or licensed practical nurses (LPNs). UAP include nurses' aides, certified nursing assistants, health aides, or other nonlicensed positions (American Nurses Association, 2012). Practice environments often include multiple services and interventions to promote the health of individuals, communities, and populations. The ability to work interprofessionally and to clearly identify the components of the delegation process is crucial to successful PHN practice. Weydt (2010) states:

> RNs are required to understand what patients and families need and then engage the appropriate care givers in the plan of care in order to achieve desired patient outcomes maximizing the available resources on the patient's behalf. Delegation is an important skill that influences clinical and financial outcomes. (para. 2)

Effective delegation is guided by three concepts the PHN must understand: *responsibility*, *accountability*, and *authority* (Weydt, 2010). The PHN has the authority to *delegate* specific tasks to individuals or groups, and these individuals or groups accept the *responsibility* for the tasks. However, at all times, the PHN retains *accountability* for the safety and quality of the outcome (Stanhope & Lancaster, 2012).

The PHN must determine when and whether delegation is appropriate. The process for determination follows the steps of the nursing process (ANA, 2012). Some tasks should not be delegated because they fall in the realm of professional nursing—for example, counseling, health teaching, and activities that require nursing knowledge, skill, and judgment based on evidence or data (American Nurses Association, 2007). Tasks that can be delegated are more often repetitive and supportive in caregiving (Williams & Cooksey,

2004). It is important to note the emphasis on individuals or communities as partners in the plan of care and the importance of communication at all phases among healthcare consumers, UAP, and PHNs. To determine whether delegation is appropriate, the American Nurses Association (ANA; 2012) has identified six care provisions (see Table 7.5).

Table 7.5   Care Provisions for Determining Effective Delegation

1. Perform an assessment of the healthcare consumer's:
   - Care needs and determine whether any cultural modifications are required;
   - Condition to determine whether it is stable and predictable; and
   - Environment where the care will be provided.

2. Develop a plan of care with the healthcare consumer and his or her family, identifying the delegable task and intended outcome as part of the overall plan of care. Involving and educating healthcare consumers and their families about appropriate expectations of the roles of care providers promotes a safer environment and improved patient outcomes. The plan of care should include:
   - Baseline status of the healthcare consumer;
   - Specific unchanging task performance steps;
   - When and to whom the UAP need to report if the baseline status changes; and
   - Documentation of expectations as appropriate.

3. Analyze the following:
   - Is the task within the delegating registered nurse's (RN's) scope of practice?
   - Do federal or state laws, rules, or regulations support the delegation?
   - Does the employing organization/agency of the delegating RN and the UAP permit delegation?
   - Is the delegating RN competent to make the delegation decision?
   - Is the UAP competent to perform the delegated task?
   - Is RN supervision of the UAP available?

4. Monitor implementation of the delegated task as appropriate to the overall plan of care.
5. Evaluate overall condition of the healthcare consumer and the consumer's response to the delegated task.
6. Evaluate the UAP's skills and performance of tasks and provide feedback for improvement, if needed.

ACTIVITY

Read the following case study and analyze how a PHN could ensure that the care provisions of delegation are followed when delegating to the family health aide. Then complete the right-hand column in the accompanying table.

Delegation Case Study

I received a referral on a 22-year-old and her 2-month-old baby. At my initial home visit, the baby appeared overweight and overfed. The young mom had started him on rice cereal in a bottle at 2 weeks. Every time he cried, she gave him a bottle, even though he often struggled and tried to pull away from the nipple. I talked with her about feeding the baby and my concern about his weight, but she responded with, "Once he starts moving around, the weight will come off."

By 4 months of age, the baby was 27 pounds. By now I was very concerned and called both the nurse and the doctor at the clinic, but no action was taken. Next I arranged a joint home visit with a nutritionist from WIC (Women, Infants and Children Supplemental Food Program). We counseled the mom to feed the baby only when he was truly hungry.

Two weeks later, I returned to do an NCAST* feeding interaction and videotaped the mom feeding the baby. We watched the tape together and talked about hunger cues and how the baby did not appear hungry. The young mother listened but continued to feed the baby whenever he fussed or cried. It was as though she had no other way to comfort him other than to feed him. I was also becoming concerned about the baby's development, as he exhibited several delays in fine motor and language when I tested him.

At this point, I started visiting every 2 weeks and placed a family health aide in the home for 2 hours at a time 1 day a week. The aide's assignment was to role-model appropriate parenting and feeding. I also arranged to get a high chair for feeding the child through a nutrition program grant. Currently, I continue to coordinate services from the clinic, nutritionist, and family health aide. At the present time, the baby's weight has stabilized, and he has not gained any more weight.

*NCAST (Nursing Child Assessment Satellite Training) is an objective and systematic assessment of interactions between parent and child (30 hours of continuing education). It can alert the nurse to areas of concern and the need for teaching. It has been used as legal documentation in court cases of child abuse.

Source: Minnesota Department of Health, Office of Public Health Practice. (2006). Wheel of public health interventions: A collection of "Getting Behind the Wheel" stories 2000–2006.

Care provisions of delegation	Example from case study
Perform an assessment of the healthcare consumer.	
Develop a plan of care with the healthcare consumer and his or her family.	
Analyze delegation factors.	
Monitor implementation of the delegated task as appropriate to the overall plan of care.	
Evaluate overall condition of the healthcare consumer and the consumer's response to the delegated task.	
Evaluate the UAP's skills and performance of tasks and provide feedback for improvement, if needed.	

Do I Need to Become Registered to Become a Public Health Nurse?

Public Health Nursing: Scope and Standards of Practice identifies the baccalaureate degree in nursing as the credential for public health nursing practice (ANA, 2013). In addition, the Association of Community Health Nurse Educators (ACHNE) assumes the minimum requirement for entry-level public health or community nursing practice is a baccalaureate nursing degree (ACHNE, 2009). There are several routes to achieving this entry-level education preference. Nurses with associate degrees may choose to enter RN-to-BSN programs, or graduates with a baccalaureate degree or higher in another major may choose an "accelerated" nursing program. *Accelerated* programs may offer a master's degree (check individual institutions) for this select group of students. For students interested in advanced studies in the area of public health nursing, the doctor of nursing practice (DNP) or the PhD are degrees that support practice and research in the field.

You can look at your state's Nurse Practice Act to determine whether a baccalaureate degree is required for the practice of public health nursing in your state. Some states require certification or registration for the title of PHN. The baccalaureate is the preferred entry into practice degree.

> *Sarah is very excited about public health nursing and asked Jennifer how she could obtain public health nursing certification. Jennifer recommended that Sarah read the Nurse Practice Act in which-ever state she practices nursing after she graduates with her baccalaureate degree in nursing. Sarah can also contact the board of nursing in that state to learn more about nursing practice guidelines specific to that area.*

Examples of Legal Requirements in Nurse Practice Acts

California, Hawaii, Iowa, Minnesota, New York, North Carolina, South Carolina, and Wisconsin require a baccalaureate degree for PHN practice.

In California, Minnesota, New York, and South Carolina, licensure acts or rules have language that defines the scope of public health nursing practice and reserves the use of the title "public health nurse" for those professional nurses who meet specific criteria.

In California, PHN certification requires training in child abuse and neglect, and a PHN certificate is needed to use the title of "public health nurse" (California Board of Registered Nursing, 2006).

Ethical Application

When working with individuals and families, PHNs often must balance acting in the professional role with building a trusting relationship. In the attempt to find this balance in working with at-risk families, a PHN might encounter tension between different ethical perspectives. If a PHN emphasizes the expert role, the client might feel inadequate or judged.

The client might need a "friend" and want to view the PHN as a friend. However, framing the relationship as a friendship implies expectations of sharing and obligation that might fall outside the professional role. Professional caring does not carry the responsibility of friendship but carries the responsibility of ethical action based on promoting good for the client, contributing to a flourishing community, and strategizing to reduce oppression for clients and families who receive public health services.

See Table 7.6 for an application of ethical perspectives to maintaining professional boundaries. Think about the related scenarios in this chapter: (a) the adolescent mother asked Jennifer to be her friend on Facebook, and (b) residents in the apartment building where Jennifer visited several elderly clients asked her how her clients were doing.

Table 7.6 Ethical Action in Maintaining Professional Boundaries

Ethical perspective	Application
Rule ethics (principles)	• Use expert public health nursing knowledge to promote good and prevent harm to clients and families. • Keep health information confidential to protect the client.
Virtue ethics (character)	• Be compassionate in recognizing the hardships and health challenges encountered by clients and families. • Use caring interactions to communicate confidence in the client's ability to make positive health decisions. • Focus on building trusting relationships as a basis for mutual goal setting.
Feminist ethics (reducing oppression)	• Connect families to resources that reduce some of the inequities they experience because of poverty. • Establish a relationship with the client that communicates valuing others as equal individuals.

ACTIVITY

For either of the two scenarios discussed earlier in the chapter (the Facebook incident or apartment residents asking about the well-being of clients), analyze the resolution to the ethical problem by answering the following questions:

Which values related to the situation do you see as important to you as a professional and as a person?

Who do you think you should be as PHN (important virtues)?

Based on your values and who you should be, what would you do in this situation?

Which ethical perspectives (rule ethics, virtue ethics, and feminist ethics) support your chosen action?

Key Points

- Nurse Practice Acts in each state and the scope and standards of public health nursing provide expectations for PHNs' professional accountability.

- The Public Health Intervention Wheel defines the independent interventions that PHNs implement in their practice.

- Professional boundaries can be more challenging to maintain in public health nursing, given the community setting and long-term relationships with clients.

- Protection of patient confidentiality can be more challenging for PHNs to ensure in rural communities, where many residents know the PHNs.

- HIPAA provides legal standards for handling protected health information.

- PHNs can use the six Care Provisions of Delegation identified by the ANA to guide their delegation responsibilities.

- Reflecting about and discussing ethical challenges in public health nursing can help the PHN practice ethically.

Learning Examples

The following learning examples can be used to expand your knowledge about public health nursing responsibilities covered in the Nurse Practice Act in your state. In addition, the examples will help you think about how to maintain professional boundaries and act ethically in public health nursing practice.

Nurse Practice Act—Locate a copy of the Nurse Practice Act from your state (Internet search). In a small group or pairs, explore implications of the Nurse Practice Act for public health nursing practice:

- How does the language in the Nurse Practice Act describe the scope of nursing practice?

- Do any requirements apply specifically to PHNs? If so, what are the requirements?

- What does the Nurse Practice Act say about delegation and supervision responsibilities of the professional nurse?

- Does the Nurse Practice Act identify any specific educational requirements?

- What does the Nurse Practice Act say about the ethical and legal accountability of nurses?

Professional Boundaries and Ethical Accountability—Analyze the following scenario from the rule ethics, virtue ethics, and feminist ethics perspectives. Do you agree with the actions taken by the students? Why or why not?

Scenario: Two students went to make a visit to a single mother and her three preschool-age children. The mother was in the final trimester of pregnancy and had severe swelling in her ankles and feet, leaving her unable to walk. She had not been able to use a cab or a bus to get to the grocery store and had no food in the apartment. The mother reported that the children had not eaten for 2 days and were very hungry. The students knew that they were not supposed to give food to their clients; however, they were very concerned about the children. They went out to their car and got their bag lunches, made sure the food was appropriate for children, and, with the mother's permission, gave lunches to the children. They also called the police and the social service agency to obtain help for the family, but first they fed the children.

Reflective Practice

Nurses who practice in healthcare organizations, such as hospitals, are constantly reminded about rules and regulations that guide their nursing practice. They are surrounded by other nursing staff and supervisors whom they can quickly ask for guidance in any situation that might seem confusing. In many situations, PHNs do not have the security of having other nurses and nursing administrators immediately available to them. School nurses are often the only nursing professionals in the building. PHNs who make home visits might feel isolated and unsure of which response comprises ethical and legal actions. PHNs must be knowledgeable about the scope of professional practice and guidelines for ethical and legal practice. They need to provide rationales that are based on ethical, legal, and professional guidelines to support their choice of nursing actions.

Read the case study and write your answers to the following questions. Then discuss them with your classmates.

Case Study: Scope of Public Health Nursing Practice

You are a PHN with approximately 40 high-risk families in your caseload. One of your clients is a 17-year-old woman, Tiffany, who has an 11-month-old baby boy whom she delivered at 34 weeks' gestation with a birth weight of 4 pounds 1 ounce. Tiffany lives in a trailer court off and on with an unemployed boyfriend who has struck her twice in the last month. She will not report the assaults, because he is on probation for selling drugs and would immediately go to prison. She states, "He has promised it will never happen again."

Your initial referral to the family was for the premature birth of Jeremy, the little boy, who had respiratory complications and spent 3 weeks in the hospital before he came home. Tiffany is estranged from her mother, reporting, "She kicked me out when she found out I was pregnant." She appears to have minimal parenting skills but is receptive to your visits and is working on developing parenting skills. She has declined your referral to Early Childhood and Family Education (ECFE) activities.

Jeremy was within normal developmental limits for the first 6 months of his life but is now starting to exhibit some delays. You suspect that his frequent illnesses are contributing to the developmental delays. He suffers from chronic upper respiratory illnesses and otitis media. Tiffany smokes a half pack of cigarettes per day and has not been receptive to discussing smoking cessation.

Tiffany just told you she took a pregnancy test last week and is pregnant again. Her smoking is putting both Jeremy and the unborn child at risk.

- How does the scope of public health nursing practice (see Chapter 1) guide the responsibilities of the PHN in this case study?

  _____

  _____

- What do you think are the most relevant interventions for the PHN to implement from the Public Health Intervention Wheel?

  _____

  _____

- What is the PHN's ethical and legal accountability for the boyfriend's domestic violence?

  _____

  _____

- What concerns do you have about maintaining confidentiality and professional boundaries in this case study?

  _____

  _____

- Which Cornerstones of Public Health Nursing do you think are consistent with supporting the PHN's interventions in working with this family?

  _____

  _____

- How would you ensure ethical practice on your part in working with this family?

  _____

  _____

Source: Adapted from a case study developed by the Minnesota Department of Health, n.d.

Application of Evidence

Jennifer, the PHN from Weaver County Health Department, has received a referral from the county's Child Protection Services. The referral was originally made by an RN who worked at the local hospital and suspected possible child abuse of a 2-year-old named Marcie who had a minor injury that required a visit to the emergency room. The child protection worker did not find any evidence of child abuse or neglect but asked to have a PHN follow up to promote positive parenting practices with the child's parents.

1. Which independent nursing interventions could Jennifer use in working with the child's parents? How are these interventions consistent with the Nurse Practice Act in your state?

2. What should Jennifer remember about maintaining professional boundaries as she meets with Marcie's parents?

3. During the visit, Jennifer discovers that Marcie attends the same community day care as one of Jennifer's children, although the two children are not in the same group. What will Jennifer need to do to maintain confidentiality in the small community setting?

4. How do rule ethics, virtue ethics, and feminist ethics guide Jennifer's interactions with Marcie's family as she balances developing a trusting relationship with the family, keeping information confidential, providing parenting guidance, and monitoring for possible child abuse or neglect?

 # Think, Explore, Do

1. Think of an ethical concern that you have encountered in your public health nursing clinical. How can you use rule ethics, virtue ethics, and feminist ethics to help you know how to act ethically in this situation? Which ethical perspective offers the most guidance?

2. Think about a situation in which you were concerned about maintaining professional boundaries. What are some strategies you could use to avoid a potential violation of boundaries?

3. How do you think Facebook should be used in communication with your peers, teachers, and clients?

4. How will you balance expectations for independent practice with collaboration to ensure that you are ethically, legally, and professionally accountable in your practice?

5. How can you create a support system for yourself to ensure that your actions are consistent with the Nurse Practice Act?

References

Aiken, T. (2004). *Legal, ethical, and political issues in nursing.* Philadelphia, PA: Davis.

American Association of Colleges of Nursing. (2013). Nurse-managed health clinics: Increasing access to primary care and educating the healthcare workforce. Retrieved from http://www.aacn.nche.edu/government-affairs/FY13NMHCs.pdf

American Nurses Association. (2007). *Registered Nurses Utilization of Nursing Assistive Personnel in All Settings.* American Nurses Association Position Statement. Retrieved from http://ana.nursingworld.org/MainMenuCategories/HealthcareandPolicyIssues/ANAPositionStatements/uap.aspx

American Nurses Association. (2010). *Nursing scope and standards of practice* (2nd ed.). Silver Spring, MD: Nursebooks.org.

American Nurses Association. (2012) *Principles for delegation by registered nurses to unlicensed assistive personnel (UAP).* Silver Spring, MD: Nursebooks.org.

American Nurses Association. (2013). *Public health nursing: Scope and standards of practice.* Silver Spring, MD: Nursebooks.org.

Association of Community Health Nurse Educators. (2009). *Essentials of baccalaureate nursing education for entry level community/public health nursing.* Wheat Ridge, CO: Author.

Barkauskas, V. H., Pohl, V. H., Tanner, C., Onifade, T., & Pilon, B. (2011). Quality of care in nurse-managed health centers. *Nursing Administration Quarterly, 35*(1), 34–43.

Beauchamp, T., & Childress, J. (1979). *Principles of biomedical ethics.* New York, NY: Oxford University Press.

Bredow, T. (2013). Personal communication. North Metro Pediatrics Clinic. http://www.northmetropeds.org/index.htm

California Board of Registered Nursing. (2006). *California nursing practice act with regulations and related statutes.* Charlottesville, VA: Matthew Bender & Company, Inc.

Clancy, A., & Svensson, T. (2007). "Faced" with responsibility: Levinasian ethics and the challenges of responsibility in Norwegian public health nursing. *Nursing Philosophy, 8*(3), 158–166.

Coddington, J. A., & Sands, L. P. (2008). Cost of health care and quality outcomes of patients at nurse-managed clinics. *Nursing Economics, 26*(2), 75–83.

Easley, C. E., & Allen, C. E. (2007). A critical intersection: Human rights, public health nursing, and nursing ethics. *Advances in Nursing Science, 30*(4), 367–382.

Evanson, T. A. (2006). Intimate partner violence and rural public health nursing practice: Challenges and opportunities. *Online Journal of Rural Nursing and Health Care, 6*(1), 7–20.

Gallop, R. (1998). Postdischarge social contact: A potential area for boundary violation. *Journal of the American Psychiatric Nurses Association, 4*(4), 105–110.

Griffith, R. (2007). Understanding confidentiality and disclosure of patient information. *British Journal of Community Nursing, 12*(11), 530–534.

Institute of Medicine. (2010). The future of nursing: Leading change, advancing change. Report Brief. Retrieved from http://www.iom.edu/~/media/Files/Report%20Files/2010/The-Future-of-Nursing/Future%20of%20Nursing%202010%20Report%20Brief.pdf

Jacobson, G. A. (2002). Maintaining professional boundaries: Preparing nursing students for the challenge. *Journal of Nursing Education, 41*(6), 279–281.

Jarrin, O. G. (2010). Core elements of U.S. nurse practice acts and incorporation of nursing diagnosis language. *International Journal of Nursing Terminologies and Classifications, 21*(4), 166–176. doi:10.1111/j.1744-618x.2010.01162.x

Keller, L. O., & Litt, E. A. (2008). Report on public health nurse to population ratio. Association of State and Territorial Directors of Nursing (ASTDN).

McGarry, J. (2003). The essence of "community" within community nursing: A district nursing perspective. *Health and Social Care in the Community, 11*(5), 423–430.

Minnesota Department of Health, Office of Public Health Practice. (2006). *A collection of "Getting Behind the Wheel Stories" 2000–2006*. Retrieved from http://www.health.state.mn.us/divs/opi/cd/phn/docs/0606wheel_stories.pdf

National Nursing Centers Consortium (2011). About nurse-managed care. Retrieved from http://www.nncc.us/site/index.php/about-nurse-managed-care

Oberle, K., & Tenove, S. (2000). Ethical issues in public health nursing. *Nursing Ethics, 7*(5), 425–438.

Przybilla, J., Johnson, A., Hooker, C. (2009). Perinatal hepatitis B prevention: Adapting public health services to meet the changing needs of a diverse community. *Public Health Reports, 124,* 454–457.

Purtilo, R. (2005). *Ethical dimensions in the health professions* (4th ed.). Philadelphia, PA: Elsevier Saunders.

Racher, F. E. (2007). The evolution of ethics for community practice. *Journal of Community Health Nursing, 24*(1), 65–76.

Robinson, K. M. (2010). Care coordination: A priority for health reform. *Policy, Politics, & Nursing Practice, 11,* 266–274. doi:10.1177/1527154410396572

Russell, K. A. (2012). Nurse practice acts guide and govern nursing practice. *Journal of Nursing Regulation, 3*(3), 36–40. Retrieved from www.journalofnursingregulation.com

Schneiderman, J. U. (2003). Exploration of the role of nurses in caring for children in foster care. (Doctoral Dissertation). University of Southern California. Los Angeles, CA.

Schneiderman, J. U. (2006). Innovative pediatric nursing role: Public health nurses in child welfare. *Pediatric Nursing, 32*(4), 321.

Scoville Walker, S. (2004). Ethical quandaries in community health nursing. In E. Anderson & J. McFarlane (Eds.) *Community as partner: Theory and practice in nursing,* 4th ed. (pp. 83–113). Philadelphia, PA: Lippincott, Williams & Wilkins.

Stanhope, M., & Lancaster, J. (2012). *Public health nursing: Population-centered health care in the community.* Maryland Heights, MO: Elsevier.

Underwood, J. M.., Mowat, D. L, Meagher-Stewart, D. M. Deber, R. B., Bauman, A. O., MacDonald, M. B., ... Munroe, V. J. (2009). Building community and public health nursing capacity: A synthesis report of the national community health nursing study. *Canadian Journal of Public Health, 100*(5), 1–13.

Volbrecht, R. M. (2002). *Nursing ethics: Communities in dialogue.* Upper Saddle River, NJ: Prentice Hall.

Weydt, A. (2010). Developing Delegation Skills. *OJIN: The Online Journal of Issues in Nursing, 15*(2). Manuscript 1. (May 31). Retrieved from http://www.nursingworld.org/MainMenuCategories/ANAMarketplace/ANAPeriodicals/OJIN/TableofContents/Vol152010/No2May2010/Delegation-Skills.html

Williams, J. K., & Cooksey, M. M. (2004). Navigating the difficulties of delegation: Learn to improve teamwork in the unit by delegating duties appropriately. *Nursing, 34*(9), 32.

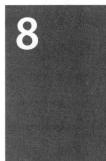

COMPETENCY #6
Effectively Communicates With Communities, Systems, Individuals, Families, and Colleagues

8

Marjorie A. Schaffer

with Raney Linck, Linda J. W. Anderson, & Rose M. Jost

Angie is a public health nursing student in a suburban public health department. Her public health nurse preceptor, Janet, asked her to create a poster for the WIC clinic (Women, Infants, and Children supplemental food program) on dental health for children. Angie had no experience with creating a poster for display in a professional setting. She also could not remember learning anything about dental health in her nursing program. What does Angie need to know to create the poster, and what steps does she need to take to create a poster that effectively communicates the importance of dental health to the population served by the WIC clinic? In addition, Janet asked Angie to assist her with creating some presentation slides to update staff on new strategies to promote oral health, such as tooth varnishing.

Angie remembered that a population-based public health nursing competency focused on communication in public health nursing. She pulled out her handout on Competency #6 to review the communication skills that would help her create a successful poster on dental health. Angie also realized she should ask more questions to assess the presentation, such as how many participants are expected, what is their predominate language, how many times will it be given, what type of equipment is available, and will part or all of it also be used for families? Then Angie can determine what kind of presentation software to use (such as PowerPoint, Keynote, or Prezi) and whether she should utilize digital tools for lecture capture, video creation, and/or online sharing.

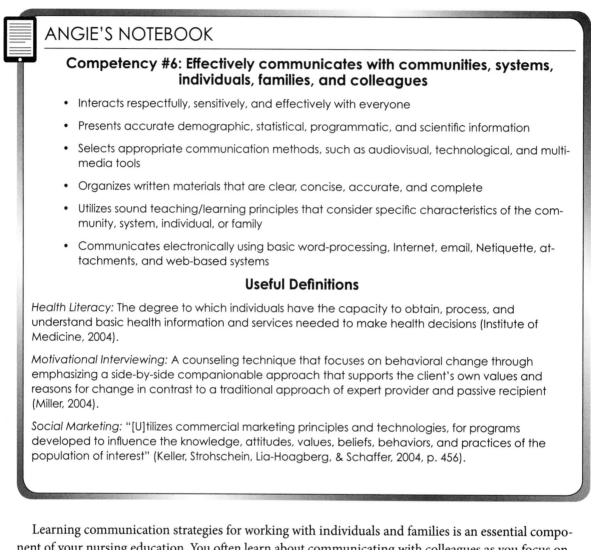

ANGIE'S NOTEBOOK

Competency #6: Effectively communicates with communities, systems, individuals, families, and colleagues

- Interacts respectfully, sensitively, and effectively with everyone

- Presents accurate demographic, statistical, programmatic, and scientific information

- Selects appropriate communication methods, such as audiovisual, technological, and multi-media tools

- Organizes written materials that are clear, concise, accurate, and complete

- Utilizes sound teaching/learning principles that consider specific characteristics of the community, system, individual, or family

- Communicates electronically using basic word-processing, Internet, email, Netiquette, attachments, and web-based systems

Useful Definitions

Health Literacy: The degree to which individuals have the capacity to obtain, process, and understand basic health information and services needed to make health decisions (Institute of Medicine, 2004).

Motivational Interviewing: A counseling technique that focuses on behavioral change through emphasizing a side-by-side companionable approach that supports the client's own values and reasons for change in contrast to a traditional approach of expert provider and passive recipient (Miller, 2004).

Social Marketing: "[U]tilizes commercial marketing principles and technologies, for programs developed to influence the knowledge, attitudes, values, beliefs, behaviors, and practices of the population of interest" (Keller, Strohschein, Lia-Hoagberg, & Schaffer, 2004, p. 456).

Learning communication strategies for working with individuals and families is an essential component of your nursing education. You often learn about communicating with colleagues as you focus on leadership strategies, teamwork, and delegation in a leadership course. However, strategies for communicating with communities and systems involve additional skills, including learning how to clearly organize and present data and health information, using technology in communication, and applying teaching-learning principles that integrate knowledge about the learner (individual or community).

How Do Public Health Nurses Interact Respectfully, Sensitively, and Effectively With Everyone?

Public health nurses (PHNs) use a repertoire of basic communication skills in all their work. Effective interpersonal communication, involving the use of self, is especially essential for counseling and health teaching interventions. The purpose of this type of communication is to benefit the clients through increasing their participation in decision-making about ways to improve their health. Keep in mind that the client might be an individual or a family. The following list contains tips for effective communication with individuals and families:

- Use active listening.

- Model "I" messages (I think. . . , I feel . . .).

- Paraphrase and summarize the client's statement to confirm its meaning.

- Pay attention to silence and nonverbal communication.

- Consider the client's comfort with degree of physical space between persons.

- Ask open-ended questions.

- Consider context of communication environment—privacy and confidentiality.

- Use touch if it enhances the communication and is acceptable to the client.

  Sources: Green, 2006; Public Health Nursing Section, 2001

Developing relationships can be challenging for PHNs in situations where clients and families may not see a need for involvement with public health nursing services. When individuals and families do perceive a need for assistance, the PHN still needs to negotiate a relationship that empowers the clients to make decisions for improving their health. In the following evidence examples, think about how the themes represent relationship development demonstrated by PHNs you observe in practice.

Evidence Examples: Developing Relationships

- Tveiten and Severinsson (2006) interviewed 13 Norwegian PHNs about their communication with families and identified four themes of building relationships through effective, client-focused communication: (1) *Building a trusting relationship* included PHN actions of listening to the needs of the family, confirming and supporting them, and being honest about one's expert knowledge and lack of knowledge. (2) *Looking beyond the current situation* involved identifying what was important to the client and revising the goal as needed to make it more realistic for the client to achieve. (3) *Creating partnership and equality* involved using communication strategies to strengthen the client's ability to make decisions that improve health. The PHN listens, affirms, and supports positive coping strategies through dialogue and conveys the belief that the client will make good decisions. (4) *Considering challenges in promoting the individual or family's best interest* included acknowledging different values and any assumptions or biases one might have about a client's lifestyle choices or cultural background. Although the PHN has expert knowledge about community resources and strategies for promoting better health, the clients have expert knowledge about their life situations and motivations for changing health behaviors.

- In a study in Japan, seven home-visit nurses described their experiences in helping clients with schizophrenia (Katakura, Yamamoto-Mitani, & Ishigaki, 2010). The researchers identified that the central theme contributing to the nurses' positive attitude toward effective visits was "having equal footing with the client" (p. 104). However, before realizing the importance of respecting and supporting the clients' abilities and wishes, the nurses (1) went through a process of recognizing their own preconceptions about clients with a schizophrenia diagnosis and (2) developed awareness of ineffective PHN communication. The nurses discovered that clients had more skills and understanding than what they had expected and that they were not paying enough attention to the clients' wishes and choices.

- In a Canadian study, researchers conducted interviews and focus groups with PHNs about their working relationships with at-risk families (Browne, Doane, Reimer, MacLeod, & McLellan, 2010). Three themes captured nurses' experiences with relationship development: (1) The PHNs understood the complexity of the families' lives and used that understanding to focus on strengths, although the situations were chaotic. They were flexible in responding to the demands of the families' lives. (2) The PHNs balanced working with family risk factors and their capacity. For the PHNs, this involved working collaboratively with families to build their capacity to manage risk situations. PHNs also needed to be self-reflective about their own judgments and assumptions. (3) PHNs managed the conflicting tensions in working with families who were also under the surveillance of child welfare due to their high-risk status. In this study, the PHNs "used their relational skills to assess and address risk—and in the process, were clear and transparent about their obligations to both intervene and prevent harm and support women and families" (p. 34).

Motivational Interviewing: A Strategy for Health Behavior Change

PHNs can use motivational interviewing to encourage positive health behaviors (Shinitzky & Kub, 2001). *Motivational interviewing* is a specific kind of counseling strategy in which the professional helps clients become aware of their values and the reasons they might have for changing their behaviors. The purpose of motivational interviewing is to encourage clients to move away from behaviors that hurt their health toward behaviors that improve their health. The collaborative approach of motivational interviewing is a dialogue, in contrast to giving advice or instruction (Harvard Medical School, 2011). The five stages of behavior change provide a framework for understanding how motivational interviewing works (see Table 8.1).

Table 8.1   Stages of Health Behavior Change

Stage	Individual action	Nurse action
1. Pre-contemplation	Has no desire or intention to change or does not understand consequences of behavior	Increase awareness and create understanding of discrepancy between behavior and health goal

2. Contemplation	Intends to take action but is not ready; is aware of benefits but ambivalent about change	Help focus on reasons for change and normalize ambivalence
3. Preparation	May have a plan for action and have made small changes; identifies goals	Affirm and explore expectations for outcomes; explore what has worked in the past
4. Action	Is making the behavior change	Praise and reinforce; ask, "What is giving you success right now in making this change?" (p. 23)
5. Maintenance	Has stopped unwanted behavior for more than 6 months	Address any relapse issues and reinforce benefits of change

Source: Richardson, 2012

PHNs can determine the relevant step of behavior change the clients are experiencing and then use motivational interviewing to encourage them to change their health behaviors. Some clients might move through these steps quickly, whereas others might remain at one step for a longer period of time. The PHN follows the clients' cues in motivational interviewing, because the emphasis is on empowering clients to make decisions that benefit their health. Empowerment results in a sense of competence, a willingness to take action, and the opportunity to make decisions (Toofany, 2006). The example in Table 8.2 illustrates the use of motivational interviewing strategies with a pregnant adolescent who smokes.

Table 8.2 Motivational Interviewing Strategies

Motivational interviewing strategy	Client statement	PHN statement
Express empathy.	I started smoking when I was 15.	It can be difficult to stop smoking, because the body is dependent on the nicotine in tobacco.
Develop discrepancies.	I know I should stop smoking.	What have you learned about why it is important to quit smoking during pregnancy or around your baby?
Avoid arguing.	I don't really think it is so bad. My best friend smoked during her pregnancy, and her baby is fine.	I'm glad to hear your friend's baby is OK. Let's take a look at how smoking might affect your baby's health.

continues

Table 8.2   Motivational Interviewing Strategies   (continued)

Motivational interviewing strategy	Client statement	PHN statement
Roll with resistance.	I just don't know if I can quit. I have so much going on in my life—smoking helps me feel more relaxed.	I would like to hear more about other things that help you relax.
Support self-efficacy.	I wish I could quit smoking.	It is your choice. What do you think you can do to have a healthy baby?

It will take practice to develop expertise and comfort with the motivational interviewing process. Pfister-Minouge and Salveson (2010) describe a tool called the Behavior Change Counseling Index that PHNs can use to evaluate interactions that will support health behavior change. See Appendix B for reference.

Evidence Examples: Effectiveness of Motivational Interviewing

- A systematic review summarizes the results of studies on the contribution of motivational interviewing to decreasing coronary heart disease risk factors that are modifiable. The authors conclude that motivational interviewing is an effective approach to changing behavior and "offers promise in improving cardiovascular health status" (Thompson et al., 2011, p. 1236).

- A proactive smoking cessation intervention program in postpartum women in Spain used motivational interviewing and relapse prevention. For recent quitters, the intervention group had a greater probability of remaining abstinent in comparison to the control group (Jiménez-Muro et al., 2013).

- Motivational interviewing to decrease alcohol use during pregnancy was tested in a pilot study. Results showed an increase in levels of autonomous motivation to decrease use of alcohol during pregnancy in a sample of 15 women (Osterman, 2011).

How Do PHNs Interpret Information in a Concise, Accessible Way?

PHNs also need to develop skills in communicating information about data for making decisions about public health interventions that improve the health of population groups and communities. PHNs are called on to translate complex concepts and information into terms that are accurate and easily understood by the general public. Health data and scientifically based information must be reduced and reformatted to enhance understanding. Simplification of both verbal and written communication of information is required. When crafting messages, PHNs need to engage members of the public to help identify their concerns. To involve the public, PHNs can recruit community members for an expert advisory group to give input on how to respond to public health data about their community (Holmes, 2008).

The evidence example that follows, written by a public health nursing student, explains the process of translating data for public understanding and decision-making. A student group completed an analysis of safe walking paths and made a recommendation for action to community decision-makers. The student project was published in the local city newspaper, and the city obtained a grant for improving walking paths.

Evidence Example: Presenting Data on Improving Walking Path Safety

We proceeded to plan how we would assess the walkability of the city, implement our plan, and eventually evaluate the results of our study. The purpose [was to identify] areas that could use improvement to increase the percentage of people who chose to walk, ultimately resulting in lower obesity rates and obesity-related health problems. We began to prepare for this project by doing background research on the problem of obesity, which health problems came from being overweight, and the role of walking in reducing these problems. After that, we planned how we would implement our study by looking at city maps and selecting the routes that we wished to walk. We also got a standardized survey to fill out as we went, which measured things such as the presence of sidewalks, behavior of drivers, and the aesthetic appeal of the route for an overall score on a scale of 1 to 30. Over a period of several weeks, we proceeded to walk each of these paths and mark down the positive and negative attributes of each as we saw them. After completing each route at least once, we began to evaluate our data. We compiled our results and came up with an average score for each of the five areas on the survey. Using these results, we were able to pinpoint a couple of areas that we thought could use the most work. More specifically, there was an overall need for more crosswalks and aesthetic appeal on several of the routes. The data were presented to a group of city officials along with our conclusions so they could have some data to help guide them in the use of their grant money. Evidence was needed to guide the use of grant money to improve the streets, hopefully increasing the physical health of the community members.

Source: Senior Public Health Nursing Student

Which Communication Methods Work Best?

Health communication involves the creation of messages that inform, motivate, and influence change for positive health behavior (Chaffee, 2000). In 2011, the Centers for Disease Control and Prevention (CDC) created a Health Communicator's Social Media Toolkit that included the following Principles for Communicating Health Messages. These principles can be applied to all communication channels, whether online or offline (see Table 8.3).

Table 8.3   Principles for Communicating Health Messages

1. Target your audience.	Describe whom you want to reach, being as specific as possible.
2. Determine your objective.	Define in S.M.A.R.T. terms (specific, measurable, attainable, relevant/realistic, time-bound).
3. Define audience communication needs.	Use market research and other data.
4. Integrate goals.	Describe how social media objectives support your organization's mission.
5. Develop the message.	Base it on target audience and objectives.
6. Determine resources and capacity.	Determine who is responsible for implementation and the number of hours these individuals can allocate.
7. Identify social media tools.	What will effectively reach your target audience and support your objectives and resources?
8. Define activities.	How will you reach your goals and objectives?
9. Identify your key partners.	Consider their roles and responsibilities.
10. Define success and evaluate.	What are your measures for success? What is your evaluation plan?

Source: CDC, 2011

Using Teaching-Learning Principles

PHNs provide health education to promote better health for their clients. Their goal is to motivate clients to learn about ways to promote their own health and then act on that knowledge. Teaching-learning principles help you assess how the learner learns so that you can plan the content and teaching method that best fits the client situation (see Table 8.4).

Table 8.4   Teaching-Learning Principles

- Target health education messages to the specific audience rather than trying to cover all information.
- Learner readiness affects what is learned—health status, health values, developmental characteristics, prior learning experiences.
- Motivation affects learning—use life goals, self-concept, responsibility, quality of life, and other factors that can "hook" and are meaningful to the learner.

- Active learning is best. Have the learner demonstrate or repeat learning.
- Use learning objectives to guide your teaching plan. Objectives should be written, clear, and measureable.
- Send a clear message that is easily understood. Avoid overwhelming the learner with excess materials. Avoid professional jargon. Use short sentences and simple, one- and two-syllable words.
- Use visuals to enhance printed materials and verbal messages.
- Create a comfortable learning environment that is free from distractions and interruptions (ask your client to turn off the TV).
- When possible, integrate a variety of learning styles to deliver content.
- Base content on best evidence—review literature for most recent evidence-based information. Give credit to information sources.
- Link information to prior knowledge.
- Allow time for interaction to apply information.
- Reinforce written materials with verbal messages.
- Use multiple methods to assess understanding of content, such as questioning and demonstration.

Sources: Clark, 2008; Kolb, 1984, 2005; Onega & Devers, 2008; Whitman, 1998

Organizing Written Educational Materials

When crafting messages, PHNs consider the health literacy of the intended target group. Health literacy is the capacity that individuals have to find and understand information about health and health services that can be used to make health-related decisions. The inability to understand health information might mean that individuals do not engage in effective self-care practices and increase their risk for hospitalization (Clark, 2008; Weiss, 2007). For groups with lower literacy, effective strategies for communicating health information include (a) using plain (nonmedical) language, (b) incorporating visuals, (c) talking more slowly, (d), limiting information to two or three key points that are repeated, (e) using a "teach-back" process when possible, and (f) encouraging questions (Black, 2008; Weiss, 2007). In a *teach-back process*, clients are asked to restate the information in their own words or demonstrate a specific skill to others, such as a peer group. To engage the reader in written information, give examples that reflect the age, gender, and culture of the targeted population group (DeBuono, 2002). You will find more information about health literacy in Appendix B.

In some settings, PHNs might work with a media or graphic design specialist to communicate clear, captivating, and motivating health messages. Effective messages result from clear and simple writing, a layout that enhances readability, and images that enhance the message (see Table 8.5 for tips to improve written messages).

Table 8.5   Tips to Improve Written Messages

- Use active voice rather than passive. For example, say, "Eat five servings of fruits and vegetables," rather than saying, "Five servings of fruits and vegetables should be eaten."
- Use subheadings.
- Use short sentences of 8 to 10 words that are varied by a few longer sentences of 12 to 15 words. Use short paragraphs.
- Summarize main points to improve understanding.
- Include no more than 5 items in a list.
- Use underlining or bold to emphasize key points rather than italics or caps.
- Use large, easily readable font.
- Avoid large blocks of information and use white space to provide a more inviting design to the reader.
- Ensure that paper and ink contrast for readability.
- Because pictures are more easily remembered, illustrate the behavior you want people to follow.

Source: Substance Abuse & Mental Health Service Administration Network, 1994

Angie is ready to design the poster. She decides to create a layout for her poster. She plans to ask a roommate who is a communication major to evaluate her planned layout. She also realizes that she needs to ask her public health nursing preceptor to evaluate her plan. She is not sure about the reading level of the population group who will be viewing the WIC poster, but she knows that her preceptor is very familiar with this population.

 ACTIVITY

Design a layout for the poster on dental health for the WIC clinic. Consider the following questions:

How could Angie learn more about the population served by the WIC clinic?

Which teaching-learning principles should Angie keep in mind as she designs the poster?

Which tips for effective written communication will you include for your poster?

Using Social Marketing Skills

Skills needed to effectively communicate health promotion messages to communities include expertise in the areas of presentation, group facilitation, and social marketing (Zahner & Gredig, 2005). PHNs are called upon to present health data to local leaders, policymakers, and community partners and to interpret the meaning of these data in relation to the community's health status (Jakeway, Cantrell, Cason, &

Talley, 2006). PHNs use group leadership and facilitation skills to bring to the table voices of all stakeholders to make decisions about community-level public health interventions.

Cultural variables—unique health beliefs, values, norms, expectations, and language barriers—influence whether the information is viewed as important (Kreps & Sparks, 2008). To increase the likelihood of successful communication, be sure to involve representatives from the cultural group in the communication strategy's design and test it to ensure readability, understanding, and appeal. Feedback mechanisms, such as consumer surveys, focus groups, hotlines, and comment cards, can help validate the strategy's effectiveness or weaknesses and provide ideas for improvement (Kreps & Sparks, 2008).

PHNs use strategies from the commercial marketing field to design health programs that "influence the knowledge, attitudes, values, beliefs, behaviors, and practices of the population of interest" (Public Health Nursing Section, 2001, p. 285). In public health, this work is known as *social marketing* (see the definition in this chapter's Notebook page), because messages are constructed to change social norms of unhealthy behaviors to create social environments that support healthy behaviors (see Table 8.6).

Table 8.6   Tips for Effective Social Marketing

- Develop a plan that includes attention to the "5 Ps"—product, price, place, promotion, and people.
- Involve opinion leaders (for example, community leaders, elders, and respected individuals whose opinions are valued by others).
- Promote active-learner involvement.
- Provide for repetition and reinforcement.
- Avoid message clutter and information overload.
- Know your audience: Consider socioeconomic factors, cultural beliefs, values, geographic location, and local norms in speech and dress.
- Use stories and anecdotes in the presentation of risk data.
- Use several approaches (written, oral, visual graphics, electronic).
- Engage the target population in the development process.
- Anticipate and manage the use of controversy and conflict.
- Avoid terminology, phrases, or visual cues that reinforce stereotypes or contradict verbal messages.

Sources: Evans & McCormack, 2008; Public Health Nursing, Section, 2001; Russell, 2009; Westdahl & Page-Goertz, 2006

Targeted health messages are developed for specific population groups. Tailored health communications are client-centered and involve customizing messages based on individuals' lifestyle, locations of residence, and consumer habits. Possible social marketing communication channels include television, radio, the Internet, social media, posters, periodicals, pamphlets, and other written material. In addition to using mass media, you need to locate opinion leaders (persons who have social influence and have adopted the desired behavior or attitude). Opinion leaders act as catalysts for behavior change. Because humans are social beings, connection to social relationships influences the adoption of healthy behavior (Levy-Storms, 2005).

Healthy People 2020 On the Healthy People 2020 website, go to 2020 Topics and Objectives, A–Z, and under "H" click "Health Communication and Information Technology." Read the "Overview" and "Objectives." Click "Interventions and Resources" and review evidence on interventions to reduce tobacco use or increase physical activity in communities. Based on the evidence, identify a health communication or information technology strategy for improving community health.

Evidence Example: Stop Smoking in Schools Trial (ASSIST)

A program in the UK used a peer nomination questionnaire to identify influential 8th graders in 30 intervention schools. ASSIST used a "whole-community" model so that the student community chose the opinion leaders, not teachers. They were then trained to disseminate smoke-free health promotion messages through their informal contacts with friends. The result was a 22% reduction in the odds of being a regular smoker when compared with students from 29 control schools (Starkey, Audrey, Holliday, Moore, & Campbell, 2009).

Evidence Example for Social Marketing: Breastfeeding on a Navajo Reservation

The Navajo Infant Feeding Project provided written and videotaped information on breastfeeding (individual and family level); created a positive view of breastfeeding through community empowerment techniques, such as radio spots, infant T-shirts, billboards, and slide shows (community level); educated healthcare providers to increase their knowledge and skills for the promotion of breastfeeding (systems level); and provided visits on the maternity unit from a native bilingual "foster grandmother" to talk about her own breastfeeding experience and its contribution to children's health (opinion leader). Measurement of outcomes showed an improvement in breastfeeding rates. Both the initiation and duration of breastfeeding increased. Fewer infants were given formula in the hospital, and the mean age at which formula was introduced increased from 12 days to 48 days (Wright, Naylor, Wester, Bauer, & Sutcliffe, 1997).

After reviewing evidence in her textbook on effective health education and social marketing techniques, Angie decides she should make a list of the next steps needed to create a dental health poster for the WIC clinic. Angie knows that the population attending the WIC clinic has a high percentage of Latino families. In addition, WIC clinics are located throughout the county. What does Angie need to think about before she begins to work on the poster?

ACTIVITY

Based on what you have learned about communicating health messages and social marketing, answer the following questions:

- What are the questions that Angie needs to consider, and which information sources does she need to explore?

- What does she need to do to create an effective poster?

- Which principles and tips for communicating health messages and using social marketing techniques did you find most useful for planning your poster?

Using Diverse Technological Tools

The Internet offers an option for broad dissemination to populations in need of health information, provided that they have access. However, information on the Internet can also be overwhelming, sometimes contradictory, and, in the worst-case scenario, inaccurate. One challenge for researchers is to determine the potential of Internet interventions to influence positive behavior change and improved health outcomes.

Evidence Example: Delivering Public Health Interventions Through the Internet

Bennett and Glasgow (2009) reviewed the evidence on effectiveness of public health Internet-based interventions, including interventions that focused on smoking cessation, increases in physical activity, weight loss, and drug-abuse prevention. Health information delivered via the Internet has resulted in positive changes in knowledge, social support, healthy behaviors, and self-efficacy. Rates of attrition as high as 40% to 50% are reported. Website use tends to drop off during the early weeks of the intervention, but improvement in website use occurred with reminders through postcards, email, and phone calls. The authors of this study suggest that support from human counselors could increase the use Internet-based interventions but would add to their cost. They also suggest that tailored messages and social networking might increase the amount of learning but note a lack of research on the contribution of social networking strategies to improved health outcomes. Most Internet interventions that have been evaluated are individually focused.

Social networking sites (SNS), such as Facebook, Twitter, LinkedIn, YouTube, Pinterest, and Instagram, offer new opportunities for public health interventions. Early studies show both opportunities and challenges. For example, a clinical trial involving more than 1,500 participants ages 16 to 25 found that exposure to Just/Us, a Facebook page with sexually transmitted infection prevention messages developed with youth input, led to a 12% increase in condom use at 2 months but made no difference at 6 months (Bull, Levine, Black, Schmiege, & Santelli, 2012). More research needs to be done to identify which aspects of SNS health messages make them more compelling and effective.

Beyond social media, many free content creation tools available on the Internet allow PHNs to create posters, infographics, videos, podcasts, and more. Nurses should type "free website builder" or "free pamphlet creator" into a search engine to explore and test software options to find which practical tools they prefer. Also, keep in mind that it is not always necessary to learn a new software program. Familiar programs, such as PowerPoint, often have untapped potential for new functionality. Simply typing "PowerPoint poster" into a search engine will provide a wide variety of templates, instructions, and videos to help a nurse use the program to create a high-quality poster.

To create a highly visual and appealing poster, Angie decides to use PowerPoint in an innovative but simple way. She changes the slide dimensions to 2[ts]3 feet under page setup and organizes all the content on a single slide, which a local retail printer can produce in full color for $30. Using free online translation tools, Angie then translates the poster text into three other languages. Angie emails the poster files in multiple languages to Janet, her preceptor, to review before printing. Janet suggests a few changes to make the English version more accessible to nonprofessionals and has native speakers help proof the translated versions. Edits are easy to make electronically. In addition to sharing the physical poster at the clinic, Angie also uploads the final version on Pinterest, a content-sharing site, which allows easy distribution to other SNS, such as Twitter and Facebook.

Janet and Angie then discuss creating a 20-minute in-service on oral health for the public health staff. Because the training room has audiovisual equipment and Internet access, Angie decides to use PowerPoint again to create a multislide presentation with graphics and some YouTube videos. Angie has accumulated a large amount of information on oral health from journal articles and government websites. However, as she is working on the presentation, Angie becomes perplexed about how to organize the content, how much information to include, and what would be most useful and interesting to staff. Then she remembers that the same principles she had used to guide her work on the poster are also applicable to creating effective messages in the PowerPoint presentation.

 ## ACTIVITY

Think about the PowerPoint presentations you have viewed. What did you like about the way content was organized and presented? What enhanced your learning? Which aspects would you like to change to increase your interest level and effective learning?

Explain how the Principles for Communicating Health Messages apply to developing the PowerPoint presentation on oral health for staff.

Which tips for improving written messages do you think are most relevant for creating the PowerPoint presentation?

Which teaching-learning principles are important to remember in your planning for the presentation?

How Do PHNs Use Interpersonal Skills in Online Communication?

Communicating effectively online requires more than technical expertise; it requires expert interpersonal skills. Online etiquette (sometimes called "Netiquette") and ethical use must be mastered. Protecting confidentiality and communicating respectfully are essential whenever you communicate online, whether it is through email, social media, websites, blogs, or even text messages.

Because much of the professional communication in the public health setting involves email, it is especially important to practice ethical and respectful email communication. Appendix B includes resources for respectful email communication. The exponential growth of social media and online communication offers many benefits to public health nurses, including expanded professional networking, improved speed and reach of communication, and dynamic new tools for professional collaboration and patient education. On the other hand, the ease and speed of posting information online can reduce time for considering appropriateness and ramifications. Any online breach of confidentiality or privacy can be instantly and broadly disseminated. The following tips discuss ways to avoid problems with social media:

- Never share or post information, including photos or video, gained through the nurse-patient relationship. Merely omitting a patient's name or limiting access to postings through privacy settings is not sufficient to ensure privacy.

- Never make disparaging remarks about patients, employers, or co-workers, even if they are not identified by name.

- Never take photos or videos of patients on personal devices, including cell phones.

- Never post content or otherwise speak on behalf of your employer unless you are authorized to do so.

- Promptly report any breach of confidentiality or privacy made by you or someone else.

- Maintain professional boundaries in the use of electronic media. Online contact with patients blurs the distinction between a professional and a personal relationship.

Source: National Council of State Boards of Nursing (2011)

When social media and electronic communication are used to send health messages, public health practitioners must also evaluate strategies for potential ethical concerns. A case study on using Facebook for concussion management revealed the following concerns: trust issues between patients and clinicians regarding privacy and confidentiality, the potential for harm given the variability in the quality of online information, and challenges in moderating the Facebook group (Ahmed et al., 2013).

In another example, employees of a county public health department evaluated the feasibility of using text messages for communication with public health audiences in light of the rules on sharing protected health information (PHI). They found that text messaging can be an effective communication channel, but it also needs to avoid the inclusion of PHI (Karasz, Eiden, & Bogan, 2013). To avoid including PHI, health department staff created the following two messages on influenza vaccine:

Message #1: Keep your child protected against the flu. Some kids need a second dose 30 days after they receive their first flu shot.

Message #2: Do you remember asking for a text message reminder for flu vaccine? It is time! Call a doctor or pharmacy to schedule an appointment (p. 619).

Although the above statements increase the likelihood that the message will be confidential and maintain privacy, the messages are also less likely to be targeted to individuals.

In using social media, PHNs must be guided by concerns for patient privacy and confidentiality and the potential for harm to individuals, families, and communities:

Nurses must always be aware of potential consequences of disclosing patient-related information via social media and mindful of employer policies; relevant state and federal laws; and professional standards regarding patient privacy and confidentiality. Patients should expect a nurse to act in their best interests and to respect their dignity. (Spector & Kappel, 2012, p. 2)

Ethical Application

When people communicate with one another, messages might be confusing, misunderstood, or responded to with a high degree of emotion, such as fear or anger. The PHN is accountable to provide professional communication that considers the consequences of this communication for individuals, family, communities, systems, and colleagues (see Table 8.7 on the application of ethical perspectives to communication).

Table 8.7   Ethical Action in Communication

Ethical perspective	Application
Rule ethics (principles)	• Maintain the confidentiality of private healthcare information.
	• Ensure the accuracy of health information, because wrong information could result in harm and/or legal liability.
	• Consider the impact of communication on others in the client's environment—evaluate whether communication could contribute to client harm.
	• When using an interpreter, explain that you expect a verbatim translation to avoid inaccurate or misleading messages.
	• Exercise caution when using social media and electronic communication to avoid harming individuals, families, and communities.

Virtue ethics (character)	• When collecting information from individuals and families and developing large data sets, collect only the information needed for decision-making. This approach respects the time of clients and staff.
	• Be respectful of the clients and build on positives if change is needed.
	• In situations of limited time or limited client capability to learn, prioritize the most important health education topics needed to avoid overwhelming the clients.
	• Consider that clients might interpret health education as a criticism of their behavior.
Feminist ethics (reducing oppression)	• Create an environment for the communication that is comfortable, welcoming, and affirming.
	• Consider client vulnerability when communicating sensitive information.

When Angie's preceptor sees the poster plan, Janet responds, "I really like the clear and simple messages. I can see that you have not overwhelmed your audience with too much information. I can see that you have emphasized the risk for 'baby bottle tooth decay.' I think that idea is very good, but what you have written sounds negative—almost critical of parents. I wonder whether you could approach this issue more positively and emphasize what the parent can do to prevent baby bottle tooth decay. I think the picture is good to include, because that helps parents know exactly which behavior should be prevented." Janet provides Angie with these additional resources:

Baby Bottle Tooth Decay—American Dental Association

Time to Stop Using Bottles—Minnesota Department of Health

 ## ACTIVITY

How can you communicate the information on baby bottle tooth decay on the poster in a way that does not blame parents but helps them understand what they can do to promote dental health for their child?

What is an example of health communication that could promote harm?

Janet suggests that it would be helpful for WIC clinic participants to have a take-away pamphlet on dental health. Angie consults with Joan, the communications specialist at the health department, about how to organize key oral health information in a simple and attractive pamphlet and use technology for creating the pamphlet. Joan uses Angie's ideas to create a draft of the pamphlet for Janet and Angie to review. Angie is excited when she sees the result. She comments, "Now, families who come to the WIC clinic can take information home with them about oral health and resources for dental health services."

Key Points

- PHNs need to develop effective communication skills at all levels of practice—with individuals, families, communities, and systems.

- Motivational interviewing is an effective strategy for promoting positive health behavior change.

- Building trust enhances healthy behavior change.

- Health education strategies are based on the characteristics and motivations of learners and on teaching-learning principles.

- Health communication messages are crafted based on the literacy level, cultural inclusiveness, and involvement of consumers in the development of messages.

- PHNs use social marketing to communicate health messages to targeted population groups.

- PHNs must exercise caution when using social media to deliver health messages to ensure confidentiality and privacy for patients and comply with laws about HIPAA.

Learning Examples for Effective Communication Strategies

The literature has many examples of activities that provide opportunities to learn about effective practices for communicating health information. In addition, interdisciplinary learning activities are helpful in preparing you for the reality of working with different disciplines. You must learn how to come to a consensus on common goals and strategies to improve population health. Here are some examples of nursing student projects that involved communicating health information to community groups:

- *Presented targeted health information at senior food commodity distribution centers* that included heart healthy recipes and samples made from the recipes (Sowan, Moffatt, & Canales, 2004).

- *Implemented a prevention project to reduce deaths from motor vehicle accidents* in a rural Appalachian county (nursing, medical, and public health students). Students interviewed key informants, worked with a community coalition on a media campaign, conducted a driver safety fair, and wrote articles for the local newspaper. The community had a reduction in automobile-related fatalities, and the state initiated an investigation on improving the roadways (Goodrow, Scherzer, & Florence, 2004).

- Created a video game on texting while driving for presentations to health classes at a local high school in Maine (Currie, 2013).

Reflective Practice

Effective communication is foundational to the implementation of all 17 interventions on the Public Health Intervention Wheel. Communication skills vary according to whether the intervention is at the individual/family, community, or systems level. Expectations for PHNs' skill base have grown with the development of communication technology. Local health departments often have staff members who are skilled in data management and analysis and have social marketing skills; however, PHNs need basic word-processing skills, the ability to work with spreadsheets and input data, and the ability to collaborate with information technology staff to develop health information materials. PHNs can bring their expertise in understanding the needs of the population, teaching-learning principles, and knowledge about health and illness to collaborate on creating effective health information messages for individuals, groups, and communities.

Use key concepts and ideas presented in this chapter to design a school campaign to decrease tobacco use among teens. You may use Table 8.8 to complete a learner readiness assessment and identify teaching-learning strategies. Then you can use Table 8.9 to develop the teaching plan including expected outcomes, key content, resources, and evaluation plan.

1. First, assess the learner or group of learners in these categories: physical, emotional, experiential, and knowledge.

2. Then match teaching-learning strategies to the learner assessment.

3. Once you have completed the learner assessment, identify behavioral outcomes (make sure they can be measured).

4. For each outcome, identify the content, resources needed, and evaluation strategy.

Table 8.8   Learner Readiness Assessment

Student _____ **Teaching Plan** _____Date _____

Educational Topic _____

Description of Learner(s) _____

Learner Readiness Assessment and Teaching Plan.

PEEK Assessment Components	Learner Strengths and Barriers (Protective and Risk Factors) Assessment Data	Teaching-Learning Approaches & Strategies Planning and Intervention
P Physical & Developmental Health Status • Cognitive Abilities • Communication Abilities (verbal, nonverbal, written) • Developmental Level • Individual • Family • Physical Environment	• What are the physical and environmental protective and risk factors that will influence the client's ability to learn and client learner outcomes? • What developmental tasks and crises will influence the client's ability to learn and client learner outcomes?	• Which communication and teaching/learning strategies could you use to build on the client's strengths or protective factors and to modify or reduce client learning barriers and risk factors? • How will you modify your teaching to fit the client's unique developmental needs? • What are the preferred time and place for teaching/ learning?
E Emotional • Current Stress, Coping, Resilience • Motivation for Learning • Readiness for Learning— Stages • Pre-contemplation • Contemplation • Preparation • Action • Maintenance	• Will the client's current stresses and coping abilities be a barrier to learning? Does the client have a history of effective coping and resilience when faced with uncertainty and need for change? • What will motivate the client to learn and change? • What is the client's readiness for learning?	• Which counseling strategies might you use to modify the client's stresses and support the client's coping abilities? • How will you modify your teaching-learning approaches to fit the client's level of motivation and readiness for learning?

E
Experiential & Social
- Culture and Languages
- Cultural Health Beliefs & Practices
- Past Experiences with Healthcare/Specific Health Topic

- What are the client's primary and secondary languages?

- What is the client's culture, and how do the client's cultural beliefs and practices affect the client's health, health beliefs, and practices?

- What are client's past experiences with the healthcare system and this specific healthcare topic?

- How will the client's past experiences influence the client's ability to learn?

- How will you modify your communication to fit the client's language abilities?

- How will you modify your teaching-learning strategies to be culturally congruent with client's culture?

- How will you build on the client's past experiences with the healthcare system and this specific health topic?

K
Knowledge
- Educational/Reading Level
- Language Literacy and Learning Style
- Language Registry (formal versus informal)
- Present Knowledge of Topic/Past Health Education
- Healthcare Literacy

- What are the client's educational and reading levels?

- Does the client use formal or informal language to discuss general or health-specific topics?

- What is the client's preferred learning style (i.e., visual/spatial, auditory, kinesthetic or physical)?

- What is the client's education and knowledge about health and the health education topic?

- Does the client understand how the healthcare system works and how to access the services and resources needed?

- How will you modify your teaching to fit the client's education and reading levels?

- Which teaching resources and materials are appropriate to use with this client?

- How might you actively engage the client in the teaching/learning process?

- How might you build on what the client already knows?

- What additional information and resources might you need to provide for the client to use the healthcare system effectively?

Source: Modified by Patricia M. Schoon (2013) from St. Catherine University, 2008. Developed by Lois Devereaux, Karen Ryan, and Patricia M. Schoon. Readiness for Learning-Stages sourced from Shinitzky & Kub (2001)

Table 8.9   Teaching Plan

Mutually Established Goal for Teaching Plan _____

_____

Priorities for Teaching Plan _____

_____

Teaching Module (note that time and pacing may be adjusted to the time frame you have for teaching)

Opening 5–10 minutes	Introduction	Confirm topic and client readiness for learning at beginning of session.		
Place/ Time/ Pacing	**Behavioral Outcomes** At the completion of this presentation, the learner will be able to:	Brief Content Outline	Teaching-Learning Strategies and Resources	Evaluation & Documentation Methods— Measures
15–20 minutes	**Outcome # 1** *Outcomes should be client-focused, behavioral, realistic, understandable, measurable, achievable, and time-specific.*	Content should be specific to outcome. Content should be listed in outline form. Amount of content should fit time available.	List strategies and resources you will use based on learner readiness assessment. Include others who will assist with teaching.	Determine whether the learner outcome was met, partially met, or not met. Describe learning activities that were effective and/or ineffective. Identify next step in learning process.
15–20 minutes	**Outcome # 2**			
Closing 5 – 10 minutes	Summarizing	Summarize what was learned. Confirm that the client's needs were met. Plan for follow-up.		

Source: Modified by Patricia M. Schoon (2013) from St. Catherine University, 2008. Developed by Lois Devereaux, Karen Ryan, and Patricia M. Schoon.

When designing the campaign, consider the following questions:

1. How will teaching-learning principles guide your campaign design (learner readiness, motivation, active learning)?

2. How will consideration of health literacy influence your plan?

3. Whom will you collaborate with to design the campaign?

4. How will you use social marketing principles to design the campaign?

5. What is the key health message that you want to convey to the teen school population?

6. What are some strategies that you can use to involve teens in planning the campaign?

7. How are the Cornerstones of Public Health Nursing reflected in the campaign's design?

 # Application of Evidence

Janet's public health department has collaborated with the local hospital and county social services to establish a suicide prevention hotline. Janet is representing the health department in the Suicide Prevention Coalition that worked to establish the hotline. The coalition is now working on a strategy for communicating the availability of the hotline to the community. The coalition members decide that they need to use multiple methods to communicate this new community resource. How can the coalition members use the evidence on effective communication strategies to reach the community?

1. How should the school nurse at the local high school communicate the availability of the suicide hotline to students, teachers, and parents?

2. Which data about suicide might motivate individuals and organizations in the community to be concerned about suicide as a health problem? How should these data be communicated?

3. Which tips for effective social marketing should be used to communicate the availability of the suicide hotline?

4. How can the coalition use electronic communication to reach a larger community audience?

Think, Explore, Do

1. Using the poster example discussed in this chapter, work through the following questions for a poster on another topic:

   a. Who will look at the poster? Will the audience be only adults, or will children be included?

   b. What are the literacy level and languages of the viewers?

   c. What are some sources of reliable information about the topic?

   d. Where will the poster be displayed?

   e. Is there room to have handouts nearby or on the poster for viewers to take?

   f. How can it be designed to grab attention and pull people in to look at it?

   g. What are the key health issues to focus on in the poster? Which key issue will you focus on, and what is the rationale for your choice?

   h. What are the two learning objectives you want your target audience to achieve?

   i. How can the poster be designed so that takeaway information is secure and firmly attached?

   j. How could the presentation be interactive for the viewer?

   k. How can the clinic environment be organized to focus attention on the poster?

   l. Whom will you collaborate with on the poster, what resources do you need, and what is your desired budget for producing the poster?

2. Practice motivational interviewing with a peer. Choose a health behavior change that your peer would like to initiate. Use the list of behavior change counseling items found in the Behavior Change Counseling Index to evaluate your effectiveness. You will find these in the following article:

   Pfister-Minogue, K. A., & Salveson, C. (2010). Training and experience of public health nurses in using behavior change counseling. *Public Health Nursing, 27*(6), 544–551. doi:10.1111/j.1525-1446.2010.00884.x

3. Review guidelines for using electronic and social media in the following sources. Read through or watch several of the provided scenarios and identify the ethical course of action in using electronic and social media (see Appendix B for list of websites):

   1. National Council of State Boards of Nursing. (2011, August). White paper: A nurse's guide to the use of social media. Chicago, IL: Author.

   2. Spector, N., & Kappel, D. M. (2102). Guidelines for using electronic and social media. Online Journal of Issues in Nursing, 17(3). doi:10.3912/OJIN.Vol17No03Man01

3. View the video *Social Media Guidelines for Nurses* found on the National Council of State Boards of Nursing website.

4. Choose a health promotion topic and search for apps related to the topic. Review three to five apps that address that topic for Android, iPad, or iPhone devices. Evaluate and compare each app based on the following criteria:

   1. Target user (professional or public)

   2. Ease of use

   3. Main features

   4. Availability on specific devices

   5. Cost

   6. Language availability

   7. Interactivity

   8. Consistency with evidence on topic

One example is breastfeeding apps, such as Breastfeeding Tabulator, iBabyLog, and iBreastfeed.

References

Ahmed, O. H., Sullivan, S. J., Schneiders, A. G., Anderson, L., Paton, C, & Crory, P. R. (2013). Ethical considerations in using Facebook for health care support: A case study using concussion management. (2013). *Physical Medicine and Rehabilitation, 5,* 328-344. doi.org/10.1016.j.pmrj.2013.03.007

Bennett, G. G., & Glasgow, R. E. (2009). The delivery of public health interventions via the internet: Actualizing their potential. *Annual Review of Public Health, 30,* 273–293.

Black, A. (2008). Health literacy and cardiovascular disease: Fostering client skills. *American Journal of Health Education, 39*(1), 55–57.

Browne, A. J., Doane, G. h., Reimer, J., MacLeod, M., & McLellan, E. (2010). Public health nursing practice with 'high priority' families: The significance of contextualizing 'risk'. *Nursing Inquiry, 17*(1), 26-37.

Bull, S. S., Levine, D. K., Black, S. R., Schmiege, S. J., & Santelli, J. (2012). Social media-delivered sexual health intervention: A cluster randomized controlled trial. *American Journal of Prevention Medicine, 43*(5), pp. 467-474. http://dx.doi.org/10.1016/j.amepre.2012.07.022

Chaffee, M. (2000). Health communications: Nursing education for increased visibility and effectiveness. *Journal of Professional Nursing, 16*(1), 31–38.

Clark, M. J. (2008). *Community health nursing: Advocacy for population health.* Upper Saddle River, NJ: Pearson Education, Inc.

Centers for Disease Control and Prevention. (2011). The health communicator's guide to social media toolkit. Atlanta, GA: Author. Retrieved from http://www.cdc.gov/healthcommunication/ToolsTemplates/SocialMediaToolkit_BM.pdf

Currie, D. (2013, July). University of Maine nursing students spread health message via lessons in local schools. *The Nation's Health.* www.thenationshealth.org

DeBuono, B. A. (2002). *Pfizer health literacy initiative*. New York, NY: Pfizer Graphic.

Devereaux, L., & Schoon, P. M. (2013). Teaching plan. St. Catherine University.

Evans, D. E., & McCormack, L. (2008). Applying social marketing in health care: Communicating evidence to change consumer behavior. *Medical Decision Making, 28*, 781–792.

Goodrow, B., Scherzer, G., & Florence, J. (2004). An application of multidisclipinary education to a campus-community partnership to reduce motor vehicle accidents. *Education for Health, 17*(2), 152–162.

Green, A. (2006). A person-centered approach to palliative care nursing. *Journal of Hospice and Palliative Nursing, 8*(5), 294–301.

Harvard Medical School. (2011). Motivating Behavior Change. *Harvard Mental Health Letter, 27*(8). Retrieved from www.health.harvard.edu

Holmes, B. J. (2008). Communicating about emerging infectious disease: The importance of research. *Health, Risk & Society, 10*(4), 349–360.

Institute of Medicine. (2004). *Health literacy: A prescription to end confusion*. Washington, D. C.: National Academy Press.

Jakeway, C. C., Cantrell, E. E., Cason, J. B., & Talley, B. S. (2006). Developing population health competencies among public health nurses in Georgia. *Public Health Nursing, 23*(2), 161–167.

Jiménez-Munro, A., Nerín, I., Samper, P., Marqueta, A., Beamonte, A., Gargallo, P., ... Rodríguez, G.(2013). A proactive smoking cessation intervention in postpartum women. *Midwifery, 29*, 240-245.

Karasz, J. N., Eiden, A., & Bogan, S. (2013). Text messaging to communicate with public health audiences: How the HIPAA Security Rule affects practice. *American Journal of Public Health, 103*(4), 617-622. doi:10.2105/AJPH.2012.300999

Katakura, N., Yamamot-Mitani, & Ishigaki, K. (2010). Home-visit nurses' attitudes for providing effective assistance to clients with schizophrenia. *International Journal of Mental Health Nursing, 19*, 102-109. doi: 10.1111/j.1447-0349.2009.00641.x

Keller, L. O., Strohschein, S., Lia-Hoagberg, B., & Schaffer, M. A. (2004). Population-based public health interventions: Practice-based and evidence-supported (Part I). *Public Health Nursing, 21*(5), 453–468.

Kolb, D. A. (1984) *Experiential learning experience as a source of learning and development*. Upper Saddle River, NJ: Prentice Hall.

Kolb, D. A. (2005). *The Kolb learning style inventory. Version 3.1*. David A. Kolb, Experience Based Learning Systems, Inc.

Kreps, G. L., & Sparks, L. (2008). Meeting the health literacy needs of immigrant populations. *Patient Education and Counseling, 71*(3), 328–332.

Levy-Storms, L. (2005). Strategies for diffusing public health innovations through older adults' health communication networks. *Generations, 29*(2), 70-75.

Miller, W. R. (2004). Motivational interviewing in service to health promotion. *American Journal of Health Promotion, 18*, A1–A10.

National Council of State Boards of Nursing. (2011, August). White Paper: A nurse's guide to the use of social media. Chicago, IL: Author. Retrieved from https://www.ncsbn.org/Social_Media.pdf

Onega, L. L., & Devers, E. (2008). Health education and group process. In M. Stanhope & J. Lancaster (Eds.), *Public health nursing: Population-centered health care in the community* (pp. 289–338). St. Louis, MO: Mosby Elsevier.

Osterman, R. (2011). Feasibility of using motivational interviewing to decrease alcohol consumption during pregnancy. *Journal of Addictions Nursing, 22*, 93-102. doi: 10.3109/10884602.2011.585723

Pfister-Minogue, K. A., & Salveson, C. (2010). Training and experience of public health nurses in using behavior change counseling. *Public Health Nursing, 27*(6), 544-551. doi: 10.1111/j.1525-1446.2010.00884.x

Public Health Nursing Section. (2001). *Public Health Interventions—Application for Public Health Nursing Practice*. St. Paul, MN: Minnesota Department of Health.

Richardson, L. (2012). Motivational interviewing: Helping patients move toward change. *Journal of Christian Nursing, 29*(1), 18-24. doi: 10.1097/CNJ:0b013.c381238c510

Russell, E. (2009). *Fundamentals of Marketing.* London, UK: Bloomsbury.

Shinitzky, H. E., & Kub, J. (2001). The art of motivating behavior change: The use of motivational interviewing to promote health. *Public Health Nursing, 18*(3), 178–185.

Sowan, N. A., Moffatt, S. G., & Canales, M. K. (2004). Creating a mentoring partnership model: A university-department of health experience. *Family & Community Health, 27*(4), 326-337.

Spector, N., & Kappel, D. M. (2102). Guidelines for using electronic and social media. *Online Journal of Issues in Nursing, 17*(3). doi: 10.3912/OJIN.Vol17No03Man01

Starkey, F., Audrey, S., Holliday, J., Moore, L., & Campbell, R. (2009). Identifying influential young people to undertake effective peer-led health promotion: The example of A Stop Smoking In Schools Trial (ASSIST). *Health Education Research, 24*(6), 977-988. http://dx.doi.org/10.1093/her/cyp045

Substance Abuse & Mental Health Service Administration Network. (1994). *You can prepare easy to read materials.* Technical Assistance Bulletin, National Clearinghouse for Alcohol and Drug Information. Retrieved from http://www.actforyouth.net/documents/YDM%20pdf6.4C%20handout.pdf

Thompson, D. R., Chair, S. Y., Chan, S. W., Astin, F., Davidson, P. M., & Ski, C. F. (2011). Motivational interviewing: A useful approach to improving cardiovascular health? *Journal of Clinical Nursing, 20*, 1236-1244. doi: 10.1111/j.1365-2702.2010.03558.x

Toofany, S. (2006). Patient empowerment: Myth or reality? *Nursing Management, 13*(6), 18–22.

Tveiten, S., & Severinsson, E. (2006). Communication—A core concept in client supervision by public health nurses. *Journal of Nursing Management, 14*(3), 235–243.

Weiss, B. D. (2007). *Health literacy and patient safety: Help patients understand.* Chicago, IL: American Medical Association Foundation and American Medical Association.

Westdahl, C., & Page-Goertz, S. (2006). Promotion of breastfeeding—Beyond the benefits. *International Journal of Childbirth Education, 22*(4), 8–16.

Whitman, N. I. (1998). Assessment of the learner. In M. D. Boyd, C. J. Gleit, B. A. Grahm, & N. I. Whitman (Eds.), *Health teaching in nursing practice: A professional model* (pp. 157–180). Stamford, CT: Appleton & Lange.

Wright, A. L, Naylor, A., Wester, R., Bauer, M., & Sutcliffe, E. (1997). Using cultural knowledge in health promotion: Breastfeeding among the Navajo. *Health Education & Behavior, 24*(5), 625–639.

Zahner, S. J., & Gredig, Q. B. (2005). Improving public health nursing education: Recommendations of local public health nurses. *Public Health Nursing, 22*(5), 445–450.

COMPETENCY #7
Establishes and Maintains Caring Relationships With Communities, Systems, Individuals, and Families

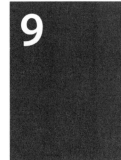

Carolyn M. Garcia

with Christine C. Andres, Maureen A. Alms, and Bernita Missal

Susan, a public health nurse (PHN) for several years, has been developing her skills as a family home-visiting nurse. She works with young families whom her supervisor has identified as high risk and has been slowly increasing her caseload. The population that Susan serves is composed of single, young mothers who need support with their parenting skills and identification of normal development for their children.

One of Susan's first families was a young mother named Julie with four children. Julie had her first child when she was 16 years old, and then she had two other children before moving to the community where Susan served as a PHN. Julie was not involved in a committed relationship and had no job. She became part of Susan's caseload when a Women, Infants, and Children's (WIC) nurse referred her for a PHN baby visit after the birth of her fourth child.

During the baby visit, Susan established the foundation for a strong nurse-family relationship. Julie was open about many issues with Susan, including the fact that the two older children were living not with her but with each of their fathers. She told Susan that she was unable to be a "good mother" to them. She was excited about the birth of her new son. Susan explored Julie's strengths and needs. It was apparent that Julie could benefit from some parenting information and anticipatory guidance for the 2-year-old and newborn whom she planned to parent. Julie was interested in the program that Susan described, which entailed monthly visits until her newborn turned 3 or until she believed she was no longer benefiting from the program.

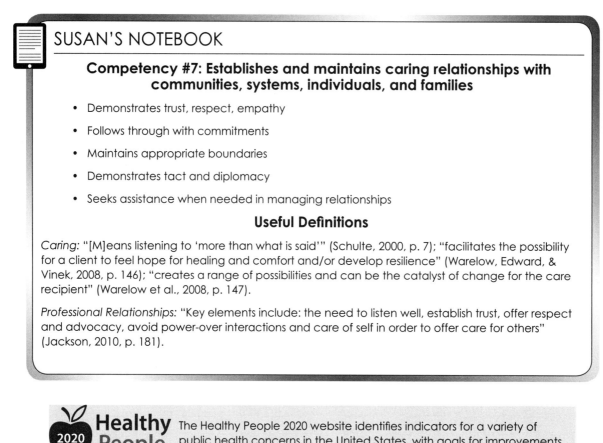

SUSAN'S NOTEBOOK

Competency #7: Establishes and maintains caring relationships with communities, systems, individuals, and families

- Demonstrates trust, respect, empathy

- Follows through with commitments

- Maintains appropriate boundaries

- Demonstrates tact and diplomacy

- Seeks assistance when needed in managing relationships

Useful Definitions

Caring: "[M]eans listening to 'more than what is said'" (Schulte, 2000, p. 7); "facilitates the possibility for a client to feel hope for healing and comfort and/or develop resilience" (Warelow, Edward, & Vinek, 2008, p. 146); "creates a range of possibilities and can be the catalyst of change for the care recipient" (Warelow et al., 2008, p. 147).

Professional Relationships: "Key elements include: the need to listen well, establish trust, offer respect and advocacy, avoid power-over interactions and care of self in order to offer care for others" (Jackson, 2010, p. 181).

Healthy People 2020 The Healthy People 2020 website identifies indicators for a variety of public health concerns in the United States, with goals for improvements by 2020. Select a health indicator and develop a public health nursing health promotion strategy that will include activities at the individual, community, and system levels. Select activities that emphasize the establishing of a caring relationship with the individual, family, or community. From your perspective, in which activities will it be challenging to establish a caring relationship? Why?

Touching Lives Without Stepping on Toes

It is probably not an exaggeration to state that most individuals who choose to become nurses have an inherent desire to care for other human beings. In some ways, caring is synonymous with nursing. As a profession, nursing is a process of assessment, planning, intervention, and evaluation delivered in a context of caring with goals of prevention, healing, recovery, or peaceful transition. As a discipline, nursing is contributing knowledge and advancing science about the complex interplay of health-environment-person-nursing (Fawcett, 2000). Much of this knowledge generation would not be possible in the absence of caring relationships.

PHNs have unique opportunities to develop caring relationships with individuals, families, and groups (e.g., communities and systems). Lillian Wald emphasized caring when she said, "Nursing is love in action, and there is no finer manifestation of it than the care of the poor and disabled in their own homes" (Ridgeway, 2010, p. 1). Although it can certainly be argued that any nurse in any environment can and should establish a caring relationship, many PHNs develop and maintain caring relationships with their clients over weeks, months, and years. This opportunity for lengthy caring relationships is not as pervasive in acute clinical settings but certainly can be observed in nursing care for the elderly (i.e., nursing homes) and the terminally ill (i.e., hospice care; Olthuis, Dekkers, Leget, & Vogelaar, 2006). Certainly, a meaningful caring relationship can be long or short, and challenges can be experienced in both situations. For new nurses, the desire to care, help, intervene, and be of benefit to an individual or family can be a great asset, but this drive can also present challenges because they are still developing knowledge of how to establish appropriate boundaries. (For information about establishing professional boundaries, see Chapter 7.) Indeed, many nurses have learned about boundaries by experiencing what happens when they are *not* established or appropriately maintained. Emotions, in moments of sickness, illness, or disease, are intense for families. Serving a family within an effective caring relationship can enable the nurse to provide support and resources that will optimally benefit the family. This chapter offers strategies for establishing and maintaining meaningful, appropriate caring relationships in public health nursing and presents challenging situations along with preventive strategies to help you avoid some of these common pitfalls as you launch your nursing career.

To appreciate the nature of a caring relationship, you need to first look at a description of caring. A thorough analysis of caring in the nursing literature has demonstrated five conceptualizations, or expressions, of caring in nursing (Morse, Bottorff, Neander, & Solberg, 1991):

1. Caring as a human trait/state

2. Caring as a moral imperative

3. Caring as an affect

4. Caring as an interpersonal interaction

5. Caring as a therapeutic intervention

In essence, caring is an attribute that, for many, is inherent to who you are as a nurse and human being. In a recent metasynthesis, caring was explored alongside the art of nursing and being present; caring was defined as "an interpersonal process that is characterized by expert nursing, interpersonal sensitivity and intimate relationships" (Finfgeld-Connett, 2008, p. 528). Caring is also a behavior or emotion that is morally mandated or expected from nurses (Morse, Solberg, Neander, Bottorff, & Johnson, 1990; Shores, 2012). In addition, caring is an action between two or more people, and it is a way to intervene or act to improve the well-being of an individual or community. These last two points—interaction and intervention—in essence reflect a "caring relationship" in nursing, because they involve the nurse and another person or group of people.

ACTIVITY

How much do you agree with the above statements regarding caring and nursing? Do you believe that it is possible to be an effective nurse and not care? Why or why not?

Do you believe it is possible to care too much? If so, how do you determine how much caring is appropriate?

Over the year that followed the initial visit, Susan saw Julie and the children monthly. The relationship flourished as Susan provided Julie with parenting support and information to understand safety and the developmental milestones of her children. Susan worked with Julie to access community resources. At times, Julie would reveal pieces of her past that included mental health issues stemming from a childhood of molestation and abuse. Susan always listened without judgment. Susan realized how much she had come to care about this family and how much Julie trusted her to care for them.

Demonstrates Trust, Respect, and Empathy

Relationships exist in every aspect of life: family relationships, casual acquaintance relationships, colleague relationships, distant relationships, and close relationships, to name a few. In public health nursing, relationships can start to build over minutes and often last for years. The variety of settings in which PHNs work is reflected in the diversity of their relationships. For example, a local public health department PHN administering flu shots might spend only 10 minutes with a client, whereas a PHN conducting weekly home visits with a pregnant mom on bed rest might be in that relationship for years. A PHN employed in a jail setting might develop an intermittent relationship with incarcerated individuals who are released and rearrested multiple times over the years. Every relationship a PHN develops, regardless of how long or deep the relationship runs, can be a caring relationship.

A caring relationship can only exist when trust is present. An effective PHN builds trust in verbal and nonverbal ways that reflect awareness of the situation and the needs of the individual, family, or community. Practically, PHNs encourage trust when their actions are consistent, dependable, nonjudgmental, and sensitive to the needs or preferences of the other person. (See Chapter 11 for more information on nonjudgmental nursing.) Professional relationship building is described in the context of a program to prevent teen pregnancy: "The daily presence of the PHN is an important program component for the kind of information nurses provide . . . as well as relationship building with a professional who can be trusted and is not judgmental about the adolescent's problems and concerns" (Schaffer, Jost, Pederson, & Lair, 2008, p. 308, 310). Often, trust is developed with time and consistency. Diane McNaughton (2005, p. 435) observes that for at-risk pregnant women, multiple nursing visits "were needed for clients to develop trust in nurses, discuss their problems, and utilize the services offered by nurses" (see the following Evidence Example).

Evidence Example: Phases of Relationship Building

McNaughton (2005) identifies phases of building relationship between at-risk pregnant women and public health nurses, including (1) Orientation Phase—Orientation (nurse assessment, women answering questions, feeling anxious); (2) Working Phase—Identification (nurse providing information, women identifying problems, asking questions); (3) Working Phase—Exploitation (nurse providing mutual support, women describe using resources provided by nurse); and (4) Resolution Phase—Resolution (problems are solved or relationship ends).

Some PHNs find themselves in situations where they are seeking to create relationships with individuals, families, or communities that might not want the relationship or simply are unsure of what they want, which can occur with vulnerable or stigmatized clients. This challenge to building relationship might occur, for example, when the PHN is working with families involved in child protection situations, necessitating thoughtful intention on the part of the PHN to develop a caring relationship. Establishing trust is critical, yet doing so can be challenging because many families are vulnerable and powerless (Jack, DiCenso, & Lohfeld, 2005; Porr, Drummond, & Olson, 2012). Often, families trust nurses more readily than they do other professionals (e.g., law enforcement or social workers), although depth of mutual trust takes patience and time and might not be achievable in every situation (Jack et al., 2005). The Evidence Example below highlights the challenges associated with establishing trust from the perspective of mothers.

 Evidence Example: Theory of Maternal Engagement With PHNs

A grounded theory study (i.e., qualitative study conducted to generate a theory about a basic social process) was conducted in Canada to describe the process of mothers engaging with PHNs as part of a home-visiting program (Jack et al., 2005). Twenty mothers participated, and data were collected using interviews and record review. Key findings demonstrate the unique feelings of those receiving home visits from PHNs: Specifically, the mothers "felt vulnerable and powerless when they allowed the service providers in their home" (p. 182). The mothers described three phases to the process: overcoming fear, building trust, and seeking mutuality. Strategies to overcome fear included "'hiding nothing,' 'trying to measure up,' and 'protecting self'" (p. 185). For example, mothers cleaned their houses and made sure their babies were looking nice before the nurse visited their homes. When fears could not be overcome, the mothers were more likely to cancel appointments, drop out of the program, or withhold information from the nurse. Trust levels ranged from no trust to tentative trust to strong trust, and the level the mother was at was largely dependent on her own characteristics and her perceptions of the PHN. The mothers wanted nurses they could relate to, thereby developing a sense of mutuality. The success of the relationship was also directly influenced by the nurse characteristics, the client characteristics, and the home-visiting context, including the frequency and duration of visits.

 ACTIVITY

What might you do to encourage a client to feel secure and comfortable during an initial visit?

How will you acknowledge the client's sense of vulnerability and work with the client to move beyond this vulnerability to establish a trusting relationship?

After this first year, Susan started to notice a change within Julie: She started to "care" less about herself and would reveal to the nurse that she was not happy. Julie reported finding it difficult to get out of bed. Susan noticed the environment of the home changing, and Julie began to miss appointments. Susan decided to have a "heart to heart," or deep conversation, with Julie, because she believed their relationship was built on trust and honesty. As Susan revealed her observations, stressing the desire to help Julie feel better, Julie stated that she did not think her depression medication was working anymore. Susan supported Julie and focused on Julie's strengths, one of which was seeking medical care when appropriate. Susan screened Julie for safety toward herself and the children. They made a plan for Julie to visit her primary care physician as soon as possible.

The next week, Julie came into the office asking for Susan. Susan was immediately concerned. Julie had pink and black hair, a pierced nose and eyebrow, and no children with her. Susan brought Julie into her office to explore her outward changes and her reasons for coming to see Susan. Julie broke down in tears, saying that she had no energy and was not sleeping and hinting that she was cutting herself. Susan had a moment of inward reflection, asking herself several questions, such as how she should respond to reflect how much she cared yet be sure to do her job of protecting Julie and her children? Susan gently explored who was watching the children when Julie was having difficulty functioning, knowing that a 3-year-old and a 1-year-old need constant supervision. Julie's answers were vague. Susan had to tell Julie that she was concerned and that if the children were not supervised or cared for, child protection could become involved with her family. This information made Julie very upset, and Susan, at that point, realized that she needed to do more. Susan put herself in Julie's shoes and relied on the trust and strength of the relationship she had with Julie to suggest immediately seeing a crisis mental health nurse working for the county. Julie stated she would if Susan believed that it would help. Susan connected them within 15 minutes, and Julie and the mental health nurse initiated a plan of safety and confirmed that the children were okay and being cared for by an appropriate person (in this case, a neighbor was watching the children while Julie visited Susan). They also scheduled a follow-up appointment within a couple of days with a mental health specialist. This meeting seemed to give Julie hope and energy. Susan felt like she had done what she needed to do, but she felt bad about upsetting Julie with her discussion of safety for the children.

Evidence Example: Public Health Nursing Practice With "High-Priority" Families: The Significance of Contextualizing "Risk"

In a study illustrating how PHNs use critical relational approaches, including providing support, building trust, and using their clinical judgment, in their work with high-priority families (Browne, Hartrick Doane, Reimer, MacLeod, & McLellan, 2010), 32 PHNs participated in interviews and focus groups that yielded three themes associated with working with families at risk: contextualizing the complexities of families' lives, responding to shifting contexts of risk and capacity, and working relationally with families under surveillance. PHNs' ability to work with families and recognize the dual influences of risk and capacity is critical to their success in establishing effective working relationships, especially with high-risk or high-priority families.

Respect is an essential component of a caring relationship. Respect in practice is more challenging than most PHNs realize due to the influences of their own cultural beliefs, values, and experiences. According to the Nurses Association of New Brunswick (2011), a therapeutic nurse-client relationship is based on respect for the dignity and worth of a client. It is really difficult, if not impossible, to establish a caring, meaningful relationship with a client or family if respect is absent. Consider how you would feel when receiving service or care for a physical need from someone who is capable of doing the job but does so in a manner that sends the message that you do not deserve the care or that you are not as important as the caregiver. Sometimes nurses send these subtle messages without realizing it; other times, they send the messages intentionally because they have established certain judgments or perceptions about specific client groups or clients with certain characteristics. Effective PHNs critically evaluate personal judgments and consider the extent to which these judgments slip into practice and make it difficult to provide respectful care and establish authentic caring relationships. In addition to reflecting on personal judgments, PHNs can also consider the assumptions they are making about clients, families, or communities and avoid doing so by understanding the diversity and differences in people and demonstrating behaviors that appreciate rather than judge or criticize this diversity. Some of these behaviors might include personalizing the care being provided, offering choices regarding care and interventions, and promoting independence to every extent possible when caring for people.

Diane Martins (2008) conducted a phenomenological (lived experience qualitative design) study to explore and understand the experiences of 15 homeless people as they accessed healthcare and highlighted the importance of respect as a value and practice among PHNs caring for all populations, including vulnerable groups, such as the homeless. Her recommendations include building on strengths rather than problems and supporting people through practical behaviors, such as recognizing and valuing that they have the right to make informed decisions about their own healthcare. A specific professional development recommendation from the study is to provide education for PHNs so that they better understand the needs of the homeless population; increasing awareness of these needs among PHNs could aid in decreasing the frustrations that can arise when providing care to this population. Finally, Martins also highlights the essential need for PHNs to advocate at the community and systems levels for social change related to complex social issues, such as homelessness; doing so in a respectful, inclusive way not only could yield positive outcomes for persons experiencing homelessness but could also strengthen individual-level interventions. Caring is the foundation for effective advocacy at community and system levels, which is discussed in Chapter 10.

In addition to trust and respect, empathy is foundational to establishing and maintaining a caring relationship. Many people confuse empathy with sympathy, which is problematic, as described by Douglas Chismar (1988, p. 257): "[B]lurring the distinction between empathy and sympathy has caused us to miss important complexities in human motivation as well as to overlook and fail to develop the unique capacity to empathize." *Empathy* is the ability to respond to someone else's emotional state by experiencing similar feelings, whereas *sympathy* goes a step further by inherently feeling positive and exhibiting lasting concern toward the other person (Chismar, 1988). For example, someone might empathize with a stranger after hearing about the loss of this person's child in a car accident and might express emotions of sadness, including crying. That same person, however, might sympathize with a sibling who has experienced the same loss, not only expressing emotions of sadness and tears but continuing to care and support the sibling over time. Empathy also includes an ability to care generally and specifically about a particular person's situation, while not necessarily agreeing with the other person's perspective. PHNs employed in jails are often asked how they care for criminals who have committed horrible crimes; empathy enables PHNs in this context to care for and even emotionally mirror the needs of an inmate while not agreeing with or supporting aspects of that individual. Table 9.1 presents distinctions between empathy and sympathy.

Table 9.1   Empathy versus Sympathy

Empathy	Sympathy
Responds to another's perceived emotional state by experiencing feelings of a similar sort	Has a positive regard or a feeling of benevolence for the person
Understands but might not agree with the other person's perspective	Agrees with the viewpoint
Senses what the other is feeling but without "mutuality"	Offers supportive response to the other's situation
Is directed toward anyone, including someone who is not necessarily liked	Is expressed toward those one feels positive about or close to
Usually occurs where no prior attachment to the person exists	Usually occurs in the context of a personal relationship or insider (from the community) knowledge
Often involuntarily experiences feelings similar to someone else's	Often voluntarily experiences feelings alongside someone else

Source: Adapted from Chismar, 1988

Despite the complex conceptualization of empathy in nursing, a scale was developed that could measure a nurse's level of empathic understanding, or ability to understand a client's emotions, feelings, and perspective (Nagano, 2000). The instrument is designed to measure nurse awareness and actions, and research is ongoing to improve its validity and reliability. The 20-item scale includes verbal (e.g., "restates important points in own words and confirms with client") and nonverbal (e.g., "looks at the client with a warm expression") elements that in many ways mirror simple yet effective nursing communication strategies.

Judeen Schulte (2000) conducted an ethnographic study exploring the perspectives of PHNs regarding building relationships with clients. These nurses believed that particular actions yielded successes in developing caring relationships, including "being a resource, detecting/asking the next questions, and making informed judgments" (p. 7), because they helped clients believe that they could openly share. Often, the nurses were conducting home visits with no particular disease or problem identified beforehand; establishing caring relationships was essential for the PHNs to accurately assess and intervene with the families. For the nurses, honesty and being direct was important to relationship building, and the nurses described needing to ignore "rude behavior" (2000, p. 7). Schulte shares comments from a participant that summarize the study:

> Felicia's words strongly communicate the link between caring and connections: "Public health nursing is more than a job. . . . When I'm out there, I care about the people, about what happens to them. I don't think I'd make a really good public health nurse if I didn't care. You get results if they know you care—they're willing to make some change. If they don't think you care at all about them, why should they take a risk for you? I think public health nursing is all about caring about people." (2000, p. 8)

For the PHNs in this study, caring meant listening to "more than what is said" (Schulte, 2000, p. 7), which is consistent with attention paid in nursing to nonverbal communication and to contextual factors in the family, community, and societal environments.

 Evidence Example: Negotiating: Experiences of Community Nurses When Contracting With Clients

Focus groups were conducted with 14 community nurses to explore the issues surrounding negotiating and establishing client care contracts (Duiveman & Bonner, 2012). The nurses' perspectives were represented by three themes: assessment of needs, education toward enablement, and negotiation. Across all themes, it was apparent that for PHNs or community nurses to deliver person-centered care, it is necessary for them to effectively assess and find a balance between the client's needs and the nurse's ability to address them. Doing so appropriately requires meaningful efforts to demonstrate care and establish a caring relationship, which can then result in successfully negotiating a plan for care.

Although much of what has been discussed thus far in this chapter is specific to nursing care for individuals or families, many of the guiding principles for establishing a caring relationship also apply to relationships at the community or systems levels. At times it can seem (and be) more challenging simply because many other people are usually involved (see Chapter 5 on collaboration). Some literature, however, does describe community-level caring in public health nursing. PHNs need to consider the importance of caring for communities, as discussed by Kathleen Chafey:

> Nurses must care about what happens to groups of citizens, as well as particular clients. . . . Although proponents of "caring" seem to have drawn a distinction between an ethic of justice and an ethic of care, this is bipolar, even antithetical. Building the health of communities requires universal application of the principles of justice. It further requires that nurses care enough about their communities and the individuals in them to do battle in political, social, and economic arenas. (1996, p. 15)

Betty Smith-Campbell (1999) developed and tested a caring model for communities (see Figure 9.1) because "nurses collectively care with and for communities" (p. 405). In the model, the foundation of caring actions is the principles discussed earlier in this chapter, including affect and moral imperative. Interaction is not only with an individual but with the "community," however community is defined. Caring actions result not only from the underlying foundation, interactions, and planning but also from the direct and indirect influences that encompass the community (e.g., economics, policies, politics, and supporting or opposing communities). For example, a parish nurse caring for the congregation will want to plan health promotion activities with an understanding of the neighborhood and other influences on those whom the PHN is serving. PHNs working in an affluent neighborhood with abundant healthcare resources can more easily develop caring relationships that involve extensive health screenings and referrals to outside resources (e.g., services for high blood pressure, weight management, and stress reduction) than PHNs serving a congregation in an impoverished neighborhood with limited healthcare options. It would be unethical and not very caring for this PHN to proceed with extensive screenings for that congregation without first establishing where they can receive care needed for identified problems. A PHN cannot effectively care for a community unless time is taken to understand and appreciate the complexity of factors (i.e., social, economic, political) in and surrounding the community.

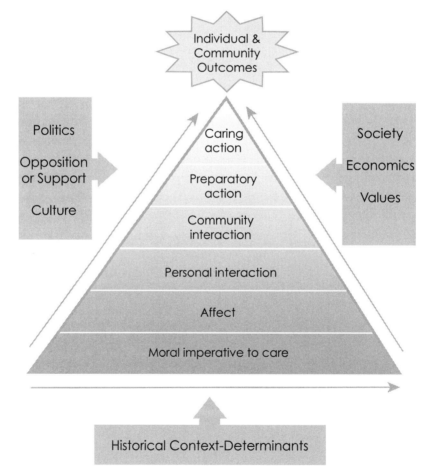

Figure 9.1. Smith-Campbell (1999) Caring Community Model (adapted with permission)

Follows Through With Commitments

PHNs cannot be trusted unless they can demonstrate consistency in care for individuals, families, and communities. Clients for whom PHNs are caring need to know that those PHNs are dependable and reliable in addition to being honest, respectful, and trustworthy. Teri Aronowitz (2005) conducted a grounded theory study to examine the ways in which adolescents develop resilience and change risk behaviors amid environmental stressors in their lives. One of the most important findings from the interviews was that the processes by which the teens felt supported were possible only within the context of a relationship with a "reliable, caring, and competent adult." These youth were able to "envision the future" when they were feeling competent and had higher expectations for their behavior. These feelings and sentiments were not apparent in the absence of a caring relationship with an adult, and notably, with a reliable adult.

The study highlights ways in which PHNs can support resiliency among at-risk youth—either by being that reliable caring adult or by supporting the development and presence of these characteristics in mentors serving adolescents. At the community level, PHNs can also advocate for strategies that make the community more supportive of at-risk youth (e.g., development of after-school programs, internship experiences, and leadership opportunities). Sometimes PHNs experience conflict in balancing attention toward community-level factors, or population health, versus individual-level care, and the establishment of a caring relationship. The following Evidence Example demonstrates this in the prevention of tuberculosis outbreaks in a population through individual-level care efforts that were sometimes not welcomed (Bender, Peter, Wynn, Andrews, & Pringle, 2011).

Evidence Example: Welcome Intrusions: An Interpretive Phenomenological Study of TB Nurses' Relational Work

In a phenomenological (lived experience) study, Amy Bender, Elizabeth Peter, Francine Wynn, Gavin Andrews, and Dorothy Pringle (2011) conducted interviews and observed nurse-client relationships (N = 9 nurses, 24 clients). The nurses were employed in a public health department in Canada and had the challenge of building caring relationships with clients who had tuberculosis while fulfilling "surveillance-type" activities to ensure population health. The nurses described experiences that were characterized into an overarching description of "welcome intrusions," with three themes identifying the relationship process: "getting through the door," "doing TB but more than that," and "beyond a professional." The nurses shared stories that demonstrated the tension between establishing and maintaining a caring relationship with TB clients and also fulfilling surveillance obligations, which can come across as intrusive and oppositional to a caring relationship. PHNs undertaking these types of core activities need to give focused attention toward establishing caring relationships, particularly when surveillance and reporting requirements are associated with the care being delivered.

Maintains Appropriate Boundaries

Boundaries can be very challenging, yet they are so important in establishing and maintaining caring relationships. If the PHNs are too personal with and close to a client, they might not garner professional respect, but if they are too distant, the PHNs might not gain the client's trust. Knowing where the boundary is and when it should be moved or adjusted takes time, experience, and practice (see Table 9.2 for example warning signs of inappropriate boundaries in a nurse-client relationship). New PHNs can benefit from the insights of experienced PHNs, who undoubtedly have numerous positive and negative examples to share. Refer to Chapter 7 for a discussion of professional boundary issues.

Table 9.2 Example Warning Signs of Inappropriate Boundaries in a Nurse-Client Relationship

- Spending extra time with one client
- Changing client assignments to give care to a specific client
- Believing that other members of the team do not understand a specific client as well as you do
- Disclosing personal problems to a client or client's family member
- Thinking about a client frequently when away from work
- Being guarded or defensive when someone questions your interactions with a client
- Spending off-duty time with a client
- Ignoring agency policies when working with a specific client
- Keeping secrets with a client apart from the health team

Adapted from Nurses Association of New Brunswick, 2011, Appendix C

When PHNs work in a community where they also live, it is important that they establish appropriate boundaries when they encounters clients in social contexts (Sundelof, Hansebo, & Ekman, 2004). Accomplishing this comes with experience and the ability to simultaneously achieve closeness and appropriate distance. Setting limits is the nurse's responsibility, not the client's, and this is particularly important when PHNs are caring for someone with whom they might have had prior personal interactions (such as might often occur in rural communities).

 Evidence Example: Caring PHN-Family Relationships

A study was conducted in Manitoba, Canada, to describe the relationships among PHNs and families they visited in their homes as part of an early childhood program (Heaman, Chalmers, Woodgate, & Brown, 2007). Twenty-four PHNs and 20 parents were interviewed. All the nurses had at least a bachelor's degree and on average 14 years of work experience. Both nurses and parents spoke about three phases of the caring relationships: establishing, maintaining, and terminating them. It was clear that the best way to end the relationship was to establish a planned exit that occurred over the last few visits. Key characteristics of caring relationships were described, including respect, support, trust, partnership, and, for the nurses, appropriate levels of supervision and evaluation. A key finding was the maintenance of professional-client boundaries and the need for the PHNs to affirm the professional nature of the relationship. Study findings emphasized the need for the PHNs to put effort into establishing relationships not only with the clients but also with colleagues, such as "home visitors" (e.g., home health aides).

Another element of maintaining boundaries is taking care of yourself to ensure personal safety when you are working as a PHN. Personal safety is important for PHNs, who can often find themselves in vulnerable or potentially harmful situations. This need for caution clearly can influence the speed at which a caring relationship is developed, but PHNs should never place themselves at risk for personal harm to advance the relationship. Instead, PHNs should creatively explore ways in which relationships can be developed and safety can be maximized. However, note that seeking to be safe does not mean seeking to be comfortable. A home environment might be uncomfortable because of the presence of head lice, cockroaches, or clutter, but PHNs caring for this family need to work amid these factors. In doing so, they gain the family's respect and trust. If the PHNs were to keep the visits short because of their personal discomfort, it might be difficult to reach the level of a caring relationship that can yield positive, lasting results with the family.

In contrast, PHNs might feel unsafe if they observe criminal activities during a visit (e.g., drug use) or if the neighborhood is known for gang violence (see Table 9.3 for factors influencing safety when conducting home visits). Patricia Fazzone, Linda Barloon, Susan McConnell, and Julie Chitty (2000) conducted a study with PHNs and other home-visiting staff and observed that the staff members believed that risks to their personal safety were high, a finding consistent with additional research on safety for staff providing care in homes, public settings, and communities (Gellner, Landers, O'Rourke, & Schlegel, 1994; Kendra, Weiker, Simon, Grant, & Shullick, 1996; Schulte, Nolt, Williams, Spinks, & Hellsten, 1998). Fazzone et al. found that the staff believed that some personal characteristics were protective in terms of safety, including "self-confidence, self-reliance, self-motivation, flexibility, 'being comfortable with the unknown,' and self-assurance about their personal judgment" (2000, p. 49).

Generally, when students are assigned a public health nursing clinical experience, faculty members ensure that appropriate safety precautions are taken (see Table 9.4). Most clinical sites also review their policies and procedures for safety during orientation with new students. If a student is unsure of what to do or feels concerned about the safety involved in a clinical experience, that student should immediately approach a clinical instructor or preceptor before proceeding. For example, many students do not feel comfortable conducting home visits alone; although it is becoming more popular to assign students in pairs for home visits or to have students accompany PHNs, many programs continue to encourage students to conduct solo home visits. When a student is uncomfortable making a visit alone, that student needs to talk through the decision with a preceptor and clinical instructor. Similarly, students might be involved in planning a community health fair but might not feel comfortable attending the fair during evening hours. Students need to address their concerns with a clinical instructor and determine a plan that meets learning goals while maintaining appropriate levels of safety. Remember, too, that feeling uncomfortable in an unfamiliar environment or climate is not the same as feeling unsafe. In many public health nursing clinical experiences, it is common to feel uncomfortable but to learn through reflecting on those feelings and experiences.

Table 9.3   Factors Influencing Safety When Conducting Home Visits

Conditions in/outside the home	Environmental conditions	Organizational factors
• People loitering around the home or street • Known felon in home • Verbal, physical, and sexual aggression • Gangs and gang activity • Police raids and drug busts • Weapons and shootings • Garbage, debris • Poor lighting or ventilation • Homes in disarray • Pests • Pets • Secondhand smoke • Mental health instability of client/family	• Night travel • Traveling in remote areas • Increase in number of garage- or home-based methamphetamine labs • Domestic and/ or neighborhood violence • Poverty • Lack of cellular phone coverage	• Absence or inaccessibility of written policies/procedures • Safety policies not enforced • Safety policies not relevant to home care issues • Staff unfamiliarity with community • Lack or delay of security assistance • Cellular phones not provided for staff • Absence of "call-in" or "check-in" systems • Lack of or minimal administrative support • Staff delay or failure in reporting incidents • Staff not always aware of violent or unsafe history with clients or families

Source: Adapted from Fazzone et al., 2000, p. 47

Table 9.4   Safety Suggestions for Student Nurses Conducting Home Visits

Know the neighborhood

- Identify safe and/or unsafe public spaces.
- Identify businesses, such as gas stations, restaurants, or grocery stores, in the neighborhood that are safe places to go for help.
- Know which roads are open and passable.
- Avoid visits after dark.

Be prepared

- Make sure your gas tank is full and that your car has appropriate supplies in case you become stranded.
- If you are taking public transportation, know the transportation schedule.
- Carry your cell phone and make sure it is charged.
- Carry valuables on your person and leave your purse at home.
- Always let someone know your schedule of visits and changes that occur (e.g., cancellations).

Demonstrates Tact and Diplomacy

In a caring, professional relationship, PHNs act in tactful and diplomatic manners. Consistent with ethical standards and expectations, PHNs strive to develop caring relationships without consideration of personal or social characteristics, such as income level or social status (Fredriksson & Eriksson, 2006). Effective PHNs are consistent in how they deliver nursing care and services, including the effort they make in seeking and obtaining resources for clients and communities. Beth Crisp and Pam Lister (2004) describe how PHNs who were working with families involved in child protection situations made an effort to see all families so that they avoided the possibility that some families would feel stigmatized. Indeed, sometimes families who receive a visit from a social worker feel stigmatized or think that they are the worst families, however "worst" is defined. When PHNs are addressing sensitive issues with families or communities, acting in a tactful or diplomatic manner enhances the potential for effective impact and enables the PHNs to be viewed as allies (Crisp & Lister, 2004).

When PHNs act in a diplomatic manner that is considerate of the opinions, beliefs, ideas, and perspectives of others, they are more likely to be successful in establishing caring relationships. Diplomacy takes time and patience as well as a willingness to listen and truly hear what others are saying. Successful PHNs know this well and protect the time they need to serve individuals, families, and communities in a diplomatic manner. Thomas Gantert, Carol McWilliam, Catherine Ward-Griffin, and Natalie Allen (2009) found that for both clients and their family members, relationship building is critical to how they perceive the actions of the staff providing care in their home (e.g., PHNs, home health aides). The relationship is not static, but rather fluid, and requires ongoing attention and determination on the part of PHNs. An established caring relationship needs to be maintained, which requires tact, respect, patience, and the ability to perceive/assess the state of the relationship on an ongoing basis. Effective PHNs do not presume that the relationship, once established, is settled and certain. Instead, they regularly take note of the relationship dynamics and make efforts with every interaction to continue to build an optimal caring relationship. In this environment, interventions are successful and lasting, as reflected in both client feedback and observed outcomes.

Seeks Assistance When Needed in Managing Relationships

Unquestionably, nurses at all levels of experience bring an inherent desire to care and respond to a moral imperative to do so. However, it is also apparent that relationship skills are honed over time as inexperienced PHNs begin to appreciate the daily struggles of clients' lives and learn to judge what does and does not work with increasing refinement (SmithBattle, Diekemper, & Leander, 2004a, p. 9).

> *Susan was still not sure of the way she handled the situation with Julie and went to her supervisor. Her supervisor listened to Susan, and together they explored other options for wordage and interventions. Her supervisor shared some of her experiences and supported Susan's desire to see this family more often to monitor the status of the mother's mental health and the interactions with her children. Susan's supervisor reassured Susan that her caring relationship appeared strong and that her actions might have initiated actions by the mother that can improve her quality of life and safety of the family unit.*

Skills in developing and maintaining caring relationships are built over time; conscientious PHNs early in their careers seek the input and guidance of experienced PHNs as they encounter challenges in developing relationships with clients and communities. Asking busy colleagues to talk through a challenging situation can be difficult, yet positive results can come from doing this. Creative solutions or ideas for addressing a barrier often result from simply talking through the challenge with someone else. More often than not, other PHNs have experienced similar situations and have a variety of strategies they have used to overcome problems and succeed in developing caring relationships. Although rare, at times a PHN is unable to establish a caring relationship with a client; in this case, the PHN should bring the matter to a manager as soon as possible so that, if necessary, the client can receive care from another PHN. If this situation occurs, the PHN should not feel ineffective, especially if a solid effort has been made to develop a caring relationship. Sometimes characteristics or experiences beyond the control of a PHN make it difficult for a client to receive care from that PHN. For example, a student who has recently been sexually abused or assaulted might find it difficult to work with a client who has been sexually abused and needs resources to heal. Similar experiences can create a degree of closeness that makes it difficult for the student, or PHN, to remain separate from the client and provide appropriate nursing care.

ACTIVITY

What might be your plan of action in a situation such as the one presented in the paragraph above, in which the student has experienced a traumatic event similar to that of the client being served? In whom should the student confide?

More often than not, PHNs experience caring relationships with clients, families, and communities. Over time, they gain experience with each new client. As SmithBattle, Diekemper, and Leander offer, "Cumulative experience provides the foundation for becoming more responsive, for appreciating the strengths as well as the vulnerabilities and suffering of clients, for becoming more open and attentive to clients needs and concerns" (2004a, p. 9). Cumulative experience develops within each PHN but can also be shared across PHNs through case reviews or at staff meetings that provide opportunities to express challenges and seek input from peers.

The emphasis here on seeking input from peers is not meant to negate the effectiveness of new PHNs. Indeed, new PHNs often bring passion, energy, excitement, and determination to their roles in ways that can inspire and recharge their more experienced peers. New PHNs also experience much success in identifying and addressing client and community needs, sometimes because their optimism levels are high and matched by their willingness to act. This is not to say that experienced PHNs are not willing or optimistic, but rather that they are more likely to "ask first" rather than "act first, apologize later." This new nurse's story about identifying an unmet community need through a caring relationship the nurse had with her client is inspiring:

> There was this gentleman who had really bad toenails. And one of the family members asked if I could trim his toenails. I was like, "Well, I guess I can. I don't know why I can't." [Laughter] So I did, after soaking his feet. And they were really bad. Turns out that after I trimmed them, he stood up and started tap dancing. And this was a really old guy who had tap danced in another life. Well, of course, word got around. They would call, "Is the foot lady there?" [Laughter] It was actually kind of a nightmare. All these people needed nail care. . . . [Eventually] we started a foot clinic and got real podiatrists in. (SmithBattle, Diekemper, & Leander, 2004b, p. 98)

Ethical Considerations

Public health nursing often occurs in the places where people live, recreate, worship, and work, and indeed, health occurs "where we live, work, and play" (Robert Wood Johnson Foundation, 2010). These are very personal settings, and PHNs are frequently alone when delivering care. Caring relationships are critical to the success of what PHNs do with their clients (e.g., assessment, planning, intervention, and evaluation). Regardless of how simple or complex the care is, PHNs can accomplish much more in the presence of caring relationships. Among many potentially challenging ethical factors, PHNs can act in a way that optimizes empathetic care. Rosalind Ekman Ladd, Lynn Pasquerella, and Sheri Smith propose ethical ideas for building relationships that are cognizant of "decision-making authority and autonomy, allow the exercise of the nurse's moral rights, and recognize the patient's relationships to significant others" (2000, p. 103). It is interesting that Ladd et al. realize both the importance of autonomy among clients and the moral rights of the nurses. This recognition is important, because it emphasizes that PHNs are not expected to simply go along with everything their clients express to maintain caring relationships. Instead, effective PHNs use judgment in every situation so that they deliver optimal care, encourage autonomy, and respect client morals. At times, this requires PHNs to maneuver between contrasting opinions and preferences among the client and family members or community members. Caring relationships and subsequent interventions are rarely straightforward, but when ethical standards are upheld, the resulting outcomes are worth the invested effort.

A framework has been developed for relational ethics (i.e., the ethics of relationships) that gives attention to what the PHN needs to do to establish or encourage the development of a trusting relationship (Marcellus, 2005). This framework includes four themes: mutual respect, engaged interaction, embodiment, and creating environment. *Mutual respect* is an interesting combination of respect and empathy; it encompasses respect for oneself and for the other, yet it also includes receiving respect from others (Austin, Bergum, & Dossitor, 2003). And, similar to empathy (described earlier in this chapter), mutual respect occurs when the PHN seeks to understand, although not necessarily agrees with, the actions or circumstances of the individual, family, or community.

Engaged interaction means being responsive and sensitive in a manner that can counteract, to an extent, the powerlessness that some clients or communities might feel in relationship with a public health professional. This level of interaction can occur only when PHNs are willing and able to truly listen to those whom they are serving. Lee SmithBattle describes this as "listening with caring" (2003, p. 369); similarly, it is important to listen to provide responsive care to clients (SmithBattle, Drake, & Diekemper, 1997). Supporting teen mothers is a common role for PHNs, and listening with care means paying close attention to the context in which the teen mother is living and supporting her by "validating strengths, joys, difficulties, learning, and development" (p. 369). When PHNs are attuned to the teen mother's situation, needs, and strengths, they can maintain a relationship that facilitates effectiveness in the care they provide. Importantly, this care at times might simply mean being silent and listening to the teen mother. In an engaged, caring relationship, PHNs will know when to teach and when not to teach, allowing the relationship to be sustained and preserved.

It is not easy to be attuned to a client's perspectives, beliefs, fears, desires, and needs, but effective PHNs seek to achieve embodiment, the third theme of the relational ethics framework. *Embodiment* can appear to be somewhat esoteric (i.e., available only to the enlightened), but it is a useful and understandable concept. Simply, PHNs demonstrate embodiment when they grasp the essence of conversations—not only the mere words but also the intertwined meanings and emotions. In a caring relationship, PHNs need to value authenticity, which requires a willingness to be influenced by the nurse-client relationship.

The fourth element in the relational ethics framework is *environment*, emphasizing the need for PHNs to be in professional environments that encourage them to reflect and work through the moral dilemmas and ethical challenges they are going to encounter when establishing and maintaining caring relationships (Marcellus, 2005). PHNs regularly encounter dilemmas that challenge their beliefs, perspectives, and, at times, best intentions. In the context of a caring relationship, PHNs use reflection to arrive at the best decision for that moment, recognizing the emotions, needs, and vulnerability of those whom their decision will affect. For example, how do PHNs report child mistreatment while continuing to provide home-visiting services to the family? This is not an uncommon scenario that PHNs face in addition to numerous similar examples of difficult yet surmountable challenges to maintaining caring relationships with individuals, families, and communities. The list below identifies common reflective questions:

- How was I feeling during this experience?

- What does that experience mean for me?

- How can I use what I have learned from this situation as I move ahead?

- Is there another way I can think about this experience?

- What other things can I learn from this experience?

- How might the outcome have been different if I had . . . ?

- What other people were affected by my actions or inactions?

Susan continued to see Julie and her two children. Julie has received mental health services along with psychological support as she dealt with past issues and her newly diagnosed bipolar disease. Julie stabilized and appreciated the day Susan made her take stronger action for herself. The issue of safety now is part of the family home visits that they share. Susan continues to be committed to the relationship by empowering this mother, building on her strengths, providing her support through education, and of course, listening. Julie continues to feel that the relationship is beneficial and supportive for her. They both recognize that boundaries must exist in maintaining a caring and ethically strong nurse-family relationship.

 ## ACTIVITY

Which Cornerstones of Public Health Nursing (see Chapter 1) do you think are consistent with supporting the PHN's interventions in working with Julie and her children?

Table 9.5   Ethical Action in Establishing Caring Relationships

Ethical perspective	Application
Rule ethics (principles)	• In relationships, realize the autonomy and the authority to make decisions regarding individuals, families, and communities. • Encourage autonomy by asking the primary client which information can be shared with others, including other family members. • Encourage shared decision-making (e.g., client and PHN, or client, family, and PHN).
Virtue ethics (character)	• Remember that respect is critical to successful caring relationships. • Act in a manner that encourages a mutually trusting relationship. • Be patient with the development of a caring relationship.
Feminist ethics (reducing oppression)	• Respect beliefs, perspectives, feelings, opinions, ideas, cultural traditions, and preferences. • Recognize that most clients come to the relationship thinking that they have little power. • Encourage shared power in the relationship by practicing mutuality and empathy.

 # Key Points

- Caring relationships are core to effective public health nursing.

- Caring relationships can be established with individuals, families, communities, and systems.

- Caring relationships are built on trust, respect, and empathy.

- A caring relationship will not last if PHNs do not follow through on commitments, maintain appropriate boundaries, and demonstrate tact and diplomacy.

- PHNs need to operate in ways that are safe for themselves and others.

- Establishing a caring relationship might require PHNs to step outside their personal comfort zones but should never require them to work in an unsafe setting.

Learning Examples for Establishing Caring Relationships

The following learning examples represent some real-life situations in which PHNs have developed caring relationships and yet experienced challenges in providing care. As you read these examples, consider how you might respond and which resources you might access to overcome the challenges:

- A PHN is proactive in breastfeeding efforts and is working to increase breastfeeding statistics within the county where she works. After receiving education on the benefits of breastfeeding, a new mother states that she wants to formula feed her new infant. The PHN confirms this decision and then assists the mother, in a caring way, to properly feed her infant with formula/bottles.

- The PHN has gone three times to a home for a visit, and the family is not present. The nurse does not take this personally and continues to try to make a connection. The PHN believes that a caring relationship exists and that the visits did not occur because it was "a bad day" for the family. When the PHN finally reaches the family, she immediately states that she has missed seeing their family and asks whether everything is okay. She does not make them feel guilty about missing her visits and listens. This demonstration of concern reflects caring toward the family. The family had personal issues unrelated to the PHN, and now the PHN can continue to serve this family. Many new PHNs make the mistake of interpreting families not being at home as a signal that families do not want to see them, so they prematurely end the nurse-family relationship.

- PHNs share stories of their experiences in the wake of the devastation of hurricane Katrina. The establishment of caring relationships was essential at all levels of structure; maintaining the infrastructure of public health (systems level), establishing essential services within communities (community level), and of course, caring for families/individuals in need (family/client level). Many online and written resources explore the caring relationships that occurred during and following this natural disaster.

 Reflective Practice

The questions below provide additional opportunities for reflecting on the challenges a PHN can experience developing or working in a caring relationship with a client.

1. As you reflect on this chapter, do you believe that a caring professional relationship can also be a friendship? Why or why not? (See Chapter 7 for discussion on professional boundaries.)

_____

_____

2. Describe possible differences in development of a caring relationship if the initial visit with the client is at the clinic versus in the client's home.

   _____

   _____

3. A PHN has been seeing a family for several visits, and then the family is not home at the next planned visit. How might you address this absence with the family in a caring manner?

   _____

   _____

4. You are going on your first PHN family home visit. Which aspects of this visit might be uncomfortable for you? How will you deal with these feelings? How are these "uncomfortable aspects" different from "safety issues"?

   _____

   _____

5. PHNs value authenticity in caring relationships with their clients. How can PHNs better prepare themselves emotionally to be willing to be influenced by the relationship as much as the client is?

   _____

   _____

6. What are some ways in which trust between PHNs and clients could be threatened?

   _____

   _____

7. What can PHNs do if trust is broken with the client and the relationship is no longer caring or therapeutic?

   _____

   _____

8. What are possible implications if PHNs find themselves unable to care for a client and they do not address this concern but continue to provide care?

   _____

   _____

Application of Evidence

1. Identify the steps you take in your current nursing practice to develop effective caring relationships with clients.

2. Describe three resources available to you in public health nursing practice for difficult caring situations.

3. What are some ways PHNs can assess the extent to which their perceptions of the client-nurse relationship are similar to or different from the client's perceptions?

4. How might you apply the relational ethics framework to a specific public health nursing situation, such as needing to do surveillance for tuberculosis?

Think, Explore, Do

1. What makes self-awareness such an important part of caring effectively for another person?

2. What are some ways in which a PHN can progress to listening to more than what is said?

3. You are discussing with another PHN student the state teen pregnancy rate and this student states, "Teen mothers are not ready to be parents; it is so sad." How might you respond to share your knowledge of a caring relationship?

4. Describe the relationships that exist in your life, such as those that exist between you and your parents, siblings, peers, and friends. Describe the caring aspects of each of these relationships. Do you need to work harder at maintaining a caring relationship with some versus others?

5. Describe a friend's strengths. Ask this friend to describe his or her strengths. How do these two perspectives compare? How can you use this knowledge to build a stronger, caring relationship with this friend?

6. Describe a time when your first impression of someone was inaccurate. How did you come to realize the inaccuracy? How did this influence the relationship you then had with this person?

7. Reflect on the last argument that you had with someone. Would you have said or done something differently after reading this chapter?

References

Aronowitz, T. (2005). The role of "envisioning the future" in the development of resilience among at-risk youth. *Public Health Nursing, 22*(3), 200–208.

Austin, W., Bergum, V., & Dossitor, J. (2003). Relational ethics: An action ethic as a foundation for health care. In V. Tschudin (Ed.), *Approaches to ethics: Nursing beyond boundaries* (pp. 45–52). Woburn, MA: Buttersworth-Heinenmann.

Bender, A., Peter, E., Wynn, F., Andrews, G., & Pringle, D. (2011). Welcome intrusions: An interpretive phenomenological study of TB nurses' relational work. *International Journal of Nursing Studies, 48*(11), 1409–1419. doi:http://dx.doi.org/10.1016/j.ijnurstu.2011.04.012

Browne, A. J., Hartrick Doane, G., Reimer, J., MacLeod, M., & McLellan, E. (2010). Public health nursing practice with "high priority" families: The significance of contextualizing "risk." *Nursing Inquiry, 17*(1), 26–37.

Chafey, K. (1996). "Caring" is not enough: Ethical paradigms for community-based care. *Nursing and Health Care Perspectives on Community, 17*(1), 10–15.

Chismar, D. (1988). Empathy and sympathy: The important difference. *Journal of Value Inquiry, 22*(4), 257–266.

Crisp, B., & Lister, P. (2004). Child protection and public health: Nurses' responsibilities. *Journal of Advanced Nursing, 47*(6), 656–663.

Duiveman, T., & Bonner, A. (2012). Negotiating: Experiences of community nurses when contracting with clients. *Contemporary Nurse: A Journal for the Australian Nursing Profession, 41*(1), 120–125.

Fawcett, J. (2000). *Analysis and evaluation of contemporary nursing knowledge: Nursing models and theories.* Philadelphia, PA: F. A. Davis.

Fazzone, P. A., Barloon, L. F., McConnell, S. J., & Chitty, J. A. (2000). Personal safety, violence, and home health. *Public Health Nursing, 17*(1), 43–52.

Finfgeld-Connett, D. (2008). Qualitative convergence of three nursing concepts: Art of nursing, presence and caring. *Journal of Advanced Nursing, 63*(5), 527–534.

Fredriksson, L., & Eriksson, K. (2006). The ethics of the caring conversation. *Nursing Ethics, 13*(1), 138–148.

Gantert, T., McWilliam, C., Ward-Griffin, C., & Allen, N. (2009). Working it out together: Family caregivers' perceptions of relationship-building with in-home service providers. *Canadian Journal of Nursing Research, 41*(3), 44–63.

Gellner, P., Landers, S., O'Rourke, D., & Schlegel, M. (1994). Community health nursing in the 1990s—Risky business? *Holistic Nursing Practice, 8*(2), 15–21.

Heaman, M., Chalmers, K., Woodgate, R., & Brown, J. (2007). Relationship work in an early childhood home visiting program. *Journal of Pediatric Nursing, 22*(4), 319–330.

Jack, S. M., DiCenso, A., & Lohfeld, L. (2005). A theory of maternal engagement with public health nurses and family visitors. *Journal of Advanced Nursing, 49*(2), 182–190.

Jackson, C. (2010). Using loving relationships to transform health care: A practical approach. *Holistic Nursing Practice, 24*(4), 181–186.

Kendra, M. A., Weiker, A., Simon, S., Grant, A., & Shullick, D. (1996). Safety concerns affecting delivery of home health care. *Public Health Nursing, 13*(2), 83–89.

Ladd, R. E., Pasquerella, L., & Smith, S. (2000). What to do when the end is near: Ethical issues in home health care nursing. *Public Health Nursing, 17*(2), 103–110.

Marcellus, L. (2005). The ethics of relation: Public health nurses and child protection clients. *Journal of Advanced Nursing, 51*(4), 414–420.

Martins, D. C. (2008). Experiences of homeless people in the health care delivery system: A descriptive phenomenological study. *Public Health Nursing, 25*(5), 420–430.

McNaughton, D. B. (2005). A naturalistic test of Peplau's theory in home visiting. *Public Health Nursing, 22*(5), 429–438.

Morse, J. M., Bottorff, J., Neander, W., & Solberg, S. (1991). Comparative analysis of conceptualizations and theories of caring. *IMAGE: Journal of Nursing Scholarship, 23*(2), 119–126.

Morse, J. M., Solberg, S. M., Neander, W. L., Bottorff, J. L., & Johnson, J. L. (1990). Concepts of caring and caring as a concept. *Advances in Nursing Science, 13*(1), 1–14.

Nagano, H. (2000). Empathic understanding: Constructing an evaluation scale from the microcounseling approach. *Nursing and Health Sciences, 2*(1), 17–27.

Nurses Association of New Brunswick (2011). *Practice Standard: The Therapeutic Nurse-Client Relationship.* Retrieved from http://www.nanb.nb.ca/downloads/Practice%20Standard%20-%20Nurse-Client%20Relationship%20-%20E.pdf

Olthuis, G., Dekkers, W., Leget, C., & Vogelaar, P. (2006). The caring relationship in hospice care: An analysis based on the ethics of the caring relationship. *Nursing Ethics, 13*(1), 29–40.

Porr, C., Drummond, J., & Olson, K. (2012). Establishing therapeutic relationships with vulnerable and potentially stigmatized clients. *Qualitative Health Research, 22*(3), 384–396.

Ridgeway, S. (2010). Lillian Wald founded public health nursing. *Working Nurse.* Retrieved from http://www.working-nurse.com/articles/Lillian-Wald-Founded-Public-Health-Nursing

Robert Wood Johnson Foundation [RWJF]. (2010). A new way to talk about the social determinants of health. Retrieved from http://www.rwjf.org/files/research/vpmessageguide20101029.pdf

Schaffer, M. A., Jost, R., Pederson, B. J., & Lair, M. (2008). Pregnancy-free club: A strategy to prevent repeat adolescent pregnancy. *Public Health Nursing, 25*(4), 304–311.

Schulte, J. (2000). Finding ways to create connections among communities: Partial results of an ethnography of urban public health nurses. *Public Health Nursing, 17*(1), 3–10.

Schulte, J. M., Nolt, B. J., Williams, R. L., Spinks, C. L., & Hellsten, J. J. (1998). Violence and threats of violence experienced by public health field workers. *Journal of the American Medical Association, 280*(5), 439–442.

Shores, C. I. (2012). Caring behaviors of faith community nurses. *International Journal for Human Caring, 16*(3), 74.

SmithBattle, L. (2003). Displacing the "rule book" in caring for teen mothers. *Public Health Nursing, 20*(5), 369–376.

SmithBattle, L., Diekemper, M., & Leander, S. (2004a). Getting your feet wet: Becoming a public health nurse, part 1. *Public Health Nursing, 21*(1), 3–11.

SmithBattle, L., Diekemper, M., & Leander, S. (2004b). Moving upstream: Becoming a public health nurse, part 2. *Public Health Nursing, 21*(2), 95–102.

SmithBattle, L., Drake, M. A., & Diekemper, M. (1997). The responsive use of self in community health nursing practice. *Advances in Nursing Science, 20*(2), 75–89.

Smith-Campbell, B. (1999). A case study on expanding the concept of caring from individuals to communities. *Public Health Nursing, 16*(6), 405–411.

Sundelof, A. E., Hansebo, G., & Ekman, S.-L. (2004). Friendship and caring communion: The meaning of caring relationship in district nursing. *International Journal for Human Caring, 8*(3), 13–20.

Warelow, P., Edward, K. L., & Vinek, J. (2008). Care: What nurses say and what nurses do. *Holistic Nursing Practice, 22*(3), 146–153.

COMPETENCY # 8
Shows Evidence of Commitment to Social Justice, the Greater Good, and the Public Health Principles

Patricia M. Schoon
with Noreen Kleinfehn-Wald and Colleen B. Clark

Erica is a new public health nurse (PHN) in a large urban county where 40% of the children live in poverty. During Erica's home visit to a young family, the mother stated that the 2- and 3-year-old children had become "slow to get things and were tripping and falling more than usual." A year ago, the family had moved from a newer apartment building into a 70-year-old building when the husband lost his job. Erica noticed paint chips on the floor and was concerned that they were from lead-based paint. She advised the mother to have her children's blood lead levels checked. The mother said she did not have health insurance and could not afford a trip to the doctor. Erica told the mother the paint should be replaced, but the mother was concerned that the landlord would not listen to her. Erica consulted with her public health nursing supervisor about what else could be done.

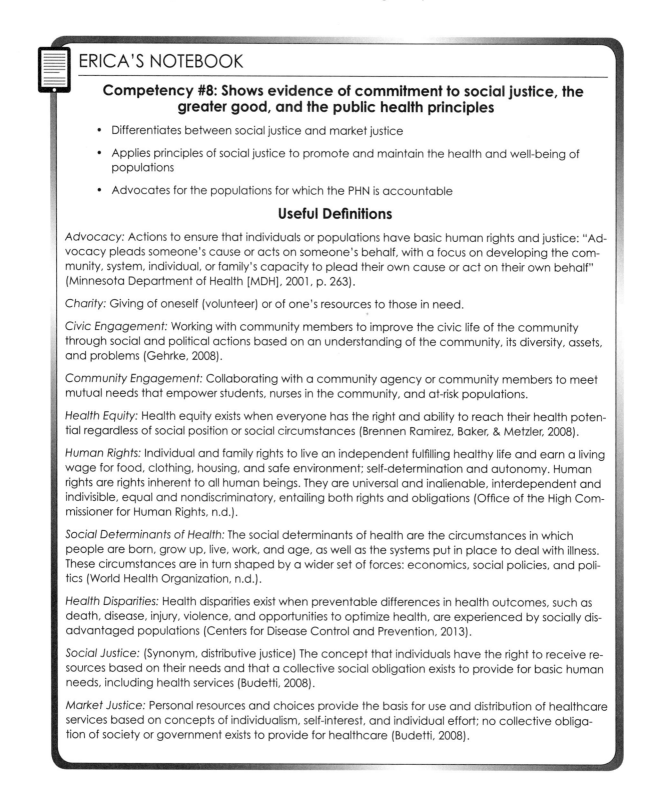

ERICA'S NOTEBOOK

Competency #8: Shows evidence of commitment to social justice, the greater good, and the public health principles

- Differentiates between social justice and market justice

- Applies principles of social justice to promote and maintain the health and well-being of populations

- Advocates for the populations for which the PHN is accountable

Useful Definitions

Advocacy: Actions to ensure that individuals or populations have basic human rights and justice: "Advocacy pleads someone's cause or acts on someone's behalf, with a focus on developing the community, system, individual, or family's capacity to plead their own cause or act on their own behalf" (Minnesota Department of Health [MDH], 2001, p. 263).

Charity: Giving of oneself (volunteer) or of one's resources to those in need.

Civic Engagement: Working with community members to improve the civic life of the community through social and political actions based on an understanding of the community, its diversity, assets, and problems (Gehrke, 2008).

Community Engagement: Collaborating with a community agency or community members to meet mutual needs that empower students, nurses in the community, and at-risk populations.

Health Equity: Health equity exists when everyone has the right and ability to reach their health potential regardless of social position or social circumstances (Brennen Ramirez, Baker, & Metzler, 2008).

Human Rights: Individual and family rights to live an independent fulfilling healthy life and earn a living wage for food, clothing, housing, and safe environment; self-determination and autonomy. Human rights are rights inherent to all human beings. They are universal and inalienable, interdependent and indivisible, equal and nondiscriminatory, entailing both rights and obligations (Office of the High Commissioner for Human Rights, n.d.).

Social Determinants of Health: The social determinants of health are the circumstances in which people are born, grow up, live, work, and age, as well as the systems put in place to deal with illness. These circumstances are in turn shaped by a wider set of forces: economics, social policies, and politics (World Health Organization, n.d.).

Health Disparities: Health disparities exist when preventable differences in health outcomes, such as death, disease, injury, violence, and opportunities to optimize health, are experienced by socially disadvantaged populations (Centers for Disease Control and Prevention, 2013).

Social Justice: (Synonym, distributive justice) The concept that individuals have the right to receive resources based on their needs and that a collective social obligation exists to provide for basic human needs, including health services (Budetti, 2008).

Market Justice: Personal resources and choices provide the basis for use and distribution of healthcare services based on concepts of individualism, self-interest, and individual effort; no collective obligation of society or government exists to provide for healthcare (Budetti, 2008).

Taking Action for What Is Right

Professional nurses have a social contract with their clients and the public to ensure that the healthcare needs of individuals, families, populations, and communities are met in a caring, nonjudgmental, just, and equitable manner. Nurses as professionals and as private citizens are guided by the rule of law that protects basic human rights and by ethical principles that undergird basic human rights and social justice, a core principle of public health. Nurses in public health are confronted with ethical issues or moral challenges surrounding human rights and social justice on a daily basis. Moral challenges are situations in which one's ethical beliefs are challenged and require critical thinking to arrive at a solution that protects the rights of individuals, families, and communities. The integration of caring, a core component of nursing, and social justice, a core component of public health, in conjunction with the moral challenge resulting when PHNs witness their clients experiencing health disparities and social injustice propel PHNs to become involved in social and political advocacy (Falk-Rafael & Betker, 2012).

As students, you will be challenged and at times conflicted by the decisions you face that require choosing between two important and good things. For example, do you decide to respect individual autonomy and confidentiality, or do you find it necessary to enforce a public health law? This chapter provides guiding principles for social justice, information about population health disparities that confront PHNs, and a framework for public health advocacy interventions to help prepare you for the difficult situations you may encounter as a student and a professional nurse. Civic engagement and community engagement are introduced as advocacy actions at the community level of practice.

Guiding Principles for Taking Actions for What Is Right

Principles of social justice and human rights provide a framework for the ethical principles of public health practice. The principles of social justice that are key to the health and well-being of populations include:

- Collective social responsibility for community members

- Responsibility of government to ensure the basic human rights and healthcare needs of its citizens

- Equitable allocation of healthcare resources based on need

- Protection of the rights of individuals and families to live safe, healthy, and fulfilling lives

Nurses are obligated by the American Nurses Association (ANA) Code of Ethics to provide fair and equal treatment that respects the "inherent dignity, worth, and uniqueness of every individual, unrestricted by considerations of social or economic status, personal attributes, or the nature of the health problem" (ANA, 2001, p. 7). Respect for human rights is a basic tenet of ethical nursing practice (ANA, 2010a; ANA, 2010b). The International Council of Nurses views healthcare as a basic right for all individuals (International Council of Nurses, 2006). Nurses have a responsibility to safeguard client rights at all times and are held accountable for both their actions and inactions. For example, a PHN might choose to have a translator present when providing health education and counseling to a woman who cannot speak English. A pregnant teen might ask her PHN not to inform her mother that she is pregnant. The PHN must honor that request, even though as the mother of a teen, she knows she would want to know if her daughter were pregnant.

The United Nations (1948) published *The Universal Declaration of Human Rights* detailing 30 articles defining human rights. The Preamble states, "Whereas recognition of the inherent dignity and of the equal and inalienable rights of all members of the human family is the foundation of freedom, justice, and peace in the world . . . a common understanding of these rights and freedoms is of the greatest importance." Articles 1 and 25 provide an international standard for health as a basic human right. Article 25 also speaks to many of the social determinants of health that have both societal and individual origins (Table 10.1).

Table 10.1   Selected Human Rights From the U.N.'s *Universal Declaration of Human Rights*

Article 1. All human beings are born free and equal in dignity and rights. They are endowed with reason and conscience and should act towards one another in a spirit of brotherhood. **Article 25.** (1) Everyone has the right to a standard of living adequate for the health and well-being of himself and of his family, including food, clothing, housing, and medical care and necessary social services, and the right to security in the event of unemployment, sickness, disability, widowhood, old age or other lack of livelihood in circumstances beyond his control. (2) Motherhood and childhood are entitled to special care and assistance. All children, whether born in or out of wedlock, shall enjoy the same social protection.

Source: United Nations, 1948

These human rights, especially those emphasizing access to living conditions that encourage health, guide much of the work that PHNs do. Sometimes advocating for the human rights of individuals and concurrently advocating for social justice for vulnerable individuals, families, or populations result in ethical conflicts. For example, laws that require reporting specific communicable diseases (e.g., sexually transmitted infections) are consistent with principles of social justice in meeting "the public good." However, mandated reporting violates the autonomy and anonymity of individuals and might interfere with the level of trust in a nurse-client relationship. Nurses have ethical responsibilities to protect the rights of individuals and to protect the health and welfare of the community. Consequently, some decisions require that nurses provide an ethical rationale for whether they choose to protect the individual or the community when protecting both simultaneously is not possible.

Public health has a code of ethics (Public Health Leadership Society, 2002) that directs public health professionals to act to protect vulnerable and at-risk populations and to work to eliminate health disparities (see Table 10.2 for principles and examples of PHN actions).

Table 10.2   Ethical Principles That Guide Public Health Professionals in Confronting Health Disparities

Principles	PHN practice examples
Public health should address principally the fundamental causes of disease and requirements for health, aiming to prevent adverse health outcomes.	• Focusing on primary prevention with individuals, families, and communities • Assessing the social determinants of health as part of the community assessment process • Sharing the data on the social determinants of health that adversely affect the health of community members
Public health should advocate and work for the empowerment of disenfranchised community members, aiming to ensure that the basic resources and conditions necessary for health are accessible for all.	• Targeting services to vulnerable and at-risk populations experiencing the greatest levels of health disparities • Advocating through the political process for funding and services for vulnerable and at-risk populations • Using an assets-based approach to collaborate with community members to empower them to manage their own healthcare needs
Public health programs and policies should be implemented in a manner that most enhances the physical and social environments.	• Providing services to the uninsured and underinsured in homes and in community and mobile clinics • Creating and providing culturally sensitive services • Collaborating with community organizations that provide safety-net services

Source: Public Health Leadership Society, 2002

 ACTIVITY
Reflect on the experiences you and your peers have participated in or observed as part of your community clinical. Were any of these ethical principles demonstrated in PHN practice?

PHN Advocacy for Population Health

Advocacy is considered a fundamental basis of nursing (Curtin, 1979; Gadow, 1999; MacDonald, 2006), while social justice is considered the fundamental basis of public health. The ANA (2013) directs PHNs to advocate for the protection of the health, safety, and rights of populations (Standard 16). To foster self-determination, facilitate empowerment, and promote self-advocacy, nurses need to create an atmosphere that supports and respects the rights of the populations they advocate for (Mallik, 1997). Nurses also need to feel and be empowered to take action (Cawley & McNamara, 2011). Table 10.3 outlines an empowerment framework for nurses.

Table 10.3   A Framework for Becoming Empowered and for Empowering Others

Definition	Components	Empowerment strategies
Personal power is the power you acquire and exercise through your informal and formal roles in your family and community.	• Personal roles: family and friends • Community roles: neighborhood, volunteer, elected official • Cultural and ethnic ties • Organizational membership: religious, political, other	• Become involved as a citizen with an issue you are passionate about. • Get to know your neighbors and community. • Identify yourself to family, friends, neighbors, community members, and stakeholders as a professional who is committed to improving the health of the community. • Participate in community or organizational meetings. Share your knowledge about healthcare. • Form linkages and networks between different groups and organizations that share common beliefs and goals. • Know your elected and appointed officials.
Professional power is the power you acquire and exercise through your formal role as a professional nurse.	• Legitimacy through licensure • Social contract with public • Professional expertise and competencies • Membership in professional organizations • Professional networks	• Find a professional and career mentor. • Join a professional nursing organization. • Attend conferences and meetings. • Continue your education through continuing education, certification, and formal higher education. • Strive to provide evidence-based care. • Develop strategies for monitoring quality and safety of care. • Role-model professional nursing practice. • Become a mentor for novice nurses.
Organizational power is the power you acquire and exercise through your formal and informal roles in your workplace and the healthcare system.	• Position and job description • Organizational communication • Coordination of care • Dispersed power of nursing throughout your organization and society	• Become involved in the work of the organization beyond patient care. • Become a member of a practice committee. • Collaborate with people in other disciplines, management, and administration. • Join an interdisciplinary group whose goal is improvement in patient care or population health. • Work with a consumer group to improve healthcare in your community. • Be politically active at the local level. Be GLOCAL: think global, act local. At some point, you may wish to become involved at the state and national levels.

Source: Schoon, Miller, Maloney, & Tazbir, Chapter 7, p. 188, from Kelly & Tazbir. Essentials of Nursing Leadership & Management (with Premium Web Site Printed Access Card), 3E. ©2014 Delmar Learning, a part of Cengage Learning, Inc. Reproduced with permission. www.cengage.com/permissions

Determining Public Health Priorities

PHNs need to identify the social justice and human rights issues they encounter in their practice to determine the actions they need to take and what their agencies' priorities should be. The following Evidence Example shows how one group of PHNs identified the common social justice and human rights issues that their clients experienced.

Evidence Example: Social Justice and Human Rights Issues Identified by Practicing PHNs

A focus-group process was used to identify social justice and human rights issues that cause staff PHNs to confront ethical dilemmas on a daily basis. Sixteen nurses working in a suburban-rural county public health agency participated in the focus group. They used storytelling to draw out examples of the social justice issues and human rights principles that were being violated. Four human rights and social justice inequities with examples emerged from this discussion, all of which had negative health status outcomes for the individuals, families, and populations involved (Kleinfehn-Wald, 2010).

Right to self-determination (human right)—Clients are in need of services but do not technically qualify according to the rules and regulations of the existing programs. For example, an elderly person might be in need of personal care attendant services but does not qualify for medical assistance, so the client remains at risk for placement in a long-term care facility.

Right to a standard of living adequate for the health and well-being of individuals and families (human right)—The working poor often work in entry-level jobs and earn salaries that make them ineligible for public services, even though their income is not enough to adequately support their families.

Autonomy (human right) versus greater good (social justice)—A client with a communicable disease chooses to break home isolation and exposes many people by going out in public. Or, parents choose not to vaccinate their child, who then becomes ill with pertussis (whooping cough) and exposes an entire classroom of children, including one child who is immuno-compromised.

Inequitable distribution of power, money, and resources (social justice)—Legal immigrants arriving in the state have received no health examination in their home country and are not provided with a health screening upon arrival in the United States. Other immigrants seeking admission to the country as refugees have a health examination prior to receiving the designation of refugee and, in addition, have a health screening upon arrival in their county of residence.

PHNs most often work with vulnerable individuals and families—those who are oppressed, marginalized, disenfranchised, or underserved and therefore at greater risk for disease, disability, and premature death. Although it is possible to improve the health status of individuals and families one by one, it is more effective, when possible, for PHNs to take actions to improve the health status of vulnerable populations as a whole:

The term "vulnerable populations" refers to social groups with increased relative risk (i.e., exposure to risk factors) or susceptibility to health-related problems. This vulnerability is evidenced in higher comparative mortality rates, lower life expectancy, reduced access to care, and diminished quality of life. Vulnerable populations are often discriminated against, marginalized and disenfranchised from mainstream society, contributing to their lower social status and lack of power in personal, social, and political relationships. (Center for Vulnerable Populations Research, n.d.)

Social Determinants of Health

The conditions that vulnerable populations experience are consistent with the World Health Organization's (WHO's; n.d.) definition of social determinants of health, "the circumstances in which people are born, grow up, live, work, and age, as well as the systems put in place to deal with illness. These circumstances are in turn shaped by a wider set of forces: economics, social policies, and politics." These social determinants of health have a significant impact on the health status of populations—often a negative one. Research has shown that interventions that address social determinants of health well in advance of identified health problems or concurrently with medical care improve health and reduce health disparities (Williams, Costa, Oduniami, & Mohammed, 2008).

The Commission on the Social Determinants of Health, established by the WHO in 2005, recommends that the focus be on creating the conditions in which health and well-being can flourish (Baum, Gollust, Goold, & Jacobson, 2007). The Commission made three recommendations for action: (1) improving daily living conditions in which people are born, grow, live, work, and age; (2) tackling the inequitable distribution of power, money, and resources; and (3) measuring and understanding the problems of health inequities and assessing the impact of action (Baum et al., 2007). The United Nations (2013), recognizing the significant impact of social determinants of health on population health worldwide, has been working on achieving eight Millennium Development Goals (MDG) for more than a decade. All are directed at reducing social determinants of health or reducing health conditions that are significantly related to the social determinants of health (Table 10.4). Look for the website in Chapter 10 Resources (Appendix B) to explore the MDGs and think about how you might be able to contribute to achieving these MDG in your own community.

Healthy People 2020 One of the Social Determinants Leading Health Indicators in Healthy People 2020 is being a student who graduates with a regular diploma 4 years after starting ninth grade. In 2007–2008, the percentage of students graduating in 4 years was 74.9%. The target for 2020 is 82.4%, or a nearly 10% increase. How might an increased graduation rate improve population health status? Which actions might PHNs or school nurses take to help increase the 4-year high school graduation rate?

Table 10.4 U.N. Millennium Development Goals (MDGs) and Examples of Social Determinant Targets and Progress

Goals	Examples of social determinant targets
Goal 1: Eradicate poverty and hunger. *Goal 2:* Achieve universal primary education. *Goal 3:* Promote gender equality and empower women. *Goal 4:* Reduce child mortality. *Goal 5:* Improve maternal health. *Goal 6:* Combat HIV/AIDS, malaria, and other diseases. *Goal 7:* Ensure environmental sustainability. *Goal 8:* Global partnership for development.	Goal 1: The number of people who live on $1/day has been halved since 1990, but 1.2 billion people still live in extreme poverty. Goal 2: From 2000 to 2011, the number of primary school age children out of school decreased from 102 million to 57 million. Goal 3: Only 2 of 130 countries have achieved gender parity at all levels of education (1990–2011). Goal 7: Global emissions of carbon dioxide have increased by more than 46% since 1990. Goal 7: More than 2.1 billion people have gained access to improved water sources, and almost 1.9 billion people have gained access to sanitation facilities since 1990.

Source: United Nations, 2013

The following Evidence Example on the Safe Motherhood Initiative describes the history of global efforts to improve the safety of pregnancy and childbirth that provides the link to MDG 5, Improve Maternal Health.

 Evidence Example: Safe Motherhood Initiative

Although maternal and infant mortality declined significantly in developed countries in the 19th and first half of the 20th centuries, it did not change in undeveloped countries. The international Safe Motherhood Initiative, launched in 1987, focused on improving infant and maternal health in developing countries. Not until 1994 did the UN International Conference on Human Rights declare the right of women to go through pregnancy and childbirth safely. This was the beginning of the movement to view maternal mortality as a human rights issue and a public health concern. Ten years after the Safe Motherhood Initiative was launched, a study of outcomes found that very little had changed. In 2008, it was estimated that 536,000 women die annually from pregnancy-related causes and that an estimated 4 million babies die during the first 4 weeks of life, of which 3 million die in the first week. Women in resource-poor countries have a 1 in 16 chance of dying of pregnancy-related causes compared to women in countries with good resources, where the risk is 1 in 4,800. Although life-saving measures and injury treatment exist for women who are pregnant and birthing, many women do not have access to these services. This lack of access is a major human rights issue that must be addressed through government policy, legislation, and service delivery (Gruskin et al., 2008).

Health Equity and Health Disparities

A major goal of public health is to achieve health equity; health equity exists when everyone has the right and ability to reach their health potential regardless of their social positions or social circumstances (Brennen Ramirez, et. al., 2008). Reutter and Kushner (2010, p. 272) outline the requirements of health equity as follows:

- Resources should be allocated equitably and fairly.

- Human rights perspective includes the right to health and its prerequisites, the right to participate fully in society, and the right to nondiscrimination.

- Access to healthcare and the social determinants of health (social, economic, material, cultural, and political structures) should be equitable.

- Health equity is shaped by politics and achieved through the political process.

- Achieving health equity requires an intersectional approach (beyond the healthcare sector).

Nurses have a mandate to promote health equity and social justice by taking actions to reduce health disparities (Reutter & Kushner, 2010). Health disparities exist when preventable differences in health outcomes such as death, disease, injury, violence, and opportunities to optimize health are experienced by socially disadvantaged populations (Centers for Disease Control and Prevention, 2013). PHNs know from experience that the populations they serve experience different levels of health status and have differing abilities to achieve their health potential. These disparities in health status are often the result of social determinants of health that negatively affect individual and family health outcomes and are not within the control of individuals and families to change. PHNs work to eliminate the social determinants of health that lead to health inequalities or health inequities:

- *Health inequalities* are differences in health disparities based on social conditions that may be temporary and reflect the level of deprivation of one group versus another group.

- *Health inequities* are systematic disparities in health and in the major social determinants of health between diverse populations with different social positions that persist over time (i.e., race, class, and advantages or disadvantages, such as wealth, power, and prestige) and are the result of long-term entrenched social practices and institutional structures.

The following Evidence Example is an illustration of health inequalities in a group of shelter-based foster children.

 Evidence Example: Immunization Rates in Shelter-Based Foster Youth

A study of shelter-based foster youth in Baltimore found that only 10.7% had documented up-to-date immunizations, only 1.2% had a documented PPD (Mantoux testing for tuberculosis) application and reading, and 13.1% had a significant delay in recommended follow-up to care. Center staff members were not aware of many of the foster youth's health needs. This study demonstrated that shelter-based foster youth had significantly less access to healthcare than non-shelter-based foster youth (Ensign, 2001).

WEB-BASED ACTIVITY

The infant death rate is a global gold standard of evaluating the quality of healthcare within a country or for a specific population. For example, the U.S. non-Hispanic Black infant death rate was 2.4 times higher than that of non-Hispanic Whites; the American Indian/Alaskan Native rate was 48% higher (Centers for Disease Control and Prevention [CDC], 2011).

Go to Chapter 10 Resources to find the websites for the following activities:

- How does your state's infant mortality rate compare with other U.S. states? You might want to use Kids Count data as well as other state data.

- Look for examples of other morbidity and mortality health disparities by race and ethnicity. You might want to use the CDC website for your search or find data from the state you live in. Identify three disparities that surprise you.

ACTIVITY

Have you observed any health disparities, health inequalities, or health inequities among the populations you and your peers are working with during your community clinical? Which social determinants of health might be involved in causing these disparities? If you wish to explore this topic in more depth, you can visit the Robert Wood Johnson websites about health disparities and social determinants of health. You can find the websites in Chapter 10 Resources (Appendix B).

A comparison of life expectancy among different social groups in the United States illustrates health disparities that may also be considered health inequalities or health inequities. For example, the gap in life expectancy between the rich and the poor and those with more education versus those with less education is widening (Congressional Budget Office, 2008). Gender and racial gaps in life expectancy continue to persist (Figure 10.1). In 2000, 83,500 more African Americans died than would have died if African Americans had not experienced differences in the social determinants of health and reduced access to healthcare services for centuries (Satcher & Higginbotham, 2008). Although gaps in life expectancy might be partially explained by lifestyle decisions and biological factors, societal factors also play a role. Those who are poor or live in poor neighborhoods have less access to healthy food, parks and public spaces, jobs, and education (p. 2). Children from low-income families are about seven times as likely to be in poor or fair health compared to children in the highest-income families (California Newsreel, 2008, p. 1). In a study of 40,000 children, obesity rates for all U.S. children ages 10 to 17 increased 10% from 2003 to 2007, while the rate increased 23% for low-income children (Singh, Siahpush, & Kogan, 2010). Extensive data on health disparities are available on the Centers for Disease Control and Prevention (CDC) website. Data comparisons by race and sex on key health disparities are presented in Figures 10.1 and 10.2.

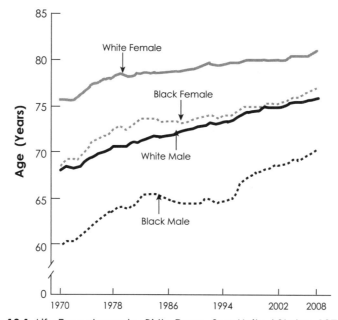

Figure 10.1. Life Expectancy by Birth, Race, Sex: United States, 1970–2008

Note: In 2008, the life expectancy for (a) non-Hispanic Black population = 73.7;
(b) Hispanic population = 81.0; (c) non-Hispanic White population = 78.4.

Source: U. S. Department of Health and Human Services, 2012

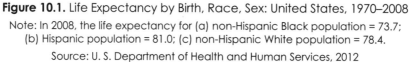

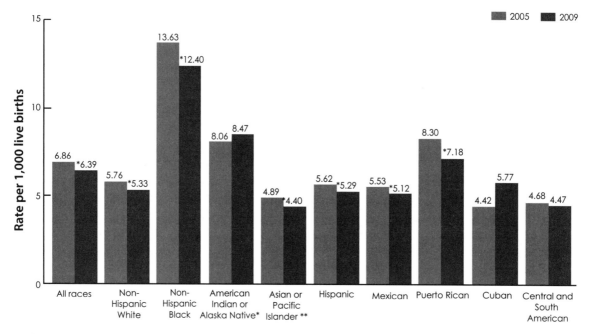

* Significant decline.

** Includes persons of Hispanic and non-Hispanic origin

Figure 10.2. Infant Mortality Rates by Race and Ethnicity of Mother: United States, 2005 and 2009

Source: U.S. Department of Health and Human Services, 2013

Dealing with the issue of health disparities often appears overwhelming. Tools to identify the disparities in specific populations and their causes help PHNs and their partners develop targeted interventions. One example is a Health Equity Assessment Tool (HEAT) developed in New Zealand (Signal, Martin, Cram, & Roberts, 2008) that provides a planning and intervention process to identify and reduce health disparities in the Maori population. Table 10.5 provides a list of 10 questions that guides the process from assessment through intervention. If you wish to view the comprehensive user's guide, look for the Health Equity Assessment Tool website in the Chapter 10 Resources (Appendix B). Note that the terms *inequalities* and *inequities* are used as synonyms in the HEAT Tool..

Table 10.5 The Ten HEAT Planning Process Questions to Reduce Health Disparities Among Maori

1. Which inequalities exist in relation to the health issue under consideration?
2. Who is most advantaged and how?
3. How did the inequities occur? What are the mechanisms by which the inequalities were created, maintained, or increased?
4. Where/how will you intervene to tackle the issue?
5. How will you improve Maori health outcomes and reduce health inequalities experienced by the Maori?
6. How could this intervention affect health inequalities?
7. Who will benefit most?
8. What might the unintended consequences be?
9. What will you do to make sure the intervention does reduce inequalities?
10. How will you know whether inequalities have been reduced?

Source: Signal, Martin, Cram, & Robson, 2008

It is also useful to look at the bigger picture of health disparities by comparing U.S. statistics with those of other countries and to examine overall global comparisons. The National Academy of Sciences (2013) reported that the United States has higher rates of chronic disease and mortality among adults and higher rates of untimely deaths and injuries among adolescences and small children than its peer countries. These differences in rates among peer countries could not be explained by racial, ethnic, economic status, or certain health behaviors, such as smoking or obesity. Multiple health determinants, including unhealthy behaviors, adverse social conditions, unhealthy environments, and healthcare system deficiencies, were identified (National Research Council and Institute of Medicine, 2013, pp. ix–x). Figure 10.3 compares the U.S. health disparity in mortality to that of other peer countries. This report suggests that it might be time to consider the dual upstream-downstream approach (discussed later in this chapter).

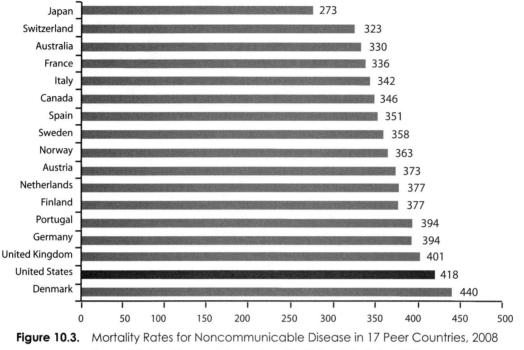

Figure 10.3.   Mortality Rates for Noncommunicable Disease in 17 Peer Countries, 2008
Source: National Research Council and Institute of Medicine, 2013

Market Justice versus Social Justice

Globally, healthcare systems vary but are generally based on principles of market justice, social justice, or a combination of the two. The U.S. healthcare system, like the rest of the U.S. economy, is based on free enterprise and the principles of market justice. An alternative healthcare system, based on social justice, is embodied in the nonprofit and governmental healthcare systems. (See Chapter 6 for a discussion of public and private healthcare systems in the United States.) Advocates of *social justice* believe that the government has a role to play in the provision of and assurance of basic health services to its citizens. Advocates of *market justice* believe that individuals and the private sectors are better prepared to meet the healthcare needs of private citizens. Social justice requires that the government be responsible and accountable for the health and well-being of its citizens. Market justice requires that individuals be responsible for their own health and well-being. Table 10.6 compares the concepts of market and social justice relative to healthcare.

Table 10.6 Market Justice versus Social Justice in the United States

MARKET JUSTICE	SOCIAL JUSTICE
People are entitled only to those valued ends, such as status, income, and happiness, that they acquire by individual efforts, actions, or abilities. The principles and beliefs include: • Individual rights and responsibility • Death and disability as individual responsibilities and problems • Minimal collective action • Freedom to act with minimal obligations for the common good • Respect for the rights of individuals • Individuals and the local private and public sector having responsibility and control over health and healthcare • Local short-term goals that are treatment oriented • Government infringement on individual rights, its inefficiency, and mistrust of it • Support for the medical model of healthcare	People in society receive benefits by belonging to a community, and the burdens and benefits of society should be fairly and equitably distributed. The principles and beliefs include: • Individual rights as members of the community • Death and disability as collective responsibilities and problems • Collective action for the common good • General obligation to protect individuals against disease and injury • Quality of life; stewardship of future • Private business's obligation to the community as a whole • Global, long-term goals that are prevention oriented • Government obligation and responsibility to protect citizens and trust that it will do the right thing • Support of a universal or single-payer model of healthcare

Source: Based on work by Keller, 2010 & Beauchamp, 2013

The United States has a dominant and enduring cultural value of individualism—a belief that individuals are able create their own destiny and that individual rights are more important than society's rights (Ludwick & Silva, 2000). This cultural belief presents a significant barrier to the development of a social justice model of healthcare. It is important for nurses in the United States to understand the cultural values of our society to determine how health equity might be achieved.

Reducing Health Disparities—Downstream versus Upstream Approach

Evidence has shown that the medical model alone, based on market justice, will not eliminate health disparities. Research demonstrates that health disparities in the United States are worsening (Iton, 2008). Based on surveillance data, an estimated 83,570 excess deaths could be prevented annually if the Black-White mortality gap could be eliminated (Satcher & Higginbotham, 2008). Social determinants of health have been identified as a major cause of health disparities; however, the medical model deals primarily with individual causes of morbidity and mortality, such as genetics, healthcare access and quality, and individual health knowledge and behaviors. When the focus of healthcare is on the individual experiencing disease (secondary and tertiary prevention), this is called the *downstream approach.* Interventions aimed at reducing these causes, although important, will not by themselves alleviate health disparities. Individuals and families do not have equal access to private healthcare systems, governmental supports, or societal resources.

Social determinants of health that are structural (i.e., income, education, housing, employment, social power, and opportunity) and those that are spatial (i.e., geographic locations within neighborhoods, cities, counties, states, and areas of the country, and concentration of poverty and race in specific neighborhoods) need to be addressed to reduce racial and ethnic health disparities. When the focus of healthcare is on modifying the social determinants of health to prevent disease and disability (primary prevention), this is called the *upstream approach.* Beauchamp (2013) argues that collective societal and governmental action based on social justice is necessary to protect the health of the public and that the burdens and benefits of these efforts should be shared equally except in situations where health disparities exist. However, there is no consensus within U.S. society for this position. Iton (2008) advocates a dual upstream-downstream approach (Figure 10.4). The dual approach involves taking an upstream approach to prevent disease and improve the health of populations while maintaining the downstream approach that treats individuals' diseases and disabilities. Figure 10.4 illustrates the dual upstream-downstream approach.

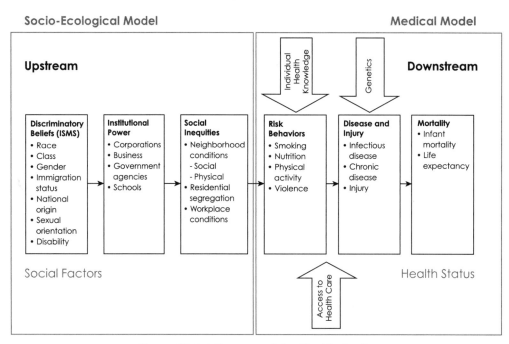

Figure 10.4. A Framework for Health Equity
Source: Alameda County Public Health Department, 2008.
Adapted from Bay Area Regional Health Inequities Initiative, 2008.

<u>ACTIVITY</u>

Discuss how you have experienced or observed the upstream versus downstream approaches to healthcare and health disparities personally and professionally. What are the costs of and benefits to each approach? Where do you see yourself as an individual citizen and as a healthcare provider fitting into the dual model approach?

Advocacy

Caring leads to advocacy, and PHNs care passionately about those experiencing health disparities. PHNs enter into the practice of "critical caring" when they recognize health disparities in individuals and families and work to change the context of people's lives to improve their health (Falk-Rafael, 2005a, 2005b; Falk-Rafael & Betker, 2012). It is not always easy to advocate for clients, either at the individual or population level of public health practice. Social justice dilemmas are part of the everyday lives of nurses. What is different for PHNs is that they often have to confront and resolve these dilemmas when they are out in the community by themselves. In an acute care setting, ethics committees can usually assist in resolving ethical issues related to autonomy, rights to self-determination, rights to refuse treatment, and rights to a safe and comfortable death. In the home and community setting, PHNs are often practicing alone, although they consult with other health team members when faced with challenging situations. Sometimes ethical decisions related to social justice and human rights need to be made during a home visit, such as placing a client who is not taking his antiviral tuberculosis medications on Directly Observed Therapy (DOT), reporting unsafe "garbage" homes to the county sanitarian, or contacting animal control about a client's pet that has just bitten a young child. Sometimes PHNs carry out advocacy interventions by themselves, and sometimes they are part of a group advocating for change.

Advocacy at the Individual/Family Level of Public Health

Nurses advocate for individuals and families by safeguarding their autonomy, acting on their behalf, and championing social justice in the provision of healthcare (Bu & Jezewski, 2006). Advocacy is aimed at building the capacity of individuals or families to manage their own healthcare needs. PHNs recognize the inequalities that exist within social determinants of health and challenge the status quo to change the social environment.

When PHNs advocate for individuals and families, they often do so within trusting relationships (MacDonald, 2006). For example, over time, nurses working with abused individuals and families often become aware of the abusive situations when they are providing trustworthy care for common physical health conditions. Trusting relationships make it possible for the clients to disclose very personal information about abuse, and then the nurses can effectively intervene and advocate for safety (Hughes, 2010; Vanderburg, Wright, Boston, & Zimmerman, 2010). (See Chapter 9 for more information on caring relationships.)

PHNs are aware that they can take actions to advocate for specific health needs of families that are related to both individual health determinants and social health determinants. They know that individuals and families can only change health determinants that are related to their own biological, behavioral, and life circumstances. They generally cannot change the health determinants that are societal in nature, or the social determinants of health. (See Chapter 1 for a discussion of health determinants, protective factors, and risk factors.) Key social determinants of health that influence access to healthcare resources and affect health and well-being include neighborhood living conditions (poverty or crime levels, housing quality), employment opportunities, community development and social cohesion, and the prevailing norms, customs, and lifestyle of the population. Table 10.7 represents the diverse health determinants Erica identifies in working with the family whose children have elevated blood-lead levels. The scenario demonstrates how Erica intervenes at the individual/family, community, and systems levels to build on the protective factors and modify the risk factors to improve the children's health. You may wish to review protective and risk factors discussed in Chapter 1.

Table 10.7 Erica's Clients: Health Determinant Analysis—Risk for Elevated Blood Lead Levels in Children

Individual/Family health determinants

Protective factors	Risk factors
• Mother exhibits health-seeking behaviors and accepts assistance from the PHN and public health resources. • Children are healthy except for increased lead levels. • Apartment owner is concerned about the tenants' health and willing to apply for funding for lead abatement.	• Exposure to lead-based paint in home • Children's developmental stages and ages • Children's liver and kidneys unable to excrete excess lead • Family's inability to afford safe housing • Lack of medical insurance

Social determinants of health—Community level

Protective factors	Risk factors
• Community volunteer resources for transportation • Faith-based resources • Community health priorities of child health and environmental health	• Older substandard housing with lead-based paint • Lack of safe, affordable housing • High poverty level due to poor economy • Downsizing of local businesses

Social determinants of health—Systems level

Protective factors	Risk factors
• Taxpayer funding of public health services • Public health nursing services available • Environmental health services available • Medicaid and CHIP funds for healthcare available for low-income, uninsured families • Local clinic willing to admit Medical Assistance clients • Free lead-level testing at local clinic • Lead-abatement funding available	• Lack of affordable private or public health insurance • Limited access to affordable healthcare • Fewer medical clinics accepting Medical Assistance clients

Erica receives a phone call from the mother of the children with high lead levels. She has been able to enroll her children in a state-run healthcare plan and is looking for a medical clinic on a bus line. The clinic she finds is no longer taking patients on government assistance. Erica knows that not many medical clinics are in the mother's neighborhood and cannot think of one on a bus line. She checks the county's database on medical clinics and the metropolitan transportation agency website to investigate bus service routes. She contacts the American Red Cross and faith-based and charitable organizations in the neighborhood for transportation assistance. These searches take an entire afternoon, but Erica is successful in finding a clinic that accepts people on government assistance and a local church that has a volunteer transportation program. Erica asks her supervisor how to code these hours on her time sheet, as she is not providing direct nursing care. Her supervisor tells Erica that she is carrying out the nursing interventions of Advocacy and Case Management by finding resources that can help her client become more self-sufficient. Erica returns to the family and draws blood from the children. Environmental Health staff has visited the family's apartment to determine whether the paint and paint chips were lead-based. Two weeks later, Erica, her PHN supervisor, and the Environmental Health staff meet to review their findings. Both children have increased blood lead levels, and a significant amount of lead-based paint has been found throughout the apartment. Erica arranges for the mother and children to be seen in the county public health clinic. Chelation therapy is recommended for the children, but the county does not provide that service. Lead abatement is recommended for the apartment building, but the owner says that he cannot afford it.

Erica knows that the human rights of the families in the apartment complex are at risk because of their exposure to lead-based paint and inability to change their living situation because of poverty and lack of affordable and safe housing. She knows that the human rights of the children cannot be met if they cannot receive the medical care they need. Realizing that the individual rights of the apartment owner are in conflict with the social justice rights of the apartment residents, Erica tries to find just solutions. Erica refers the family to a social worker to apply for the state Medicaid/ Medical Assistance program and Children's Health Insurance Program (CHIP) services. She thinks funding is available for medical treatment for the children through these programs. Erica also refers the apartment owner to a state program that provides financial assistance for lead abatement. The apartment owner is relieved to know that he can get financial assistance for lead abatement to provide a safer environment for his tenants.

Erica reflects on the positive health outcome for the two children with increased lead levels and the lead abatement of the apartment building that is scheduled for next month. She remembers that she had been in a hurry on the home visit and was impatient when the mother started talking about her children rather than responding to the questions Erica was asking. Luckily, Erica managed to focus on the mother's concerns rather than her own. She knows that if she had not taken the time to listen carefully, she might have missed the mother's comments about the children's symptoms and might not have noticed the paint chips. Erica renews her commitment to listen to clients telling her what their priorities and needs are. She decides she will be more observant when assessing the homes and neighborhoods of children in her caseload. Erica knows that collecting data and reporting her findings are the first steps in advocating for change.

Advocacy at the Community and Systems Levels of Public Health

To reduce health disparities, PHNs need to be engaged in interventions at both community and systems levels of practice. PHNs spend most of their time working with individuals and families to modify their health determinants (i.e., reduce their risk factors and strengthen their protective factors) and empower them to manage their own healthcare needs. PHNs are interested in reducing health disparities among populations as well. To do this, PHNs must understand the multiple causes or health determinants that influence populations' health statuses. Individuals and families within populations that experience health disparities suffer consequences even if their personal behaviors and biological/genetic factors encourage health. Thus, PHNs must advocate for change in the societal causes of population health disparities by working at the community and systems levels of practice. Working with individuals and families to help them change their own behaviors and risk factors cannot by itself eliminate health disparities at the population level. In a perfect world, health resources would be infinite, and everyone would have access to all the healthcare they need. Unfortunately, this is not the case, and much of the time people cannot even agree on the type of healthcare that is needed. It is important for PHNs to work with other community members to create a sustainable community partnership to work to achieve health equity. Figure 10.5 illustrates the components of a community partnership model to achieve health equity.

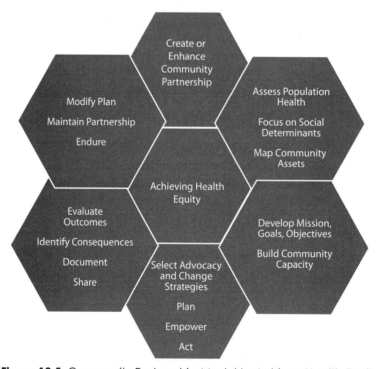

Figure 10.5. Community Partnership Model to Achieve Health Equity

Source: Modified from *Promoting Health Equity: A Resource to Help Communities Address Social Determinants of Health*, Brennen Ramirez, et al. 2008, p. 33

Civic Engagement as Social Justice Intervention

As advocates for social justice, PHNs by necessity must be involved in the civic life of their communities to have an impact on the social determinants of health. Nurses have both professional and citizenship obligations to the communities in which they work and live as part of the collective responsibility for social action to improve population health. Civic engagement involves working to improve the civic life of communities in partnership with community members. Nursing students who participate in civic engagement develop knowledge, skills, values, and motivations to make a difference (Gehrke, 2008, p. 53–54). Many nursing students are comfortable volunteering in their communities as a form of charity. These actions are commendable, but volunteering is not considered civic engagement. Charity is downstream action—an adaptive response to ameliorate the outcomes of societal inequities and health disparities. Civic engagement involves more than charity. It is a means to achieve social justice through upstream actions—changing the social structure that creates health disparities. It involves social and political advocacy. Like others, you might tend to prefer to carry out acts of charity and avoid political engagement (Gehrke, 2008; Iton, 2008). However, it is important that you participate in civic engagement at some point in your nursing education and career. Civic engagement may occur at the local, national, and international levels (see Chapter 13 for information on political advocacy).

 Evidence Example: National Association of School Nurses: Speaking Up for Children

The National Association of School Nurses (NASN) advocates for child health and the resources needed to promote health and safety among school children. School nurses are aware of the significant number of children coming to school with preventable physical and mental health conditions. School nurses work hard to obtain the needed health and social services for these children, but they know that they cannot solve the problem of inadequate resources by working one nurse to one child at a time. NASN has a history of lobbying for school health resources to meet children's needs. To more effectively lobby at the national level, NASN moved its headquarters to Washington, D.C., in 2005. The NASN Annual Conference in 2005 brought hundreds of school nurses to Washington, D.C.; prepared them for lobbying efforts; and provided opportunities for the nurses to meet with their elected representatives to talk about child and school health issues, explain the role of the school nurse, and discuss the positive impact school nurses have on child health. The NASN 2007 policy agenda, Capital Investment for Children, was an effort to secure a place at the national policy-making table for school nurses so that they could advocate for children with unmet health needs. NASN continues its efforts to work with national, state, and local officials to achieve its goal of achieving a ratio of school nurses to students in each school that can adequately meet their health needs (Denehy, 2007).

Community Engagement as Advocacy

Nursing students carry out their public health nursing clinicals in the community setting. More and more often, their clinicals include providing services to at-risk or vulnerable clients in community safety-net agencies and programs. The primary goal of healthcare safety-net programs is to ensure that no citizen's access to essential health services, regardless of the individual's socioeconomic condition, falls below a certain level (Redlener & Grant, 2009). You may work with these agencies as a volunteer, or you may wish to become involved in community engagement, an advocacy intervention. Community engagement involves collaborating with a community agency or community members to meet mutual needs that empower students, the community, and the at-risk population. These learning activities are often structured as service-learning experiences in which the students learn public health nursing by providing a needed service—a win-win situation for students, the safety-net organization, and the at-risk population it serves. The services and interventions you provide should enrich the healthcare abilities of the agency and build organizational capacity. By acknowledging and building on the strengths that already exist, you are adding to the community's assets and strengthening its ability to manage its own healthcare needs. Public health nursing advocacy involves empowering vulnerable populations and their communities through capacity-building.

When you participate in a community engagement clinical activity, your public health nursing instructor may structure the learning activity as a service-learning experience, which includes three components: preparation, community service, and reflection. Table 10.8 provides a checklist to determine whether your community engagement project will be successful.

Table 10.8 Checklist for Successful Community Engagement

_____ Research the community, the community safety-net organization, and at-risk populations.

_____ Develop trust relationships with the safety-net organization and diverse at-risk populations.

_____ Identify public health nursing activities beneficial to the organization, at-risk populations, and students.

_____ Collaborate with the safety-net organization to plan, implement, and evaluate public health nursing activities.

_____ Develop culturally sensitive public health nursing services that are respectful of diverse populations.

_____ Create public health nursing services that are asset-based, building on the strengths of the safety-net organization, community resources, and at-risk populations.

_____ Be flexible in developing and implementing public health nursing services.

_____ Provide public health nursing services that strengthen an ongoing relationship with the safety-net organization.

Source: Builds on work of Broussard, 2011; Schoon, Champlin, & Hunt, 2012.

Care and a passionate commitment to social justice drive PHNs to practice advocacy to create social change and improve well-being at the systems and community levels of practice (see Table 10.9). Some students also become so committed to their community engagement activities that they plan to continue involvement after graduation. This scenario is a win-win for the students and their communities. The following are examples of a few collaborative community engagement projects under development that students chose to continue:

- A support group for parents with children with Attention Deficit Hyperactivity Disorder

- "Get Moving Program" (physical/nutritional community youth program)

- A community garden to ensure access to fruit and vegetables

- An action plan for concussion intervention for traveling youth sports teams

Table 10.9 Public Health Nursing Interventions at the Community and Systems Levels of Practice That Include and Support Advocacy

Advocacy: Florence Nightingale demonstrated advocacy throughout her nursing career. As superintendent of a London hospital for impoverished women, she successfully had the hospital policy changed from admitting only those who belonged to the Church of England to admit women of all faiths. Her nursing leadership of 38 nurses in Ottoman, Turkey, during the Crimean War was directed primarily at improving the plight of the wounded (Selanders & Crane, 2012).

Community Organizing: A community action model was used in California to increase the community's capacity to address the social health determinants of tobacco-related health disparities to take action to develop local policies to eliminate or weaken smoking-related social health determinants (Lavery et al., 2005).

Collaboration: PHNs in Alberta, Canada, who were concerned about the incidence of postpartum depression initiated a demonstration project in which they collaborated with a group of obstetricians and a group of midwives to have pregnant women referred to PHNs for psychosocial screening, health education, referral, and follow-up. Of the 150 women assessed, 37% had a history of postpartum depression, and 33% had a family history of depression. They accessed 93 services. Of the 75 women who participated in the program evaluation, 68% reported that the PHN intervention was helpful. The outcomes were so positive that the collaborative program was continued (Strass & Billay, 2008).

Policy Development and Policy Enforcement: Barriers that limit access to healthcare in the uninsured elderly population were explored in a journal article in a special health policy feature. Key barriers were lack of transportation, lack of insurance, complexity of the healthcare system, poverty, lack of family support, culture, communication, and race and ethnicity. Recommendations included improvements to health insurance coverage, use of the case management model of care, outreach services, improvements to transportation, and cultural competency and communication. Many of these recommendations were directed toward needed changes in federal healthcare policy (Horton & Johnson, 2010).

Erica has been with the county public health agency for a year. She is committed to social justice and wants to improve her ability to advocate for vulnerable individuals and families. She wants to be able to support agency initiatives to improve population health in her community. Erica has noticed that agency nurses in management positions frequently carry out community-organizing, coalition-building, and policy-development interventions. Sometimes she supported these agency initiatives. Erica makes a list of the opportunities she participated in and the opportunities she missed (outlined in Table 10.10).

Table 10.10 Erica's List of Agency Initiatives

Opportunities taken	Opportunities missed
Brief conversation with a county health board member. Told a client story about a teenage mom who benefitted from the existence of a Healthy Families Collaborative. (Coalition Building)	In the past legislative session during a debate on a ruling regarding preservatives in vaccines, I could have written a personal letter to my legislator. (Policy Development)
Articulated several "talking points" from the state department of health policy on vaccines and autism at the early childhood meeting for parents to motivate parents to encourage other parents to have their children vaccinated. (Community Organizing)	Did not attend a meeting organized by city hall regarding hiking and biking trails in my community. I could have been a voice for obesity prevention in my community. (Community Organizing)
Led a focus group with Cambodian immigrants on cultural competency in services for the elderly in their community. Provided a summary report to the Cambodian community and service providers. (Collaboration)	Missed an opportunity for PHN team case study discussion to identify unmet health needs among their case loads. I could have learned how my case load was similar to or different from other PHNs' case loads and how this influences our decision-making and priority-setting processes. (Collaboration)
Represented the agency on a task force organized by the state health department to develop guidelines on blood lead and healthy housing. (Policy Development)	Missed a meeting with a senior coalition to lobby county commissioners to extend green light walking time to allow seniors to walk across streets safely. I could have learned more about this health risk for the elderly. (Coalition Building)
Met with the OB nurse manager, Newborn Nursery nurse manager, and the Infection Control nurse at the local hospital to discuss Tdap vaccination of staff as a means to prevent pertussis in newborn infants. (Collaboration)	Did not return a survey regarding vending machine policies in the school district. I could have helped with the data-collection process. (Policy Development)

Ethical Application for Social Justice and Nursing Advocacy

PHNs often make ethical decisions related to social justice and human rights. Most of the time these decisions are related to the health status of individuals and families, but sometimes they are clearly related to the health status and health disparities of diverse populations. You need to be able to identify and describe the ethical principles based on social justice and human rights that guide you. It is also important to understand how your ethical beliefs and the ethical beliefs of others affect your capacity to act when confronted with health disparities. You need to have a strong sense of your own ethical beliefs. We all bring personal biases to our ethical decision-making, and we have differing abilities and skills to take action. Consider your level of *moral courage*, the ability to confront moral challenges based on steadfast commitment to fundamental ethical principles despite potential risks (Edmondson, 2010; Gallagher, 2011; Lachman, 2010; Murray, 2010). Think about the *ethical environment* that surrounds you, the social environment consistent with principles of human rights and social justice that is supportive of individual or collective actions of moral courage (Edmondson, 2010; Gallagher, 2011; Lachman, 2010; Murray, 2010). Do you have the personal and professional resources you need as a student and future nurse to be the advocate you want to be?

 ACTIVITY

Consider the following case study: A PHN making a home visit to a recently paroled inmate of the local jail notes on the referral that the man is PPD positive on repeat testing and needs to start antibiotic medications for TB. The man has the medication with him but is not taking it. The PHN considers her options:

Should she start DOT?

Should she notify his physician or parole agent of his noncompliance?

What is the ethical dilemma, and how would you resolve it?

Review the ethical principles listed in Table 10.11, and use them to resolve the ethical dilemma.

Table 10.11   Ethical Principles and Actions in Advocacy

Ethical perspectives	Examples
Rule ethics (principles)	• Public health resources and services are allocated based on need, so they might be distributed unequally—maximizing utility.
	• Identify individuals, families, populations, and communities who are vulnerable and experiencing health disparities.
	• Provide public health nursing services to those who are most vulnerable, at greatest health risk, and experiencing health disparities and health inequities, focusing on equal access to goods.

continues

Table 10.11   Ethical Principles and Actions in Advocacy   (continued)

Ethical perspectives	Examples
Virtue ethics (character)	• Make ethical decisions based on social justice and human rights. • Focus on fair procedures rather than outcomes. • Provide support for individuals, families, populations, and communities who advocate for themselves. • Be caring and compassionate. • Select advocacy goals and actions that are culturally congruent with the racial and ethnic diversity of individuals, families, and populations within the community.
Feminist ethics (reducing oppression)	• Advocate for the health and well-being of individuals, families, populations, and communities. • Include and partner with clients in priority setting, goal setting, and advocacy actions. • Empower clients to manage their own healthcare needs. • Increase capacity of individuals, families, populations, and communities to manage their healthcare needs. • Take actions to address social injustice at all levels of public health nursing practice. • Focus on ensuring equal access to resources. • Focus on traditions and practices in a community.

Table based on work by Racher, 2007, and Volbrecht, 2002

Key Points

- Social justice and human rights serve as the foundation for public health nursing advocacy.

- Public health priorities and actions are directed at vulnerable populations experiencing health disparities.

- To reduce health disparities at the local, national, and global levels, it is necessary to eradicate the social determinants of health that create negative health outcomes.

- PHNs advocate for health equity and justice for individuals, families, populations, and communities at all three levels of practice—individual/family, community, and systems.

- PHNs bear professional accountability to advocate for vulnerable individuals, families, populations, and communities experiencing health disparities.

- Civic and community engagement are strategies that students and PHNs may use to empower communities to manage their own healthcare needs.

Advocating for Justice in the Digital Age

Today's students are comfortable being members of the "digital age." Therefore, using digital technology for advocacy activities to promote health fits student interests and expertise. Suggested activities (Galer-Unti, 2010) include the following:

- *Friending and Social Networking*—Use such websites as Facebook and Tumblr to promote social justice issues and advocacy activities. Link to other participants' pages or create your own page with a health promotion and advocacy theme.

- *Real-Time Communications*—Use a newsletter blast or email list for advocacy alerts; use Twitter for sending advocacy alerts, issuing press releases, mobilizing people for demonstrations, and increasing awareness of a specific health issue through a planned advocacy campaign.

- *Advocacy Channel*—Develop portals for reporting the news and educating the public on health issues (e.g., website, blog, Twitter, YouTube channel, BlogTalkRadio show, photographs and videos, widgets).

 ## Reflective Practice

It is difficult to think about the bigger picture on a daily basis when providing nursing care to vulnerable individuals and families. The annual review period is a good time to compare your professional goals with actual practice to determine the congruence between goals and practice and to identify future opportunities for professional growth and development.

Think about your experiences in your public health nursing clinical and the advocacy competencies you developed during it:

- Which vulnerable populations have you worked with as a student nurse?

_____

_____

- How did you know whether an individual, family, or population was experiencing a health disparity?

_____

_____

- Which health disparities did you identify in your community?

  _____

  _____

- How did you explore the causes of health disparities in your community?

  _____

  _____

- Which unmet health needs did you identify in your community?

  _____

  _____

- Which clients did you advocate for as part of your public health clinical?

  _____

  _____

- Which advocacy actions did you observe or participate in during your public health nursing clinical?

  _____

  _____

- What worked and what did not? What would you do differently?

  _____

  _____

- If you were going to develop an intervention at the community or systems level of practice for an unmet health need, what would it be? How would you start?

  _____

  _____

Refer to the Cornerstones of Public Health in Chapter 1. Which of these cornerstones support the social justice approach of achieving health equity through community partnerships? Does this cornerstone also support social justice as a foundation of public health nursing?

Erica is preparing for her annual review with her supervisor. She decides that one of her goals for the following year will be to begin developing her advocacy skills at the community and systems levels of practice. She believes that her values and perspectives are consistent with social justice and the mission and goals of the county public health agency. She believes that she has been effective in advocating for individuals and families, such as the family whose children had increased blood lead levels. She now understands that she has to intervene at all three levels of practice to create change sufficient to improve population health. Erica is ready to work on her ACTIONS!

Application of Evidence

Think about how Erica developed and demonstrated public health nursing advocacy competencies as she worked with the two young children with increased blood lead levels and their mother, analyzed her own practice, and set the goal of developing additional advocacy competencies. Discuss the following questions with your classmates.

1. Which values and perspectives motivated Erica to act in a socially just manner?

2. Which aspects of the situation required Erica to take actions for this family?

3. Which ethical conflict between social justice and individual human rights did Erica have to resolve? How did she resolve it?

4. Why was it important for Erica to include others and work as part of a team?

5. Which health determinants required Erica to take actions at the systems level of practice?

6. Which advocacy actions did Erica take to help the family and owner of the building?

7. What were the health outcomes of her actions and the team's actions?

8. Which future civic engagement or community engagement actions might Erica participate in to protect children from environmental hazards?

Think, Explore, Do

1. How will you prepare to work with diverse vulnerable populations in your public health clinical? Consider the following suggestions:

   - Review health status data and scientific literature on vulnerable populations, health disparities, social justice, advocacy, and community resources.

   - Use the Internet to learn more about health disparities and social determinants of health.

   - Find the websites for the following presentations in the Chapter 10 Resources in Appendix B:

     - Providers Guide to Quality and Culture: Presentations on healthcare disparities and quality and culture.

     - Unnatural Causes website: California Newsreel social determinants of health

     - Review some of the cultural assessment and intervention tools at the National Center for Cultural Competence.

2. How can you take advantage of the learning opportunities available to you during your public health clinical? Consider the following suggestions:

   - Participate in a variety of community experiences so that you gain broad exposure to the diverse community populations, their health priorities, their needs, and their strengths.

   - Observe an activity where community members partner with healthcare providers to solve community health problems.

   - Identify social justice issues in your public health clinical setting.

   - Use nonjudgmental therapeutic listening to understand your clients' perspectives, health needs, and health priorities.

   - Empower your clients by providing them with information, community resources, and access to support networks.

3. Think about the public health activities you have participated in or observed during your clinical. Would you classify these activities as examples of charity, civic engagement, or community engagement?

4. Which advocacy actions might you take at the systems and community levels of practice?

5. Which advocacy competencies would you like to develop in the future? What should be your first step?

6. Read the following story and reflect upon upstream versus downstream thinking:

   Two people were walking by a river. Suddenly, they observed babies floating down the river. They ran to the river to pull out as many babies as they could possibly reach. One of the rescuers yelled, "I'm going upstream to find out how these babies are getting into the river." This rescuer climbed the pathway up the side of the river, found where the babies were being thrown into the river, and immediately prevented more babies from being thrown into the water. This is upstream thinking and action in contrast to downstream action. Falk-Rafael (2012) explains how downstream approaches that are aimed at meeting the needs of individuals and families must be paired with upstream approaches that aim to change power in societal relationships and structures to give voice to those with poor health and social disadvantages.

7. Think of a health disparity you would like to see decreased in a specific population. How would you use upstream thinking to achieve your goal? Do you think a dual approach of combining upstream and downstream strategies might work? What would you propose?

References

Alameda County Public Health Department (ACPHD). (2008). A framework for health equity. *Life and death from unnatural causes—health and social inequity in Alameda County.* Oakland, CA: ACPHD, p. 4. Retrieved from http://www.acphd.org/media/53628/unnatcs2008.pdf

American Nurses Association (ANA). (2001). *Code of ethics for nurses with interpretive statements.* Washington, DC: Nursesbooks.org.

American Nurses Association (ANA). (2010a). *Guide to the code of ethics for nurses—Interpretation and application.* Silver Springs, MD: Nursesbooks.org

American Nurses Association (ANA). (2010b). Nurses human rights. ANA position statements on ethics and human rights. Silver Springs, MD: Nursing World. Retrieved from http://www.nursingworld.org/MainMenuCategories/EthicsStandards/Ethics-Position-Statements.aspx

American Nurses Association (ANA). (2013). *Public health nursing: Scope & standards of practice.* Silver Springs, MD: Nursesbooks.org.

Baum, N., Gollust, S., Goold, S., & Jacobson, P. (2007). Looking ahead: Addressing ethical challenges in public health practice. *Journal of Law, Medicine, and Ethics, 35*(4), 657–667.

Bay Area Regional Health Inequities Initiative (BARHII). (2008). Health Inequities in the Bay Area. San Francisco, CA: BARHII. Retrieved from http://www.barhii.org/press/download/barhii_report08.pdf

Beauchamp, D. E. (2013). Public health as social justice . In M. T. Donohue (Ed.), *Public health and social justice* (pp. 11–19). San Francisco, CA: Jossey-Bass/John Wiley & Sons, Inc.

Brennen Ramirez, I. K., Baker, E. A., & Metzler, M. (2008). *Promoting Health Equity: A Resource to Help Communities Address Social Determinants of Health.* Atlanta, GA: U.S. Department of Health and Human Services: Centers for Disease Control and Prevention.

Broussard, B. B. (2011). The bucket list: A service-learning approach to community engagement to enhance community health nursing clinical learning. *Journal of Nursing Education, 50*(1), 40–43. doi:10.3928/01484834-20100930-07

Bu, X., & Jezewski, M. A., (2006). Developing a mid-range theory of patient advocacy through competency analysis. *Journal of Advanced Nursing, 57*(1), 101–110.

Budetti, P. (2008). Market justice and US healthcare. *Journal of the American Medical Association, 299*(1), 92–94.

California Newsreel. (2008). Backgrounders from the unnatural causes health equity data base. *Unnatural Causes.* Retrieved from http://www.unnaturalcauses.org/assets/uploads/file/primers.pdf

Cawley, T. & McNamara, P.M. (2011). Public health nurse perceptions of empowerment and advocacy in child health surveillance in West Ireland. *Public Health Nursing, 28*(2), 150–158. doi:10.1111/j.1525-1446.2010.00921.x

Center for Vulnerable Populations Research. (n.d.). Who are the vulnerable? Los Angeles, CA: University of California, Los Angeles, School of Nursing. Retrieved from http://nursing.ucla.edu/site.cfm?id=388

Centers for Disease Control and Prevention. (2011). CDC health disparities and inequality report – United States, 2011. *Morbidity and Mortality Weekly Report Supplement, 60.* Retrieved from http://www.cdc.gov/mmwr/pdf/other/su6001.pdf

Centers for Disease Control and Prevention. (2013). CDC Health Disparities & Inequalities Report (CHDIR), 2013. *Morbidity and Mortality Weekly Report Supplement, 62*(3), 1-187. Atlanta, GA: U.S. Department of Health and Human Services. Retrieved from http://www.cdc.gov/minorityhealth/CHDIReport.html

Congressional Budget Office. (2008). Growing disparities in life expectancy. *Economic and Budget Issue Brief.* Retrieved from http://www.cbo.gov/publication/41681

Curtin, L. (1979). The nurse as advocate: A philosophical foundation for nursing. *Advances in Nursing Science, 1*(3), 1–10.

Denehy, J. (2007). National Association of School Nurses: Speaking up for children. *Journal of School Nursing, 23*(3): 125–127.

Edmonson, C. (2010). Moral courage and the nurse leader. *Online Journal of Issues in Nursing, 15*(3). doi:10.3912/OJIN.Vol15No03Man05.

Ensign, J. (2001). The health of shelter-based foster youth. *Public Health Nursing, 18*(1), 19–23.

Falk-Rafael, A. (2005a). Speaking truth to power: Nursing's legacy and moral imperative. *Advances in Nursing Science, 28*(3), 212–223.

Falk-Rafael, A. (2005b). Advancing nursing theory through theory-guided practice—The emergence of a critical caring perspective. *Advances in Nursing Science, 28*(1), 38–49.

Falk-Rafael, A., & Betker, C. (2012). Witnessing social injustice downstream and advocating for health equity upstream. *Advances in Nursing Science, 35*(2), 98–112. doi:10.1097/ANS.0b013e31824fe70f

Gadow, S. (1999). Relational narrative: The postmodern turn in nursing ethics. *Scholarly Inquiry for Nursing Practice: An International Journal, 13*(1), 57–70.

Galer-Unti, R. (2010). Advocacy 2.0: Advocating in the digital age. *Health Promotion Practice, 11*(6), 784–787.

Gallagher, A. (2011). Moral distress and moral courage in everyday nursing practice. *Online Journal of Issues in Nursing, 16*(2). doi:10.3912/OJIN.Vol16No02PPT03

Gebrke, P. M. (2008). Civic engagement and nursing education. *Advances in Nursing Science, 31*(1), 52–66.

Gruskin, S., Cottingham, J., Hilber, A. M., Kismodi, E., Lincetto, O., & Roseman, M. J. (2008). Using human rights to improve maternal and neonatal health: History, connections and a proposed practical solution. *Bulletin of the World Health Organization, 86*(8), 589–593.

Horton, S., & Johnson, R. J. (2010). Improving access to health care for uninsured elderly patients. *Public Health Nursing, 27*(4), 362–370.

Hughes, J. (2010). Putting the pieces together: How public health nurses in rural and remote Canadian communities respond to intimate partner violence. *Online Journal of Rural Nursing and Health Care, 10*(1), 34–47.

International Council of Nurses. (2006). The ICN position statement on nurses and human rights. Geneva, Switzerland: Author. Retrieved from http://www.icn.ch/images/stories/documents/publications/position_statements/E10_Nurses_Human_Rights.pdf

Iton, A. B. (2008). The ethics of the medical model in addressing the root causes of health disparities in local public health practice. *Journal of Public Health Management Practice, 14*(4), 335–339.

Keller, L. O. (2010). Table: Comparison of value structure. Unpublished, personal correspondence.

Kleinfehn-Wald, N. (2010). Social justice and human rights issues identified by practicing public health nurses. Unpublished research.

Lachman, V.D. (2010). Strategies necessary for moral courage. *Online Journal of Issues in Nursing, 15*(3). doi:10.3912/OJIN.Vol15No03Man03.

Lavery, S. H., Smith, M. L., Esparza, A. A., Hrushow, A., Moore, M., & Reed, D. F. (2005). The community action model: A community-driven model designed to address disparities in health. *American Journal of Public Health, 95*(4), 611–616.

Ludwick, R., & Silva, M.C. (2000). Nursing around the world: Cultural values and ethical conflicts. *2000 Online Journal of Issues in Nursing, 5*(3). Retrieved from http://www.nursingworld.org/MainMenuCategories/ANAMarketplace/ANAPeriodicals/OJIN/Columns/Ethics

MacDonald, H. (2006). Relational ethics and advocacy in nursing: Literature review. *Journal of Advanced Nursing, 57*(2), 119–126.

Mallik, M. (1997). Advocacy in nursing—A review of the literature. *Journal of Advanced Nursing, 25*(1), 130–138.

Minnesota Department of Health (MDH). (2001). *Public health interventions—Application for public health nursing practice.* St. Paul, MN: MDH.

Murray, J.S. (2010). Moral courage in healthcare: Acting ethically even in presence of risk. *Online Journal of Issues in Nursing, 15*(3). doi:10.3912/OJIN.Vol15No03Man02

National Research Council and Institute of Medicine. (2013). *U.S. health in international perspective: Shorter lives, poorer health.* Washington, D.C.: The National Academies Press, p. 32. Retrieved from http://www.nap.edu/catalog.php?record_id=13497

Office of the High Commissioner for Human Rights, United Nations Human Rights. (n.d.). Retrieved from http://www.ohchr.org/EN/Issues/Pages/WhatareHumanRights.aspx?Pages/WhatareHumanRights.aspx

Public Health Leadership Society. (2002). *Principles of the ethical practice of public health.* Version 2.2. Retrieved from http://phls.org/CMSuploads/Principles-of-the-Ethical-Practice-of-PH-Version-2.2-68496.pdf

Racher, F. E. (2007). The evolution of ethics for community practice. *Journal of Community Health Nursing, 24*(1), 65–76.

Redlener, I., & Grant, R. (2009). America's safety net and health care reform—What lies ahead? *New England Journal of Medicine, 361*(23), 2201–2204. doi:10.1056/NEJMp0910597

Reutter, L., & Kushner, K. E. (2010). "Health equity through action on the social determinants of health": Taking up the challenge in nursing. *Nursing Inquiry, 17*(3), 269–280.

Satcher, D., & Higginbotham, E. J. (2008). The public health approach to eliminating disparities in health. *American Journal of Public Health, 98*, 400–403.

Schoon, P. M., Champlin, B., & Hunt, R. (2012). Developing a sustainable foot care clinic in a homeless shelter within an academic-community partnership through curricular integration and faculty engagement. *Journal of Nursing Education, 51*(12), 714–718. doi:10.3928/01484834-20121112-02

Schoon, P. M., Miller, T. W., Maloney, P., & Tasbir, J. (2012). Chapter 7: Power and politics. In P. Kelly, & J. Tazbir (Eds.), *Essentials of leadership and management* (pp. 186–208). Clifton Park, NJ: Delmar/Centage.

Selanders, L. C., & Crane, P. C. (2012). The voice of Florence Nightingale on advocacy. *Online Journal of Issues in Nursing, 17*(1), 1–10. doi:10.3912/OJIN.Vol17No01Man01

Signal, L., Martin, J., Cram, F., & Robson, B. (2008). *The Health Equity Assessment Tool: A user's guide.* Wellington, New Zealand: Ministry of Health.

Singh, G. K., Siahpush, M., & Kogan, M. D. (2010). Rising social inequalities in US childhood obesity, 2003–2007. *Annals of Epidemiology, 20*(1), 40–52. http://dx.doi.org/10.1016/j.annepidem.2009.09.008. Retrieved from http://www.sciencedirect.com/science/article/pii/S104727970900324X

Strass, P., & Billay, E. (2008). A public health nursing initiative to promote antenatal health. *Canadian Nurse, 104*(2), 29–33.

United Nations. (1948). The universal declaration of human rights. Geneva, Switzerland: Author. Retrieved from http://www.un.org/en/documents/udhr/

United Nations. (2013). *The Millennium Development Goals report–2013.* Geneva, Switzerland: Author. Retrieved from http://www.un.org/millenniumgoals/pdf/report-2013/mdg-report-2013-english.pdf

U.S. Department of Health and Human Services. (2012). United States life tables, 2008. *National Vital Statistics Report, 61*(3), 3. Retrieved from http://www.cdc.gov/nchs/data/nvsr/nvsr61/nvsr61_03.pdf

U.S. Department of Health and Human Services. (2013). Infant mortality statistics from the 2009 period—Linked birth/infant death data set. *National Vital Statistics Report, 61*(8), 1.

Vanderburg, S., Wright, L., Boston, S., & Zimmerman, G. (2010). Maternal child home visiting program improves nursing practice for screening of woman abuse. *Public Health Nursing, 27*(4), 347–352.

Volbrecht, R. M. (2002). *Nursing ethics—Communities in dialogue.* Upper Saddle River, NJ: Pearson Prentice Hall.

Williams, D. R., Costa, M. V., Oduniami, A. O., & Mohammed, S. A. (2008). Moving upstream: How interventions that address social determinants of health can improve health and reduce disparities. *Journal of Public Health Management Practice. 14*(Suppl), S8–S17. doi:10.1097/01.PHH.0000338382.36695.42

World Health Organization. (n.d.). Social determinants of health—Key concepts. Retrieved from http://www.who.int/social_determinants/thecommission/finalreport/key_concepts/en/index.html

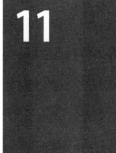

COMPETENCY #9
Demonstrates Nonjudgmental and Unconditional Acceptance of People Different From Self

Carolyn M. Garcia
with Christine C. Andres and Bernita Missal

Josie is a public health nursing student completing her final clinical hours before graduating. She and a classmate have been volunteering in a school-based clinic. The school nurse has invited Josie to join her on a home visit to check up on a student who has just given birth. Josie uses the GPS on her smartphone to find the apartment; it is located in a part of the city she normally avoids. She carefully locks her car and joins the school nurse in the apartment lobby. The client answers the buzzer, and they are invited upstairs to the apartment. The unfamiliar hallway lighting and smells cause Josie to proceed cautiously. She hopes to focus on what the school nurse accomplishes rather than on her own feelings of discomfort. What are some of the fears or worries Josie might be experiencing in this, or other, situations that are different for her? What are some things that might have helped Josie prepare for the "discomfort" that can often be experienced during home visits? What does Josie need to know or understand to help her work with clients who do not live like she does?

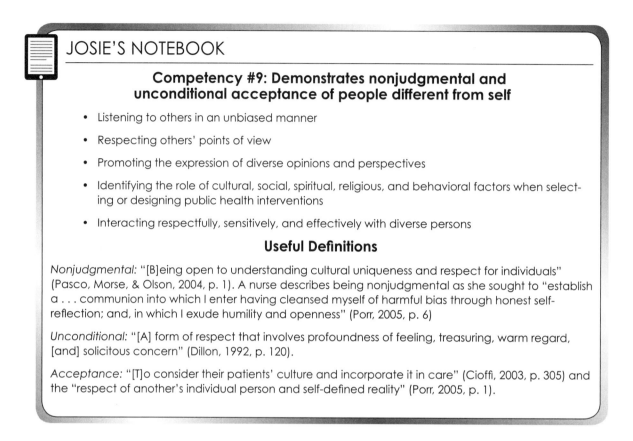

JOSIE'S NOTEBOOK

Competency #9: Demonstrates nonjudgmental and unconditional acceptance of people different from self

- Listening to others in an unbiased manner

- Respecting others' points of view

- Promoting the expression of diverse opinions and perspectives

- Identifying the role of cultural, social, spiritual, religious, and behavioral factors when selecting or designing public health interventions

- Interacting respectfully, sensitively, and effectively with diverse persons

Useful Definitions

Nonjudgmental: "[B]eing open to understanding cultural uniqueness and respect for individuals" (Pasco, Morse, & Olson, 2004, p. 1). A nurse describes being nonjudgmental as she sought to "establish a . . . communion into which I enter having cleansed myself of harmful bias through honest self-reflection; and, in which I exude humility and openness" (Porr, 2005, p. 6)

Unconditional: "[A] form of respect that involves profoundness of feeling, treasuring, warm regard, [and] solicitous concern" (Dillon, 1992, p. 120).

Acceptance: "[T]o consider their patients' culture and incorporate it in care" (Cioffi, 2003, p. 305) and the "respect of another's individual person and self-defined reality" (Porr, 2005, p. 1).

They Do Not Live Like I Do

Public health nursing is similar to other areas of nursing when it comes to valuing the ability to deliver nursing care in a nonjudgmental, accepting manner. A public health nurse (PHN) is often in the client's context, such as in the home, and this situation provides endless opportunities for a nurse's acceptance of others to be tested, confirmed, or challenged. A PHN might work with a faith community to offer blood pressure screening, which might require the nurse to work alongside others with different values or beliefs. It is important to recognize that some people or populations, due to their past experiences, have a heightened level of stigma consciousness (i.e., perception or awareness of being stigmatized) and expect to be judged, which can present a challenge for nurses (Porr, Drummond, & Olson, 2012). Similarly, nurses might also have past experiences that have contributed to their development of biases or prejudices that need to be addressed so that they can truly provide nonjudgmental or unconditional care. This chapter explores the ways in which a PHN can demonstrate nonjudgmental or unconditional acceptance of people. It also provide examples of how PHNs have worked to develop acceptance for individuals, families, and communities across difficult situations. Finally, the chapter concludes with suggestions for assessing your own acceptance of others and ways to develop yourself as a nonjudgmental person and a nurse.

A nurse can be nonjudgmental yet at the same time disagree with something that is observed or said. This distinction is subtle but important; a nurse should be able to discern whether a behavior is healthy or harmful yet should also be able to make these assessments in a manner that is nonjudgmental. For example, it is important to note that there are instances when a nurse must act on a duty to report apparent abuse that might be "acceptable" in that personal or cultural context by the individual or family but violates a law in the United States. In these very difficult situations, the effective nurse will carefully intervene, realizing at the time that the interventions might not appear to be nonjudgmental. In attitude and behavior, the nurse can strive to be as nonjudgmental as possible, even in difficult situations that must balance legal and ethical obligations to individuals/families and society. A PHN caring for someone who has committed a violent crime is likely to feel strongly about the crimes that have been committed. This nurse will regularly face the challenge to provide nursing care that is equal to the care provided to a non-prisoner, care that is not conditionally based on what the person has done or not done. The nurse's clients will perceive the care being provided as nonjudgmental and unconditional when the nurse demonstrates a sincere desire to learn more about the client through unbiased listening and asking of questions, respect, and openness.

Another example in which PHNs might be confronted with a challenge of being nonjudgmental is when they are providing nursing care to a generation very different from their own. This challenge is often encountered within the context of changing cultural trends. For example, a current cultural trend seen in late adolescence and young adults is expression through the form of body tattooing. Nurses displaced by several decades from this population group might have negative perceptions of tattooing. Those PHNs have the challenge of trying to "fit" into this generation and to understand the current trends and values and their importance. PHNs can be more successful in building nonjudgmental, ongoing relationships when they respect possible cultural generational differences. In the case of tattooing, respecting differences might mean not addressing the issue of whether someone is getting a tattoo but rather promoting safe tattooing practices.

Diversity is reflected in numerous ways, which might include:

- Culture.
- Lifestyle preferences.
- Religion.
- Socioeconomic position.
- Age.
- Race.
- Physical appearances.
- Sexual orientation.

- Education level.
- Neighborhood.
- Geographic region.
- Language use.
- Immigration status.
- Health status.
- Beliefs.
- Values.

It is increasingly important to be aware of diversity, because the U.S. population will shift to a multiracial/multiethnic majority in the next few decades (see Table 11.1).

Table 11.1   U.S. Population, Actual and Proejcted: 2005 and 2050

	2005	2050
Population (in millions)	296	438
Share of total		
Foreign born	12%	19%
Racial/Ethnic Groups		
• White	67%	47%
• Hispanic	14%	29%
• Black	13%	13%
• Asian	5%	9%
Age Groups		
• Children (17 and younger)	25%	23%
• Working age (18-64)	63%	58%
• Elderly (65 and older)	12%	19%

Note: All races modified and not Hispanic; American Indian/Alaska Native not shown.

Source: Passel & Cohn, Pew Research Center, 2008

This population transformation will occur in some areas of the country sooner than others. Figure 11.1 demonstrates state and regional differences.

Some of the ways that nurses demonstrate nonjudgmental and unconditional public health nursing might include:

- Listening to others in an unbiased manner.

- Respecting others' points of view.

- Promoting the expression of diverse opinions and perspectives.

- Identifying the role of cultural, social, spiritual, religious, and behavioral factors when selecting or designing public health interventions.

- Interacting respectfully, sensitively, and effectively with diverse persons (e.g., diverse by culture, socioeconomic position, educational level, race, ethnicity, gender, sexual orientation, religious background, health status, age, and lifestyle preferences).

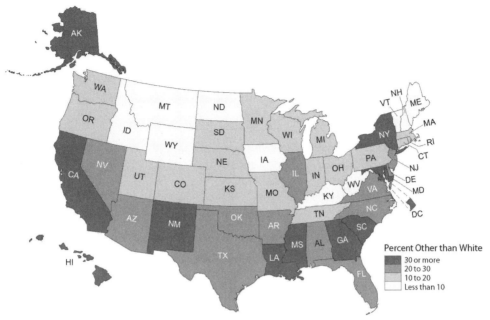

Figure 11.1. Population Percent Other Than White by State: 2000 Census
Source: U.S. Census Bureau, 2013

Listening to Others in an Unbiased Manner

Have you watched yourself in a mirror to observe your nonverbal cues and signals when you are reacting to what someone else is saying? Do you smile? Do you nod cautiously or in positive support for the other person? Do you scowl quickly when something you do not agree with is said? Effective listening is a combination of verbal and nonverbal responses to the person with whom you are talking; another concept that is growing in popularity is that of deep listening, which is a process of listening to learn (Center for Spirituality and Healing, 2013). When you listen deeply, you do not generate what your response is going to be to what is being said or relayed nonverbally. Instead, deep listening is reflective listening in which you listen to learn, you listen for understanding rather than agreement, and you ask powerful questions (CSH, 2013). Listening in an unbiased manner takes effective listening to a higher level, because it requires you not only to listen in a way that helps people who are talking believe that they are being heard but also to listen in a manner that expresses acceptance for those people.

As with most communication attributes (refer back to Chapter 8, which is devoted to communication), verbal and nonverbal listening cues can vary by culture, developmental age, and other factors. Therefore, you need to know the clients you are working with and understand what conveys listening and support to them. Do not presume to know. The following are some broad categories that serve as examples of the many ways in which we express listening, support, inattention, or boredom (see Table 11.2).

Table 11.2   Nonverbal and Verbal Listening Cues

Nonverbal	Verbal
—Eye contact (not too little, not too much)	—Supportive sounds (uh huh, ah)
—Facial expressions (smile, stare, frown, grimace)	—Timing and pace (responding quickly indicates active listening rather than distraction)
—Gestures (head nod, hand motions)	—Voice tone (angry, supportive, authoritarian)
—Intensity (the amount of energy you exude to the other person can support or bother that individual)	
—Movements and posture (leaning toward someone indicates interest)	
—Space (closeness and proximity to the other person/people)	
—Touch (hand on shoulder, hug)	

Source: Segal, Smith, & Jaffe, 2013.

You must adequately prepare for interactions with clients and families so that your nonverbal actions are consistent with their cultures. Learning about your clients' beliefs and value systems through open-ended questions will support your knowledge of appropriate interactions. For example, in some cultures it is not appropriate to pat a child on the head, and in others it is not acceptable to look people in the eye. Importantly, remember that differences often exist within a culture as well, so awareness of a nonverbal behavior that is acceptable or not to some people in a culture should not be automatically assumed as universal to everyone in that cultural group.

Respecting Others' Points of View

Are you quick to defend your own views or beliefs? Is it hard for you to listen to someone argue for a value that is not your own? It can be difficult to respect others' points of view when they do not naturally align with your own. However, this skill is critical to being a nonjudgmental nurse. The key is demonstrating respect for another point of view regardless of whether you concur. You can express respect verbally and nonverbally. For example, when a PHN visits a mother who has recently delivered her fifth child, the nurse is likely to explore birth control or child spacing plans with the mother. If the mother expresses a view that opposes family planning or use of birth control, the nurse needs to respect that view. One way you can show respect is through offering relevant information in an unassuming manner and choosing to respect the client's autonomy for maintaining a different perspective. This respect can be particularly difficult to project when you perceive client, family, or community views as unhealthy.

Promoting the Expression of Diverse Opinions and Perspectives

Do you seek others' opinions before making a decision? Do you welcome multiple perspectives, or do you find them annoying? Nurses are often in situations that require advocacy for families and communities, and each family and community includes multiple perspectives and opinions. Effective PHNs can assess the situation and intervene in a manner that helps everyone express an opinion. For example, a PHN visiting a family with a hospice client might encounter many opinions from that family about how to best help their loved one go through the dying process. It is very helpful when the nurse can learn who is the spokesperson for the family or community, if one has been identified and agreed upon. Even though it might be impossible to act upon each opinion, the nurse can assist family members in expressing their perspectives and, ultimately, in coming together to make many difficult decisions.

Identifying the Role of Cultural, Social, Spiritual, Religious, and Behavioral Factors When Selecting or Designing Public Health Interventions

Have you thought about how a nursing action might look different if you are caring for someone with a lot of money versus someone with very little? Do you enjoy learning about other cultures? Throughout this book, you have been reminded that PHNs consider multiple factors when providing care for individuals, families, and communities. Nonjudgmental PHNs carefully consider the particular clients being served when specific interventions are being planned. For example, when PHNs implement a child-obesity prevention program, they need to consider the cultural perceptions that might impede or support the program. A recent refugee population might view additional weight on a child as a positive, healthy attribute because they are comparing this to the poverty and malnourishment experienced by many children in their home country. Sociocultural expectations can also influence the success of public health nursing interventions if PHNs are not proactive. For example, in some immigrant communities, the community leaders are consulted by their members about issues of concern. Effective PHNs assess the extent to which these cultural patterns exist within a community and act in accordance with the sociocultural standards to gain entry and intervene. Similarly, PHNs, including those who serve as parish nurses, carefully consider the religious or spiritual implications of certain interventions. For example, PHNs might need to schedule a health promotion intervention around certain holidays or celebrations so that attendance and involvement are optimal.

Interacting Respectfully, Sensitively, and Effectively With Diverse Persons

Are you comfortable having a conversation with an individual who is homeless? Do you enjoy learning about cultures different from your own? Do you believe you are deserving of good things, maybe more so than other people? Do you see the person serving you in a store or a restaurant, or do you see through them? Ultimately, your success as a PHN depends on your ability to establish a meaningful relationship with the individual, family, or community you are serving. You cannot establish that relationship unless you can interact with diverse people in a nonjudgmental and accepting manner. You are going to find it easier to be nonjudgmental toward some people more than toward others, so you should engage in learning activities or reflective exercises to help you recognize and address preconceived stereotypes you might have about certain groups of people. Certainly, your worldview provides, in essence, a cultural filter for how you view and interact with others. Over time and with experience, you will learn more about yourself, including your reactions to those who are different from you. You might find that you are very accepting toward certain people and communities, whereas with others you struggle to feel nonjudgmental. Becoming nonjudgmental is a process that takes time. Practically, you can begin to implement behaviors helpful in your development toward being a nonjudgmental and accepting nurse: understanding specific personal beliefs and values; being respectful to everyone; interacting in a sensitive, responsive manner (rather than an overbearing, assuming one); and developing effective verbal and nonverbal communication skills. For example, you might reflect on what you choose to wear in your professional role as a PHN, and how others might view your attire; this perception is particularly important because PHNs often do not have required uniforms or scrubs. You can practice these behaviors in a variety of settings and begin to learn about the environments, situations, or moods that make being accepting more difficult for you. Most important are your willingness to learn, your reflections on personal behavior and thinking, and your attempts at new skills that enhance your acceptance of others.

Empathy is an important attribute that can contribute to a PHN's ability to practice in a nonjudgmental manner (Porr et al., 2012). In essence, *empathy* is an ability to accurately perceive the emotions, feelings, and thoughts of others; often, people can express empathy more easily when they have experienced something similar to what is occurring and resulting in another person's current emotions, feelings, or thoughts. A nurse's ability to express empathy can encourage a client to feel cared for, heard, and accepted rather than judged. Similarly, the concept of *mutuality*, or the ability to get into someone else's "shoes," is valuable. This sense of mutuality encourages empathy, because the nurse purposefully works to understand as closely as possible what the client is experiencing. Mutuality is a skill that can be developed as you regularly take the time to reflect on what you would be feeling or thinking if you had just experienced what the other person has had happen. Challenge yourself to try this exercise in work and personal settings and reflect on how your ability to connect with, respond to, or support that other person strengthens with greater levels of mutuality and empathy.

It is interesting to look back in history and examine how some people worked to encourage nonjudgmental attitudes, particularly in such eras as the early 1970s, which followed the civil rights efforts in the 1960s. Interestingly, in the 1970s, the language about being nonjudgmental might not have been as sophisticated as it has become in the 21st century. Yet the principles are timeless, and what was explored in 1970 regarding stigma and judgments toward African Americans, the poor, and college students is relevant to nurses today, who work with diverse populations ranging from those in poverty to ethnic minority groups to adolescent parents. Below are steps to help you work toward becoming nonjudgmental, although you should remember that "becoming nonjudgmental is hard work and a lifetime process" (Goldsborough, 1970, p. 2340):

1. Recognize judgmental feelings. (Becoming nonjudgmental begins with openness to yourself, even though it might be painful to acknowledge your judgmental feelings.)

2. Accept your judgmental feelings for what they are. (Without acceptance, you will be unable to move toward changing the feelings.)

3. Explore the origin of the judgmental feelings, maybe with a friend or colleague. (Where did they come from?)

4. Take steps to change. (Realize that there will always be another person and another judgment to work through over the course of your life and nursing career.) (Goldsborough, 1970)

ACTIVITY

Have you ever experienced someone acting judgmental toward you? How did you feel? How did you react?

What do you wish you would have done differently?

What could that person have done to express his or her opinion or beliefs in a nonjudgmental manner?

Do you believe that a person can change from being judgmental to become nonjudgmental? How do you think this change happens? How can you encourage this process in your life and in the lives of those around you?

Josie and the PHN enter the apartment and find they are in a cheery, well-decorated but modest home for the teen, her newborn daughter, and the teen's mother. Josie continues to absorb the surroundings as she hears the school nurse ask the teen about her baby and her healing body. She is surprised that the apartment is so clean and organized. She considers her reaction and tunes out the conversation. "Why am I surprised this apartment is so nice? Do I expect that if you are poor, you are dirty or unkempt? Where is this opinion coming from? Did my facial expressions portray discomfort when I walked through the door?" Josie reflects on her reaction and compares it to that of the PHN, who appears to be at ease and enjoying her interaction with the new mom and baby. At this point in the visit, Josie is questioning her reaction and the judgments her thoughts have revealed. This reflection is critical to growing toward an unconditional acceptance of others. It is an example of mindful nursing practice, which is simply being aware, present, and in the moment with those you are serving or caring for.

Healthy People 2020 The Healthy People 2020 website identifies indicators for a variety of public health concerns in the United States, with goals for improvements by 2020. Select a health indicator and develop a public health nursing health promotion strategy that will include activities at the individual, community, and system levels. Identify activities that will emphasize nonjudgmental acceptance of others and will minimize the barriers that various groups often encounter. What are some things the PHN can do when working with populations that are different from his or hers?

Evidence-Based Practice for Acceptance of Others in Public Health Nursing

A logical question, now, is where in public health nursing practice can we observe acceptance of others and how this improves outcomes for individuals, communities, or systems. In the following section we explore the existing research at these three levels of care delivery for public health nurses.

Individual

Much of the research supporting the need for PHNs to be nonjudgmental and accepting when working with individuals, families, or communities focuses heavily on relationship building. This focus makes sense because, in essence, when a nurse is nonjudgmental and accepting, the client-nurse relationship is likely to be positive and healthy, which leads to more successful interventions and more meaningful interactions for everyone. The Evidence Example below demonstrates positive results experienced by PHNs working with new moms.

 Evidence Example: Nurse-Mother Relationship—What Moms Want and Nurses Can Offer

In a qualitative study, moms and nurses were interviewed to understand how the nurses engage the mothers in a way that is empowering so that the mothers can more effectively bear and raise children (Aston, Meagher-Stewart, Sheppard-Lemoine, Vukic, & Chircop, 2006). In this study, a researcher observed the interactions between the PHN and the mother during a home visit with the new mom (baby born 2–3 weeks prior). Following this observation, the researcher interviewed the mother and PHN to talk about how the home visit had gone. This information helped identify key themes in the relationship, many of which are directly relevant to the PHN's ability to be accepting and nonjudgmental. For example, the mothers identified key attributes of the PHNs that made them feel comfortable, at ease, and positive toward the nurses, including being "full of confidence . . . gentle . . . quiet" (Aston et al., 2006, p. 63). The nurses also talked about the importance of their actions in encouraging the moms to feel comfortable and competent, including "respect, trust, listening, confidence, and communication" (p. 63). At a time when women feel incredibly vulnerable and incompetent, these nurses were able to express acceptance in a way that facilitated feelings of confidence in the new moms.

Few scenarios can demonstrate the challenges that a PHN might face in providing nonjudgmental and accepting nursing care better than poverty. Caroline Porr (2005) is a PHN who reflected on her interactions with clients in poverty and specifically challenged herself to answer the following question: "By all accounts I was thorough, or was I? I certainly 'dealt with' Karen and her family in scrupulous fashion but did I adequately 'dwell with' Karen; that is, did I understand her lived experience as a lone parent enduring the margins of society due to poverty?" (p. 190). Poverty is something that every PHN is going to encounter when serving individuals and families in a variety of contexts (e.g., home visits, case management, case finding).

How PHNs respond to a family in poverty influences the relationship and, subsequently, the outcomes of the care provided. PHNs might, without thinking, consider the poverty as more central to the problems and solutions than the individual or family living in poverty perceives it to be. PHNs therefore need to seek to understand how the individual or family perceives the experience of poverty. After gaining this understanding, PHNs can then effectively support and accept the individual or family. Rather than focusing simply on the reason for the visit (e.g., a home visit to provide education), nonjudgmental and accepting PHNs can dig deeper and appreciate the clients simply for who they are, not as they exist within the narrow context of their situations (e.g., poverty). Similarly, PHNs need to identify and examine the strengths in the situation within the individual, the family, and potentially the community. As Porr concludes, "I had once thought that client assessment and intervention were sufficient until I became curious about *who is* the Other sitting across from me. It was then that I realized that I did not know this mother and thus could never appreciate the uniqueness of her human existence and of her experiences in the world" (2005, p. 194).

The following Evidence Example describes the development of a quantitative tool that clients could use to assess the level of empathy they perceive from the PHNs caring for them. This is quite different from a qualitative approach, in which open-ended questions might be used to learn the clients' perspectives.

Evidence Example: Quantitatively Assessing Empathy

A scale was developed to assess the level of empathic understanding that a nurse has demonstrated (Nagano, 2000). Although the scale is intended to provide an opportunity for a client to give feedback about a nurse, it can also be useful in self-reflection by the nurse regarding verbal and nonverbal behaviors. Examples on this scale include the following:

"The [nurse] summarizes the client's emotions or feelings by saying, 'It seems that you are feeling this. . . .'

The [nurse] looks at the client with a warm expression (eyes, facial expression).

The [nurse]'s voice and rate of speaking are calm, slow, and relaxed.

The [nurse] faces the client and shows interest in the client" (p. 26–27).

Community

Culture is an area in which many PHNs are regularly faced with opportunities or challenges to be nonjudgmental and unconditionally accepting. Realizing that every PHN has a distinct cultural background is fundamentally important when engaging with diverse communities in health promotion or disease-prevention activities. In nursing, much time is spent examining culture in the context of providing care, but what exactly is culture? Broadly defined, *culture* is a set of beliefs (learned or shared), norms, and practices that guide the thoughts, decisions, and actions of a group (Leininger, 1978). This definition presents some challenges, because any cultural group, or community, always has a range of "patterned ways" that are not necessarily consistently similar. So on the one hand, culture might cause a community to share some behaviors or norms that are distinct from other groups, but on the other hand, culture is colorful and inherently diverse, which requires commitment and time to gain understanding. Effective PHNs working with communities understand that effective interventions begin with investments of time and themselves.

For example, a PHN might have opportunities to promote the health of individuals and families who are part of a religious community. Often the support of religious leaders can foster trust of the PHN among the community members. However, if the leaders are not supportive of the PHN's specific priorities, this situation can be challenging, especially if the religious leaders are primary decision-makers and members do not have high levels of autonomy. The PHN in this case needs to respectfully and carefully work with the religious leaders to achieve mutual goals related to health promotion or disease prevention.

The culture of the poor, or those in economic poverty, provides an example of how PHNs rise to provide respectful, quality care amid differences. Public health nursing research on providing care to the poor can be traced back to the first year, 1984, that the *Public Health Nursing* journal was published. A multidimensional model of poverty has been developed that considers individual/group and environmental factors influencing the person experiencing poverty (Pesznecker, 1984). In this model, a person in poverty is cared for with careful consideration of how that person is dealing with his or her specific situation and how he or she is feeling about it (e.g., depressed, powerless, incapable).

ACTIVITY

As a new PHN, you need to learn to carefully reflect on why people might be reacting the way they are when you are trying to intervene. What are they going through? How are they handling their situations?

When the response you are receiving is cautious or unwelcoming, how can you determine whether it is because of the situation and not necessarily specific to you?

Consider how you might incorporate strategies into your practice that convey the message to those you are serving that you come open-minded and open-handed.

Certainly, PHNs are in a work environment that values nursing efficiency. Yet many of the cultural groups that PHNs serve have overarching values that conflict with efficiency. For example, in the culture of generational poverty, time is valued differently than in the middle-class culture. Poverty often necessitates that people view the present time (i.e., in the moment) as most important and make decisions based on immediate feelings or survival needs, whereas those in stable economic situations often value future time as most important and make their decisions with more consideration of future ramifications (Payne, DeVol, & Smith, 2001). PHNs who clearly understand this distinction are going to allow some flexibility in scheduling visits or appointments. You might view an efficient nurse as one who has carefully planned the week with full days of scheduled, often back-to-back, appointments. However, this efficiency might be challenged as the week unfolds and the PHN finds that several of the clients are not home at their scheduled visit times. How can the PHN incorporate and respect the time value for this poverty culture and still implement effective nursing interventions? The PHN might incorporate some time in the schedule each week for same-day home visits or might have a time each week when families can "drop in" for in-office visits. This aspect of scheduling can be very distressing to new PHNs, as many view such client behavior as a sign of disrespect or a lack of desire to see them. This perspective often changes with a deeper appreciation, understanding, and acceptance of the unique value of time for each person.

Systems

At the systems level, demonstration of acceptance of others is most often reflected in policy or program-level strategies. Commonly there can be challenges in achieving continuity of care across organization systems, such as collaboration across clinical care and community-based care settings (e.g., hospital or clinic care transferred to a PHN agency). PHNs need to be aware of the diversity of perspectives that can emerge due to the setting in which they work. As described by Helleso and Solveig Fagermoen (2010), a nurse's assessment and the information obtained for a patient are influenced extensively by the patient's situation, the context in which the nurse works, and the nurse's character. Being aware of differences can enhance nonjudgmental exchanges across organizational systems to improve the continuity of care of populations. In addition to setting differences across various healthcare organizations, multigenerational conflict can arise among healthcare professionals within and across these organizations. Multigenerational conflict occurs when the values and practices of healthcare professionals vary across the different generations (i.e., the new PHNs versus the "old guard" PHNs; Kupperschmidt, 2006). Key to addressing or minimizing multigenerational conflict is a commitment to respecting one another and exhibiting that respect within and across healthcare organizations.

Policies that support interpreter services for those who do not speak English well are an ideal example. Much research has shown that the quality of healthcare is better when interpreters are available for Limited English Proficiency (LEP) persons. The following Evidence Example summarizes recent studies on interpreter services and healthcare quality.

Evidence Example: Interpreter Services and Healthcare Quality

In a broad critical review of literature about interpreter services and healthcare quality, many studies showed that when needed interpreter services were not provided, the quality of that healthcare was low and not ideal (Flores, 2005). The review also clarified the importance of using trained professional interpreters rather than informal interpreters, such as friends or family members. The evidence exists to support systems-level policies that require professional interpreter services. When these services are provided, clients are more likely to receive better quality care and are likely to feel respected, and accepted, for who they are. Pam Garrett (2009) has proposed a cultural empowerment model for an interpreter service policy that can serve as a guide for healthcare organizations that need to implement such a policy. The model identifies key attributes that promote cultural empowerment, including (a) facilitating language; (b) negotiating family involvement; (c) understanding patient beliefs, experiences, and constructions; (d) compassionately respecting patient and human rights; (e) negotiating the care partnership; and (f) providing systems so that providers can be competent. These types of models can be useful when organizations are not sure where to begin creating their own policies.

The use of cultural brokers, or community health workers, in providing health education, outreach, support, and resources to others in their community is another example of systems realizing the need to provide culturally relevant care and outreach (Mack, Uken, & Powers, 2006; O'Brien, Squires, Bixby, & Larson, 2009). Although PHNs need to carry out many responsibilities, others can be appropriately delegated to paraprofessionals, such as community health workers. In many situations, community health workers can be important liaisons for families navigating the complex United States healthcare system. It is important to note, though, that PHNs can serve diverse cultural groups and effectively care for those who are different from them. This is the essence of this competency—namely, realizing that PHNs need to develop acceptance of others, which can go far in reaching clients and communities. Policies that support unconditional PHN care, and such approaches as using community health workers when appropriate, can promote optimal delivery of nursing care.

The following example illustrates the impact that can be made when a policy does not exist to support particular activities and when a policy is changed without considering its impact on others. In a community with a large population of African immigrant families, Personal Care Attendants (PCAs) were providing care for men who lived alone. As part of their home care, the PCAs were cooking meals because the men had no knowledge or experience preparing meals. The law changed with respect to the PCAs' scope of practice, preventing them from preparing meals for these clients. No organizational policy was in place to support this informal job duty the PCAs had been performing. As a result of this change, the community had to generate creative options to address the gap in care. Although the community did come up with alternative solutions (e.g., cooking classes for the men, a meal delivery service), in the short term, the men lost valuable care and services because a reimbursement law changed.

Broadly, it is important to recognize the societal practices, values, and standards that influence the delivery of public health nursing care in an accepting manner. Society is always changing, and with these changes come challenges or solutions that support or impede what you are trying to do. For example, many "groups" in the United States have endured societal oppression that directly and indirectly influences how they receive services, such as public health nursing care. Being respectful of where people have been or come from, and what they have experienced in the past, or recently, is imperative to being a successful PHN. Even if you are a very accepting person, you are going to have barriers to overcome if you are providing care to someone who has experienced discrimination or judgments from a person who looks or acts in ways that are similar to you. You need to maintain awareness of the societal climate, federal and state policies, and local sentiments within which you are working as a PHN. When you do this, your care is going to be attuned, aware, and, ideally, effective and meaningful.

Intra-Agency

Finally, PHNs must also demonstrate acceptance of each other and of their colleagues in the workplace. This can be difficult but is critical as workforce diversity expands in healthcare, nursing, and public health. Coworkers might experience differences in work ethics, time management, and opinions concerning how a nursing procedure should be done. Experiences in practice or in the field certainly contribute to opinions regarding how things should be done in PHN practice, and it is not uncommon for two experienced nurses to differ in their opinions about what should or should not be done. These differences represent another reason why evidence-based practice is so important to guide practice—with growing bodies of evidence, some of these disagreements can be minimized.

Some studies addressing healthcare work environments offer relevant research findings. For example, although it was conducted with nursing assistants rather than PHNs, an important study examined organizational respect and emotional exhaustion, or burnout (Ramarajan, Barsade, & Burack, 2008). Organizational respect was measured using such statements as "staff members respect each other," "cultural diversity of staff is valued," and "staff members are treated with dignity." Not surprisingly, when nursing assistants reported higher levels of organizational respect the first time they were interviewed, when they were later re-surveyed, they were less likely to report feeling emotional exhaustion than their colleagues who had initially reported feeling that organizational respect levels were low. PHNs need to be in a work environment that respects and values them. This respect is very important because without it, a PHN might be less satisfied with work, might be more emotionally exhausted, and might choose to leave public health nursing. Because the need for PHNs is so great across the United States, workplace environments need to be supportive and accepting. If you feel judged by coworkers, consider the following strategies:

- Confront the person making you feel this way. Explore with that person why the differences exist (i.e., Are you from different generations, cultures, experiences?).

- Reflect on the situation with your supervisor (or another appropriate person) to clarify your feelings and actions that you should take.

- Approach human resources staff for assistance.

Similarly, new PHNs need to be in an environment that supports their learning and growing in new roles and experiences. Experienced nurses might find it difficult to adapt to the next generation of PHNs, but the effort needs to be made to understand each other and grow together. In this way, the public health nursing workforce can remain strong and express acceptance of one another and of clients being served. Following are some specific techniques to gain trust at the individual, community, systems, and intra-agency levels. Regardless of the level, keep in mind three overarching strategies to establishing trust: (1) Ensure clear boundaries for the relationship and comfort among all with these boundaries, (2) be authentic, and (3) create an optimal environment for interactions (i.e., comfortable, safe, relaxed; Falk-Rafael & Betker, 2012).

Table 11.3 Techniques to Gain Trust at Individual, Community, Systems, and Intra-Agency Levels

Individual level: Find a commonality with which you can connect to the individual or family.
• Respect the client's time schedule and availability. For example, clearly state your intended length of visit at the time you set the appointment, or upon arrival, so that you provide an opportunity for the client to make any necessary adjustments. This practice builds trust through mutual investment in the commitment.
• Respect the client's "home rules" that might be different than your own, such as shoe removal, where to park, or which door to use to enter the home. If you are not sure, ask.
• Whether you are seeing a specific client or an entire family, include and interact with additional family members present at the home visit. This inclusion allows you to develop a trusting atmosphere that expresses the understanding that they function within the context of their family unit.

continues

Table 11.3   Techniques to Gain Trust at Individual, Community, Systems, and Intra-Agency Levels   (continued)

Individual level: Find a commonality with which you can connect to the individual or family.

- Ask easy, open-ended questions on the telephone or at initial home visits with a genuine interest, allowing the client/family to share information. This action is essential to developing a trusting, nonjudgmental relationship. Recognize that a trusting relationship might not develop until the client sees that you keep your word and maintain confidentiality and trust, which might require many visits to demonstrate.

- Initially, focus on positive aspects and strengths of the client or family unit. Until you establish a trusting relationship, interventions are going to be less effective when they lack emphasis on assets and focus solely on problems to be addressed or fixed.

- Ask whether you can share information prior to providing it. This approach allows respect and trust to develop.

- Communicate with basic language, avoiding medical or technical language/terms.

- Avoid using a laptop or a tablet in the home if it is apparent that the clients/family do not trust that data will not be shared (because of prior experiences they might have had).

Community level: Find a fit with the members' goals (e.g., working with churches).

- Invest time in building professional relationships with key community members and in understanding the goals and missions of other community agencies that are serving the community. This outreach can lead to the establishment of trusting collaborative efforts to serve community population segments.

- Be honest and provide accurate, consistent messages to the community about health-related situations that might arise (e.g., a pertussis outbreak).

Systems level: Ensure that policies are accepting and do not ostracize.

- Implement policies and programs that meet the needs of the population being served. For example, if women utilizing the Women, Infants, and Children (WIC) program, a supplemental nutrition program, are surveyed in the community and 25% indicate that they could only come to the office to receive their food vouchers between 4 and 6 p.m., it would be appropriate to have some evening hours available and to establish a policy supporting this within the agency. This act displays openness and acceptance to the needs of this WIC population segment.

- Use community-based participatory research methods so that communities have an opportunity to participate in planning, implementing, and evaluating interventions or policies.

> **Intra-agency level: Show acceptance of coworkers within and across disciplines.**

- Openly share and discuss evidence-based nursing practice in a nonthreatening way that encourages group reflection. This approach can lead to a more unified nursing force based on mutual respect and trust in research and in each other's nursing practice.

- Engage in reflective supervision and/or reflective practice groups. This process goes beyond reflection and journaling and has become increasingly popular in evidence-based home-visiting protocols/models. Simply, reflective supervision provides PHNs with feedback they can use to examine the patterns they might be using in caring for their clients and to readjust patterns that are not optimal.

Ethical Application

Feminist and virtue ethics provide excellent principles with which to examine this competency. Feminist ethics emphasizes that actions should not oppress others. This competency focuses on accepting others and not being judgmental. By respecting the clients you are working with, you demonstrate acceptance, and you do not oppress. Similarly, virtue ethics emphasizes tolerance and justice as two leading principles. When you are tolerant of others' experiences, beliefs, or perspectives, you are achieving this competency and acting as an ethical nurse. Finally, when you act in a just manner, you express to other people that they have worth and dignity. Imagine the positive influence you, the PHN, can have in the diverse lives and communities you serve when you ethically provide care. This positive influence might come from something as simple as maintaining appropriate confidentiality, facilitating a nonjudgmental environment in a home visit or a community screening event, and expressing acceptance in verbal and nonverbal ways. With regard to the importance of maintaining appropriate confidentiality, PHNs care for clients in vulnerable states and complex situations. PHNs, therefore, need to be very conscientious to respect their clients and the confidentiality of the nurse-client relationship by refraining from talking about clients to other people beyond what is necessary for care coordination purposes. In the case study in this chapter, you have observed Josie addressing many preconceptions regarding the client she is visiting. You have noticed how easy it can be to make judgments and how challenging it can be to provide nursing care in a nonjudgmental manner. Yet, when nursing care is nonjudgmental, it is much more likely to be effective and promote lasting change (see Table 11.4).

Table 11.4   Ethical Action in Providing Nonjudgmental and Unconditional Care

Ethical perspective	Application
Rule ethics (principles)	- Nonjudgmental public health nursing should simultaneously encourage beneficence and promote the good of families and communities.
	- Encourage autonomy by listening respectfully and showing verbal and nonverbal respect for the opinions of those being cared for.

continues

Table 11.4   Ethical Action in Providing Nonjudgmental and Unconditional Care   (continued)

Ethical perspective	Application
Virtue ethics (character)	• Be respectful in actions and words. • Be persistent in showing tolerance and creatively promoting health. • Be accepting and aware of how responses and actions can promote or discourage those being served.
Feminist ethics (reducing oppression)	• Conduct assessments in a manner that appreciates strengths while also identifying areas for intervention. • Respect everyone. • Advocate for individuals and community groups that might have less power because they are regularly judged (e.g., homeless youth).

Key Points

- Even the most experienced PHNs can struggle with being nonjudgmental and accepting of other people.

- People and communities can be different from each other on multiple levels, including social, economic, geographic, religious, behavioral, age, ethnicity, race, or sexual orientation.

- Acting in a nonjudgmental manner does not mean that PHNs are accepting of everything.

- PHNs can increase the potential for program or intervention success by carefully examining the key cultural or social beliefs or practices within a community.

- Reflecting on your own reactions toward those who are different from you is a critical starting point toward achieving this competency.

- Remember that policies can promote acceptance or judgment of people or groups and that they should be made with input from diverse stakeholders.

Learning Examples for Strategies to Increase Acceptance of Others

This is one of those competency areas that is not so easily translated into a set of experiences or exercises that can ensure that you develop into a more accepting person or nurse. However, you can undertake some experiences that are likely to encourage reflection on how you react in an uncomfortable or unfamiliar setting or among people who differ in their beliefs, culture, or behaviors. Becoming culturally competent or proficient is a lifelong learning process, but you can start by gaining appreciation of diverse cultures, learning about other health practices, and being meaningful in your desire to increase your competent care of others. In a pilot project, students from two nursing schools in two different states, primarily operating in urban and rural settings, shared their community health assessments through videoconferencing (Pirkey, Levey, Newberry, Guthman, & Hansen, 2012). This method allowed students to increase their cultural awareness by gaining exposure to diverse populations they would not typically have encountered through their educational programs.

For some, being culturally competent is possible only when they can be cultural brokers, which includes language fluency and deep cultural understanding. Although many PHNs might not be "competent" in that way, they can be culturally respectful and responsive. Most important is your willingness to evaluate yourself with respect to how nonjudgmental or accepting you are and, based on that evaluation, to identify things you might do to enhance acceptance. The following examples will help you increase your acceptance of others:

- Engage in self-reflection via journaling or simple thought, because "this is an opportunity . . . to expose [your] biases" (Porr, 2005, p. 192). Sample journal questions include the following: "What do I believe contributes to my own health status?" "How am I different from other students, family members, neighbors?" "How am I similar?" "When I felt uncomfortable in a recent experience in the community, why did I feel that way?" "How have I been made to feel comfortable in a group or with someone different from myself?"

- Engage in activities that develop *perceptual* (nurse's ability to make relevant observations) and *conceptual skills* (ability to give meaning to observations). Examples include role-playing and observing and analyzing DVDs of actual family/nurse interactions (Wright & Leahey, 2005, p. 184–185). Engaging in these activities allows observation and analysis of interactions that might impede or increase your acceptance of others.

- Invest in developing virtues essential to good nursing character, such as compassion, integrity, fidelity, courage, justice, mediation, self-confidence, resilience, and practical reasoning (Volbrecht, 2001, p. 102). This development increases not only your acceptance of clients but the client's acceptance of you.

- Invest time in reading and developing background knowledge pertaining to aspects of the client, population, or system that you are serving as a PHN.

- Consider visiting a setting that is not familiar or comfortable to you and reflectively journal about how you felt and what you experienced (e.g., a religious ceremony, a cultural event, a shelter, or a nursing home).

- Read books that challenge your perspectives and deepen your understanding. Examples include *The Spirit Catches You and You Fall Down* by Anne Fadiman (1998, Fararr, Straus and Giroux); *Nickel and Dimed* by Barbara Ehrenreich (2002, Holt); and *A Thousand Splendid Suns* by Khaled Hosseini (2008, Riverhead Trade).

- Watch an episode of *Call the Midwife* and describe observed examples (or not) of empathy and being nonjudgmental.

Reflective Practice

Considering what you have learned in this chapter, identify what Josie might do next to act on her reflections during the home visit and her realization that her preconceived judgments are not only inaccurate but also not helpful in providing optimal care for the teen and her new baby. After writing your responses to the following reflective questions, compare the questions and strategies you identify with those noted at the end of the chapter:

1. What does Josie need to understand about being nonjudgmental and accepting?

   _____

   _____

2. What are some additional reflective questions that Josie needs to ask herself, and which information sources might be useful to her in growing more accepting of others?

   _____

   _____

3. How will Josie know that her efforts to be increasingly accepting of diverse people and communities are successful?

   _____

   _____

4. How might the Cornerstones inform Josie's efforts to be accepting and nonjudgmental?

   _____

   _____

Application of Evidence

1. Which ethical considerations are important to think about in responding to individuals, families, and communities in a nonjudgmental manner?

2. How might you work with colleagues to process judgmental feelings and work toward becoming more nonjudgmental?

3. What might you do to contribute to a work culture that supports nonjudgmental and unconditional acceptance of people?

Think, Explore, Do

1. What might you ask yourself before you go on a home visit or meet with a client?

2. Where is the neighborhood? Have you been there before? What do you think about it?

3. What is something that you have in common with the family you are visiting?

4. Does the policy you are enforcing encourage acceptance of others' beliefs, cultures, etc.?

5. How might you change a policy in your department so that it is nonjudgmental?

6. Which resources might you use to learn about a new cultural group you are serving?

7. What are the key issues you need to consider when outreaching to an elderly group?

8. What are two things you can do to create a welcoming, accepting physical environment?

9. How might you show that you value another person or community?

10. When designing a health promotion activity for a religious audience, such as cholesterol screening, what are some things you want to consider so that the screening is most successful?

11. How can you show acceptance to your coworkers and interdisciplinary colleagues?

12. When you see someone acting in a judgmental manner, which steps might you take to model acceptance?

References

Aston, M., Meagher-Stewart, D., Sheppard-Lemoine, D., Vukic, A., & Chircop, A. (2006). Family health nursing and empowering relationships. *Pediatric Nursing, 32*(1), 61–67.

Center for Spirituality and Healing [CSH]. (2013). *Deep Listening.* Retrieved from http://cityhill.org/media.php?pageID=96

Cioffi, J. (2003). Communicating with culturally and linguistically diverse patients in an acute care setting: Nurses' experiences. *International Journal of Nursing Studies, 40*(3), 299–306.

Dillon, R. (1992). Respect and care: Toward a moral integration. *Canadian Journal of Philosophy, 22*(1), 105–132.

Falk-Rafael, A., & Betker, C. (2012). The primacy of relationships: A study of public health nursing practice from a critical caring perspective. *Advances in Nursing Science, 35*(4), 315–332.

Flores, G. (2005). The impact of medical interpreter services on the quality of health care: A systematic review. *Medical Care Research Review, 62*(3), 255–299.

Garrett, P. (2009). Healthcare interpreter policy: Policy determinants and current issues in the Australian context. *Interpreting and Translation, 1*(2), 44–54.

Goldsborough, J. D. (1970). On becoming nonjudgmental. *American Journal of Nursing, 70*(11), 2340–2343.

Helleso, R., & Solveig Fagermoen, M. (2010). Cultural diversity between hospital and community nurses: Implications for continuity of care. *International Journal of Integrated Care, 10,* e036.

Kupperschmidt, B. R. (2006). Addressing multigenerational conflict: Mutual respect and carefronting as strategy. *Online Journal of Issues in Nursing, 11*(2).

Leininger, M. (1978). Transcultural nursing theories and research approaches. In M. Leininger, (Ed.), *Transcultural Nursing* (pp. 31–51). New York, NY: Wiley.

Mack, M., Uken, R., & Powers, J. (2006). People improving the community's health: Community health workers as agents of change. *Journal of Health Care for the Poor and Underserved, 17*(1), 16–25.

Nagano, H. (2000). Empathic understanding: Constructing an evaluation scale from the microcounseling approach. *Nursing and Health Sciences, 2*(1), 17–27.

O'Brien, M. J., Squires, A. P., Bixby, R. A., & Larson, S. C. (2009). Role development of community health workers: An examination of selection and training processes in the intervention literature. *American Journal of Preventive Medicine, 37*(6), s262–s269.

Pasco, A. C. Y., Morse, J. M., & Olson, J. K. (2004). The cross-cultural relationships between nurses and Filipino Canadian patients. *Journal of Nursing Scholarship, 36*(3), 239–246.

Passel, J., & Cohn, D. (2008). U.S. Population Projections 2005–2050. Retrieved from http://www.pewhispanic.org/files/reports/85.pdf

Payne, R. K., DeVol, P. E., & Smith, T. D. (2001). *Bridges out of poverty: Strategies for professionals and communities.* Highlands, TX: aha! Process, Inc.

Pesznecker, B. L. (1984). The poor: A population at risk. *Public Health Nursing, 1*(4), 237–249.

Pirkey, J. M., Levey, J. A., Newberry, S. M., Guthman, P. L., & Hansen, J. M. (2012). Videoconferencing expands nursing students' cultural realm. *Journal of Nursing Education, 51*(10), 586–590.

Porr, C. (2005). Shifting from preconceptions to pure wonderment. *Nursing Philosophy, 6*(3), 189–195.

Porr, C., Drummond, J., & Olson, K. (2012). Establishing therapeutic relationships with vulnerable and potentially stigmatized clients. *Qualitative Health Research, 22*(3), 384–396.

Ramarajan, L., Barsade, S. G., & Burack, O. R. (2008). The influence of organizational respect on emotional exhaustion in the human services. *Journal of Positive Psychology, 3*(1), 3–18.

Segal, J., Smith, M. A., & Jaffe, J. (2013). *Nonverbal communication skills: The power of nonverbal communication and body language.* Retrieved from http://www.helpguide.org/mental/eq6_nonverbal_communication.htm

U.S. Census Bureau. (2013). U.S. Population Other Than White by State: 2000. Retrieved from http://www.census.gov/geo/maps-data/maps/pdfs/thematic/pct_otherthan_white_2000.pdf

Volbrecht, R. M. (2001). *Nursing ethics: Communities in dialogue.* Upper Saddle River, NJ: Prentice Hall.

Wright, L. M., & Leahey, M. (2005). *Nurses and families: A guide to family assessment and intervention,* 4th ed. Philadelphia, PA: F. A. Davis.

COMPETENCY #10

Incorporates Mental, Physical, Emotional, Social, Spiritual, and Environmental Aspects of Health Into Assessment, Planning, Implementation, and Evaluation

12

Carolyn M. Garcia
with Christine C. Andres, Maureen A. Alms, and Karen Goedken

Maria has just finished her 6-month orientation at a local public health department in the Maternal Child Health division. She has received her nursing license just 7 months ago after spending a decade in business management as a supervisor of a large customer service and sales department. Maria is concerned about how she can possibly assess all aspects of health in high-risk populations. One weekend, Maria receives a referral from the local hospital involving a child who needs to be seen by a public health nurse (PHN). Maria is excited and nervous about this first case. The only information she receives is that the family has a 2 year-old boy who is being released from the hospital after suffering an asthma attack. Newly diagnosed with asthma, the boy and his family need education and a home assessment.

Maria calls the mother to set a time for the visit. While driving to the home, Maria mentally reviews everything she knows about asthma. She anticipates that education will be easy, because she has a son with asthma and is familiar with the disease process and management. Upon arrival at the home, she becomes slightly uneasy with the multiple dogs and cats roaming the yard. She knocks several times on the trailer door before a man answers and lets her inside the home. Maria enters the kitchen, and everyone exchanges introductions. Marcus, the boy with asthma, is quiet in his mother's arms. His brothers, 1 and 5 years of age, are running around the kitchen table, trying to open Maria's nursing bag, jumping on her, and attempting to take her pen. It is very chaotic. Maria has to overcome her anxiety as she realizes that completing a nursing assessment is going to be a challenge.

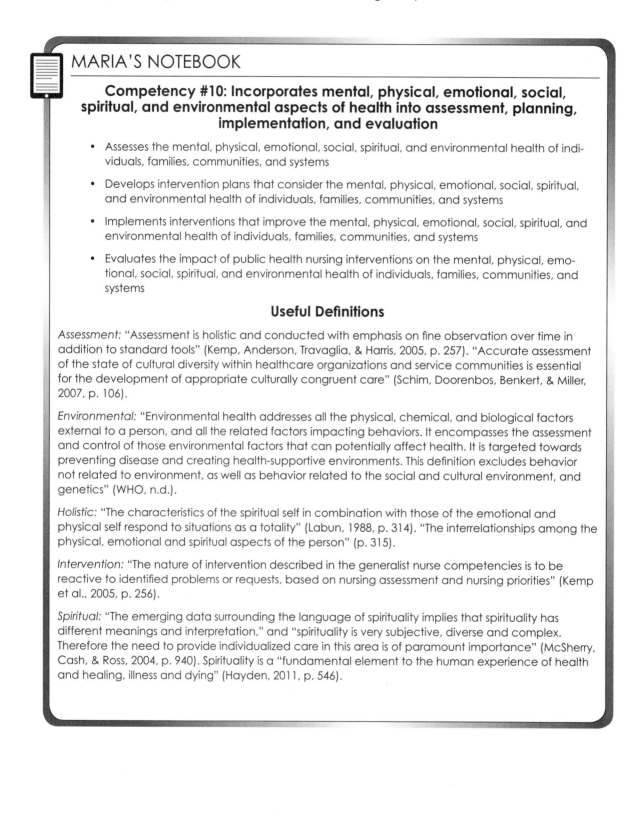

MARIA'S NOTEBOOK

Competency #10: Incorporates mental, physical, emotional, social, spiritual, and environmental aspects of health into assessment, planning, implementation, and evaluation

- Assesses the mental, physical, emotional, social, spiritual, and environmental health of individuals, families, communities, and systems

- Develops intervention plans that consider the mental, physical, emotional, social, spiritual, and environmental health of individuals, families, communities, and systems

- Implements interventions that improve the mental, physical, emotional, social, spiritual, and environmental health of individuals, families, communities, and systems

- Evaluates the impact of public health nursing interventions on the mental, physical, emotional, social, spiritual, and environmental health of individuals, families, communities, and systems

Useful Definitions

Assessment: "Assessment is holistic and conducted with emphasis on fine observation over time in addition to standard tools" (Kemp, Anderson, Travaglia, & Harris, 2005, p. 257). "Accurate assessment of the state of cultural diversity within healthcare organizations and service communities is essential for the development of appropriate culturally congruent care" (Schim, Doorenbos, Benkert, & Miller, 2007, p. 106).

Environmental: "Environmental health addresses all the physical, chemical, and biological factors external to a person, and all the related factors impacting behaviors. It encompasses the assessment and control of those environmental factors that can potentially affect health. It is targeted towards preventing disease and creating health-supportive environments. This definition excludes behavior not related to environment, as well as behavior related to the social and cultural environment, and genetics" (WHO, n.d.).

Holistic: "The characteristics of the spiritual self in combination with those of the emotional and physical self respond to situations as a totality" (Labun, 1988, p. 314). "The interrelationships among the physical, emotional and spiritual aspects of the person" (p. 315).

Intervention: "The nature of intervention described in the generalist nurse competencies is to be reactive to identified problems or requests, based on nursing assessment and nursing priorities" (Kemp et al., 2005, p. 256).

Spiritual: "The emerging data surrounding the language of spirituality implies that spirituality has different meanings and interpretation," and "spirituality is very subjective, diverse and complex. Therefore the need to provide individualized care in this area is of paramount importance" (McSherry, Cash, & Ross, 2004, p. 940). Spirituality is a "fundamental element to the human experience of health and healing, illness and dying" (Hayden, 2011, p. 546).

From the Seen to the Unseen

One of the reasons that nursing is such an exciting profession is the breadth and depth of nursing practice. Nurses work in so many different arenas and engage in a range of health promotion, intervention, and healing or transition process activities. Public health nursing is no exception, and to an extent, it sets a precedent for the diversity of nursing practice. In public health nursing, one can be employed in a local public health department, a manufacturing plant, a school, a church, or a prison. PHNs care for people where they work, recreate, worship, and live. An appreciation for this complexity informs this public health nursing competency. Indeed, competent PHNs can holistically assess numerous aspects of health and then intervene in creative, meaningful ways. This chapter explores the 10th Henry Street Consortium Competency, with particular emphasis given to those aspects of health that can be subtle and perhaps more challenging to consider for a beginning PHN. Rather than overwhelm, we hope this chapter informs and encourages you to consider the range of possibilities in public health nursing as viewed through a holistic lens.

Assessing the Mental, Physical, Emotional, Social, Spiritual, and Environmental Health of Individuals, Families, Communities, and Systems

Assessment gives PHNs an understanding of what is going on, including what might be contributing to or preventing solutions and how they can assist or intervene. In preparation for becoming a nurse, you spend numerous hours learning and practicing assessments. In a clinical assessment for heart disease, nurses might take a blood pressure, measure cholesterol, run a stress test, and take a verbal personal and family history. In a public health nursing assessment, these objective and subjective types of data are also collected, yet the scope is often broader in that PHNs conduct assessments at the community and systems levels. At all levels, the nurses' emphases on objective and subjective data remain similar. PHNs systematically observe, document, and summarize data to support assessment findings. These data are quantitative (e.g., rates of disease, symptom frequency, number of risks, number of assets, costs) and qualitative (e.g., personal experiences of those affected, expressed opinions, photographs that demonstrate risks/assets). Most important is that an assessment is carefully planned and thoroughly implemented so that results are useful and can be acted upon.

At the individual level, examples of direct care assessment include examining a newborn for signs of healthy development, screening a new mother for postpartum depression, and determining the spiritual state of someone recently diagnosed with terminal cancer. In the home setting, PHNs consider the environment in which a family is living by assessing home safety (e.g., loose rugs that might cause an elderly client to trip or lead paint flakes a toddler could ingest) and the social environment, such as neighborhood safety (e.g., crime levels) or access to healthy food sources.

Another type of assessment is conducted when individuals are asked how they might be best supported by a PHN. Fifty mothers who had gone through drug dependency court were asked in a study how they could be best supported by PHNs in their treatment and reunification with their children (Somervell, Saylor, & Mao, 2005). In interviews, the mothers suggested they would like PHNs to serve as a bridge of information to them, reporting on the health and well-being of their children while those children were in foster care. This needs assessment provided the PHNs with clarity of what the mothers wanted, and did not want, in services, knowledge that was useful in planning their activities while working with these mothers.

Family-level assessment expands the individual-level focus to the family unit, which can be large. The family is viewed as an interactional system, with its holistic health determined by such factors as family dynamics and relationships, family structure, and family functioning (Friedman, Bowden, & Jones, 2003). This approach is particularly useful when PHNs try to manage a health condition that is somewhat dependent on the family setting. For example, a school nurse might work with a student to manage asthma, but without adequate family assessment, the nurse might miss risk factors in the home that are aggravating the asthma (e.g., smoking family members, dust, presence of rodents). Assessment of family-level risk behaviors can also contribute to a family-level intervention, such as efforts to increase the activity level of all family members to reduce obesity and risks for diabetes. Holistic public health nursing at the family level might use family strengths theory, a theoretical approach that emphasizes building on existing strengths within the family, as a guide to assessment and intervention planning and implementation (Sittner, Hudson, & Defrain, 2007).

 Evidence Example: Holistic Public Health Nursing Care for the Family

The following are some helpful clinical examples of holistic public health nursing care for the family unit (Sittner et al., 2007, p. 357):

- Consider assessing a family's strengths when planning nursing care for the family.
- Help families cope with stress and crises effectively by providing consistent information.
- Be sure to listen and work toward establishing a trusting relationship with the family.
- Acknowledge the family members' individualized spiritual perspective and implement nursing interventions that promote their spiritual needs.
- Help the family understand that enjoyable time together during an illness is important.
- Encourage the family to be physically close and celebrate occasions.
- Encourage family members to express appreciation for assistance during an illness.
- Help nursing students understand the family strengths perspective.

Maria starts with a simple focused assessment of Marcus. He has no temperature and no apparent difficulty breathing. His lung sounds are clear. When she asks about using the nebulizer, the parents respond, "What nebulizer?" Maria calls the hospital triage nurse and, after multiple transfers, reaches a nurse who discovers that the order was never placed but that it would be delivered immediately, with arrival expected yet that day. In the meantime, Maria wants to start addressing some of the asthma triggers present in the environment. The floor is coated with food crumbs, and dishes in the sink have flies hovering over them. The windowless room where the boys sleep has three mattresses on the floor with dirty blankets and pillows without coverings. The bathroom has a strong air deodorizer smell; it is also where the parents smoke. Maria starts to feel an itchy sensation on her legs and assesses the children's ankles and legs. They are covered with little red marks, and Marcus's legs feel rough like sandpaper. She mentions the bites on the children, and the mother states that they have a flea problem but have not had the money to do anything about it. Maria feels overwhelmed. How can she help a family with so many needs?

Table 12.1 offers an example of a home safety checklist that a PHN might use during a home visit with an elderly person, which would differ from one used with a family with young children, for example. Home safety checklists can assist PHNs in identifying potential strengths or risks in a home environment; findings at this individual level can also inform community- or systems-level strategies (e.g., promoting removal of throw rugs for the elderly population after observing the risks at the individual level in homes).

Table 12.1   Example Home Safety Checklist for an Elderly Person

Home Safety Checklist
Living Room and Family Room
1. Can you turn on a light without having to walk into a dark room?
2. Are lamp, extension, or phone cords out of the flow of foot traffic?
3. Are passageways in this room free from objects and clutter (papers, furniture)?
4. Are curtains and furniture at least 36 inches from baseboard heaters or portable heaters?
5. Do your carpets lie flat?
6. Do your small rugs and runners stay put (don't slide or roll up) when you push them with your foot?
Kitchen
7. Are your stove controls easy to see and use?
8. Do you keep loose-fitting clothing, towels, and curtains that might catch fire away from the burners and oven?
9. Can you reach regularly used items without climbing to reach them?
10. Do you have a step stool that is sturdy and in good repair?
Bedrooms
11. Do you have working smoke detectors on the ceiling outside of bedroom doors?
12. Can you turn on a light without having to walk into a dark room?
13. Do you have a lamp or light switch within easy reach of your bed?
14. Is a phone within easy reach of your bed?

continues

Table 12.1   Example Home Safety Checklist for an Elderly Person   (continued)

Bedrooms

15. Is a light left on at night between your bed and the toilet?

16. Are the curtains and furniture at least 36 inches from your baseboard heater or portable heater?

Bathroom

17. Does your shower or tub have a nonskid surface, such as a mat, decals, or abrasive strips?

18. Does the tub/shower have a sturdy grab bar (not just a towel rack)?

19. Is your hot water temperature set to 120° or lower?

20. Does your floor have a nonslip surface or does the rug have a nonskid backing?

21. Can you get on and off the toilet easily?

Stairways

22. Is there a light switch at both the top and bottom of inside stairs?

23. With the light on, can you clearly see the outline of each step as you go down the stairs?

24. Do all stairways have sturdy handrails on both sides?

25. Do handrails run the full length of the stairs, slightly beyond the steps?

26. Are all the steps in good repair (not loose, broken, missing, or worn in places)?

27. Are stair coverings (rugs, treads) in good repair, without holes and not loose, torn, or worn?

Hallways and Passageways

28. Do all small rugs or runners stay put (don't slide or roll up) when you push them with your foot?

29. Do your carpets lie flat?

30. Are all lamp, extension, and phone cords out of the flow of foot traffic?

Front and Back Entrances

31. Do all entrances to your home have outdoor lights?

32. Are walkways to your entry free from cracks and holes?

Throughout Your House

33. Do you have an emergency exit plan in case of fire?

34. Do you have emergency phone numbers listed by your phone?

35. Are there other hazards or unsafe areas in your home not mentioned in this checklist that you are concerned about? If so, what?

Making Your Home Safer

What home safety changes do you want to make?

1.

2.

3.

Provided by: California Department of Aging, Senior Housing Information and Support Center
Adapted from: "Home Safety Checklist Summary"
Developed by: Community and Home Injury Prevention Project for Seniors (CHIPPS)
Sponsored by: Community Health Education Section, San Francisco Department of Public Health

The following evidence example provides a picture of a unique, holistic approach to assessment at the individual level but focused on past experiences and how those experiences might influence adulthood health and well-being.

Evidence Example: Minnesota Department of Health Adverse Childhood Experiences (ACE) Project

In 2011, the Minnesota Department of Health (MDH, 2013a) used questions developed by the Centers for Disease Control and Prevention (CDC) to understand the scope and influence of adverse childhood experiences (ACE) on adult health and well-being. The ACE questions focus on exposure to such experiences as emotional, physical, and sexual abuse; substance use; and family disruption. Results of the 2011 survey revealed that many Minnesotan adults report experiencing multiple ACEs in their childhood (before age 18). Many of these adults also reported current social and health problems, including higher rates of chronic illnesses than adults who reported no ACEs in their childhoods. Additional research is needed, but as more states ask the ACE questions, there is greater understanding of the influence of ACE on health and well-being into adulthood. Such research strongly supports the need for holistic assessment and health promotion efforts. The role of resilience in offsetting adverse experiences and promoting well-being despite adversity is also recognized and demonstrated in this research. PHNs can play an important role in identifying risk factors as well as protective factors in all aspects of an individual, family, and community.

> ### 🍏 Healthy People 2020
>
> The Healthy People 2020 website identifies indicators for a variety of public health concerns in the United States, with goals for improvements by 2020. Select a health indicator and explore how a PHN might work to improve health while paying attention to all aspects of an individual's or community's health. Identify possible collaborators who might work with the PHN to achieve intervention goals and also promote health in a comprehensive holistic manner (i.e., working with a local religious institution or partnering with mental health professionals).

Community assessment broadens the public health nursing perspective to consider the health of a group. Remember that community can be defined in many different ways, as a group of people connected by geography, age, ethnicity, spiritual beliefs, or health and risk behaviors. PHNs working with a community need to earnestly examine the strengths and needs in that community before engaging in health promotion or disease prevention activities. For example, a parish nurse might assess the need for a cardiovascular or diabetes screening program and determine the presence of existing resources or gaps in resources in the parish and surrounding community. The PHN in this case is also going to want to know the extent to which a cardiovascular or diabetes screening program might be a priority health concern for parish members. A detailed assessment contributes to the increased likelihood of a successful, accepted program.

An occupational PHN might assess the needs and preferences of workers prior to starting a health promotion intervention. This assessment is necessary because without it, the PHN cannot have a clear picture of the needs and problems and how possible solutions are going to be received. Oxygen delivery drivers might benefit from an intervention that teaches them stretching and ways to prevent repetitive motion injuries, but assessment can inform the PHN whether the drivers have any interest in such a program. Without the drivers' interest or some level of motivation, the intervention could be a significant waste of time, energy, and other resources.

PHNs in local public health departments have often undertaken large-scale geographic community assessments, driving through cities and documenting risks (e.g., crime, abandoned buildings, manufacturing plants) and assets (e.g., police, recreation, grocery stores). It is more common in today's environment with constraints on resources (e.g., time, finances) to see PHNs conducting focused or targeted community assessments to inform specific initiatives or activities. However, especially if PHNs are new to a setting, they might conduct more thorough community assessments to drive their or their agency's priorities and goal setting. Often an assessment helps decision-makers determine how best to use limited funds and resources by prioritizing the greatest areas of need. The following are the basic steps of a community health assessment (also see Chapter 3, which is devoted to assessment in public health nursing).

Note that this process is not intended to be linear and that many aspects of an assessment might be "combined, rearranged, or worked on simultaneously" (MDH, 2013b):

1. Organize.

2. Plan assessment in partnership.

3. Gather and analyze assessment data.

4. Document and communicate findings (MDH, 2013b).

The systems level is often more difficult to understand with respect to the nursing process and public health nursing. If you think about the system comprising many of the larger, overarching policies and governmental/societal forces that influence health, then it might be easier to grasp this concept of "system." PHNs employed with the local public health department must work within the guidelines of local-, state-, and federal-level policies, rules, and regulations (see Competency #4, Chapter 6). Assessment at the systems level, then, can be useful when PHNs believe that a particular policy or regulation is needed or should be eliminated. An example of this situation is the assessment that took place across the United States that resulted in a realized need for indoor antismoking regulations. PHNs worked with many colleagues to assess the potential impact of an indoor smoking ban, including its costs, ethics, and health implications. Systems-level assessment is complex, yet it is so important, because when policies or laws are made, they have the potential for extensive, long-lasting influence.

PHNs can often contribute to the successes of statewide screening programs. When PHNs are directly involved in the assessment, planning, implementation, and evaluation of infant screening programs, they are more likely to be successful (Kemper, Fant, & Clark, 2005). Specifically, PHNs work directly with infants, parents, and families, and this experience is valuable when large-scale efforts are planned. The PHNs are ideally prepared, for example, to develop the screening tools that can be used not only in the home but also in common healthcare settings, such as clinics (Kemper et al., 2005). Another example is the Follow Along Program (FAP), a Minnesota statewide screening method for young children that is intended to ensure early and continuous screening for health concerns and developmental and behavioral delays. This screening is a cooperative arrangement between the Minnesota Department of Health Children and Youth with Special Health Needs and local FAP agencies, which are typically public health agencies. The PHNs use a computerized tracking program to holistically screen all aspects of a child and to work with families as concerns arise to ensure access to appropriate child and family interventions and support. When the early screening data were evaluated in 1999, the counties with an FAP identified many more children who were eligible for early intervention than those counties that did not have an FAP (MDH, 2009).

See Table 12.2 for an example of assessment at the individual, community, and systems levels for primary, secondary, and tertiary intervention strategies.

Table 12.2   Example of Assessment Addressing Adolescent Substance Use

Levels of assessment and intervention	Individual	Community	Systems
Primary	Assess risk and protective factors that might influence substance use decision-making. School nurses might screen/survey all students to determine which prevention messages might be ideal based on existing beliefs, assets, and risks among peers, families, and neighborhoods.	Assess community-level attitudes and ideas regarding substance use among adolescents. PHNs might partner with local schools, religious institutions, community parks and playground facilities, and healthcare organizations to conduct focus groups, walk-along interviews, and community assessment to identify key points of intervention—attitudes, behaviors, knowledge, or infrastructure.	Identify the laws and policies that support prevention of substance use among adolescents. PHNs might advocate for stricter penalties for bars selling to underage drinkers if this is a problem in the particular area/city.
Secondary	Assess adolescent substance-use behaviors, including risk and protective factors. PHNs might screen a pregnant teen during a home visit to determine substance-use behaviors and plan risk-reduction intervention.	PHNs might assess substance-use behaviors among homeless adolescents to determine incidence and prevalence of drug use and help guide the development of interventions. PHNs might screen homeless youth seeking healthcare and offer cessation programs for those reporting use.	Assess level of substance-use treatment programs available to adolescents in the state. PHNs might work with health insurance providers to ensure that coverage includes adequate time for adolescent participation in a cessation program.

| Tertiary | Assess adolescent's level of willingness to participate in efforts to reduce risk behaviors during pregnancy. PHNs might provide case management and support for pregnant adolescent trying not to use during the pregnancy and explore resources with her that promote self-worth, including emotional and spiritual resources. | Partner with community members to assess readiness for change in a community where many adolescents are already using or abusing substances. | Assess the scope of existing resources to serve/treat adolescents who are using/abusing substances. PHNs might collaborate with local community organizations to support or establish treatment centers that can reach and target adolescents. |

ACTIVITY

Using the table above, construct a similar table for a new health problem or condition you have discussed in class or observed in clinical.

Develops Intervention Plans That Consider Mental, Physical, Emotional, Social, Spiritual, and Environmental Health

At some point, the assessment findings are used to prioritize possible interventions and inform decision-making. The next step, then, is to develop an intervention plan for the target individual, family, community, or systems (see Figure 12.1 for this process). PHNs often work with a family, for example, so that together they consider the findings from the assessment and arrive at a plan to address concerns. Sometimes the intervention plans are very narrow and focused, driven by an assessment that obviously leads to a clear problem and solution. Other times, the intervention plans are broad and encompass several goals and strategies to reach those goals. Regardless of whether the intervention plan is narrow or broad, it can and should be holistic and address multiple aspects of an individual, family, community, or system.

For example, a PHN might conduct home visits with a newborn and mother for the first few postpartum months. Assessment might indicate healthy newborn development but a risk of postpartum depression. The intervention plan is likely to consider all aspects of health for that mom and baby, yielding a multilayered strategy that might include mom breaks (mental), medication for depression or regular walks outside (physical), friend connections (emotional and social), yoga or meditation (spiritual), and housecleaning help (environmental). In this way, a focused intervention to prevent or minimize postpartum depression encompasses, or has the potential to encompass, every aspect of health.

At the community level, the parish nurse might conclude that a cardiovascular screening program is needed and desired. The resulting intervention plan might include a variety of activities that consider varied aspects of health, including stress evaluation (mental), blood pressure or cholesterol measures (physical), stress levels (emotional), relationships (social), prayer practices (spiritual), and access to exercise outlets/recreation (environmental). In this example, the screening program is holistic and will lead to relevant, individualized interventions.

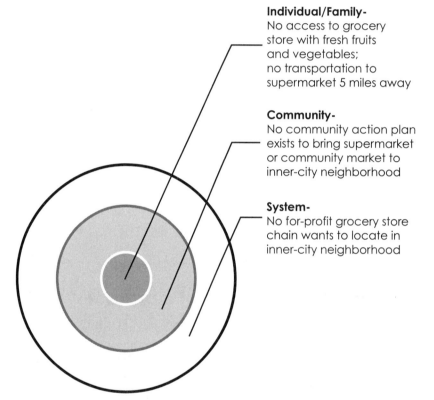

Individual/Family-
No access to grocery store with fresh fruits and vegetables; no transportation to supermarket 5 miles away

Community-
No community action plan exists to bring supermarket or community market to inner-city neighborhood

System-
No for-profit grocery store chain wants to locate in inner-city neighborhood

Figure 12.1. Public Health Nursing Process

Maria goes back the next day to review with the family what is important to them and how to prioritize and develop a plan of care. Maria and the parents agree that managing Marcus's asthma is a top priority. Maria completes hands-on education on utilizing the nebulizer. The flea infestation and environmental asthma triggers are considered important, so Maria and the parents plan together how and when they can treat the home to get rid of the fleas, minimize dust, and so forth. Maria addresses some safety issues, such as having the bedroom with no window and hearing Marcus at night if he is having an asthma attack. The father appreciates her help in getting connected to a company that supplies an alarm system that flashes lights instead of producing noise.

Implements Interventions That Improve Mental, Physical, Emotional, Social, Spiritual, and Environmental Health

After an intervention plan is identified, the PHN needs to identify resources and arrange the logistics (i.e., details) for implementing the plan. This might include collaborating with colleagues, finding community partners, or leveraging financial resources to ensure success. Careful planning is necessary to ensure successful intervention implementation.

 Evidence Example: Health Department Partnerships to Prevent Obesity Among Cognitively Challenged Persons

Health and wellness for the cognitively challenged population has become an important policy issue for the State of Minnesota and Hennepin County. Millions in taxpayer dollars are spent on hospital and nursing home stays for this population each year because of poor nutrition and lack of exercise. Karen Goedken, a PHN for Hennepin County, learned that public health nursing students were involved in promoting the health of communities and initiated a relationship that would involve students in the health promotion of cognitively challenged clients, specifically focusing on nutrition and prevention of obesity. Over the next 12 months, a collaboration was developed that included cognitively challenged clients and staff from Minnesota Life College, a nonprofit semi-independent living setting in Hennepin County; program managers and nutritionists from Hennepin County; the PHN; and teams of public health nursing students from the University of Minnesota School of Nursing. To date, students have conducted baseline assessments for 12 aspects of the cognitively challenged population in the program, including weight, height, waist circumference, body mass index (BMI), blood pressure, and pulse. The students have also experimented with developing a mHealth application (i.e., app) that clients could use when they shop at a grocery store. The app would guide them to the ingredients for recipes for several healthy meals. Minnesota Life College has also developed a program titled "Emerging Leaders" that promotes health and wellness by encouraging cognitively challenged clients to work out at the YMCA, attend lectures on health and wellness, participate in work and community health activities, and help design a community garden. Minnesota Life College staff have benefited from program planning with the county nutritionists as well as parents and community support members who have been included in health and wellness project training, such as healthy meal preparation. Outcomes of this practice-based collaborative health promotion intervention are promising. One participant has lost 20 pounds, another 12, and another 10. All participants have modified their diets, greatly reduced their intake of sugary drinks, reduced frequent trips to nearby fast food restaurants, and increased their willingness to cook healthy meals once or twice a week. The collaboration is ongoing, with plans to broaden the collaborative efforts to include more clients, family members, caretakers, and staff. Nursing students will continue to be engaged, promoting various ways to keep the emphasis on healthy eating and steady routine exercise sessions. Ongoing evaluation efforts will help determine new ways to enhance health promotion efforts for the developmentally disabled throughout Hennepin County and the State of Minnesota.

A PHN working with the mother and baby in the case study can implement the intervention by carefully discussing the approach with the mother in an empowering manner. It would be overwhelming to recommend and implement every part of the plan immediately. Instead, the nurse and mother can work together to prioritize parts of the intervention and determine achievable goals. For example, access to asthma medication might be an initial goal, and the PHN can help the mother contact and work with her child's primary care provider to arrange a prescription and teach her how to contact the insurance provider to confirm that coverage is available. The PHN can also provide the mother with resources that she feels might be beneficial for her and her family, such as a community center offering yoga classes or a nearby babysitting service that has drop-off options for moms who need an urgent break. Depending on financial resources, the PHN might explore housecleaning services or might put the mom in touch with youth willing to do this service for needy families at little to no cost. The PHN does not simply give the mother a to-do list but instead works with the mother in a thorough and thoughtful manner to appropriately implement the intervention plan and assess the process and the acceptability to ensure that the mother is not overwhelmed and that she is empowered and building self-efficacy skills to care for herself and her family.

A case management intervention, where the PHN intervenes to address many health needs over the course of many visits, has been shown to be effective (see the following Evidence Example).

Evidence Example: PHN Prenatal Care Case Management

A study was conducted to evaluate the effectiveness of case management by PHNs for prenatal care, as compared to programs offering limited prenatal assessment and/or referral programs (Ricketts, Murray, & Schwalberg, 2005). The PHN prenatal care case management was provided to more than 3,500 women. Key findings for the women receiving the prenatal care case management were that many of them decided to reduce risk behaviors that could lead to poorer birth outcomes. For example, mothers who acted on PHN advice to quit smoking during pregnancy or to gain enough weight had fewer low-birth-weight babies than did mothers who did not address these risks. Consistent with case management practices, women who had more than 10 visits were more likely to reduce their risks than those who received fewer visits. The study demonstrated the particular value of PHN case management in helping reduce risks during pregnancy and to promote healthy pregnancy outcomes and the well-being of newborns.

At times, PHNs have insights and experience that are also helpful to colleagues working with the family. PHNs are often valuable resources and sources of support to colleagues addressing child protection or abuse concerns with families (Crisp & Green Lister, 2004). The issues surrounding child protection situations are complex and require intention toward understanding multiple factors (e.g., social, emotional, spiritual, and environmental) rather than simply carrying out mandated reporting requirements. (See Competency #4, Chapter 6.) Indeed, PHNs have an important role in helping link the public health and child welfare systems so that optimal care is provided to the families in an integrated, comprehensive way (Schneiderman, 2006). When integration occurs, children in the foster care system, for example, can more easily have their healthcare needs met because PHNs can provide a critical link for the families to the healthcare system while being aware of the foster care requirements and restrictions. In another example of prenatal care, PHNs conducted a demonstration project in which they assessed each referred pregnant woman to identify psychosocial risks and to increase her awareness of local community resources available during the pregnancy (Strass & Billay, 2008). The key to the success of this intervention was the effort of the PHNs to assess and consider the diverse psychosocial risks rather than to focus solely on the physical nature of the pregnancy. Healthcare providers making referrals to the PHNs wanted them to continue providing the service, demonstrating support for, and the value of, this public health nursing intervention.

At the community level, a PHN planning a cardiovascular screening program as a parish nurse needs to organize a team of individuals, depending on the number of people who will be screened and how frequently the screenings will occur. The PHN arranges the logistics, organizes volunteers, and provides leadership for the screening program (see Table 12.3). The most successful intervention is one that is carefully planned and considers all the possible influencing factors for success or failure. Key factors include the time of day, day of the week, conflicting local activities (e.g., holidays, meetings), ease of the registration process, adequate trained staff, child care options, refreshments, signs, the presence of multiple events or screenings in one large room, and privacy, to name a few.

Evidence Example: Community-Based Holistic Care

At the systems level, PHNs can be influential in bringing together community partners to implement interventions that affect the way current healthcare systems function and care for people. Healthcare reform provides the context for new innovative models of holistic care. For example, in Philadelphia, a PHN led efforts to create a transdisciplinary, nurse-managed health center in partnership with the community, bridging the efforts of the local university and the community (Gerrity, 2010). The underserved community desired a "place of their own where healthcare was delivered in response to their identified needs" (p. 62). The center's holistic approach to create health includes primary care by nurse practitioners, integrated behavioral health, dental care, chronic disease management, health promotion, and wellness services, including a variety of complementary integrative therapies. PHNs can be involved in many aspects of this intervention as they advocate for new healthcare systems to support the development of healthy communities. Creating and implementing this healthcare system change to improve health outcomes requires trust between the community and providers and support from government agencies as well as collaboration between many community partners.

Table 12.3 Setting Up a Screening Clinic

IN ADVANCE

—Assess risk to determine the need for a screening clinic.

—Identify screeners (e.g., determine whether you will use volunteers, paid staff, people from the community or outside the community). Conduct interviews/application process as needed. Note that screeners might need criminal background or reference checks, depending on their activities.

—Train screeners (e.g., screening equipment, process).

—Establish protocol and schedule for screening, referrals, and follow-up.

continues

Table 12.3   Setting Up a Screening Clinic   (continued)

DAY OF THE EVENT

—Focus on logistics (i.e., details specific to the event, such as signage, refreshments and supplies, and the staffing schedule).

—Offer child care options.

—Convey a clear communication and decision-making structure.

—Plan for adequate, supportive, and thorough follow-up and referrals.

 ACTIVITY

Reflect on how you might conduct a holistic screening event in your community.

Identify how you would set up the event and which interventions you would offer to address physical, emotional, and spiritual needs or concerns.

Maria develops a strong relationship with this family, especially the mother and children, over the next year. She spends time following up on past referrals and interventions. Maria monitors the emotional, physical, environmental, and spiritual health of this mother through tough times that include multiple housing moves, relationship issues, and a period of homelessness. The mother ends her marriage in a bitter divorce that results in many crises for this family. Throughout, Maria helps the mother monitor Marcus's asthma. As Maria continues to monitor the children's development, she becomes concerned about the youngest son and helps the mother access local services, including early childhood education and parenting groups.

 ACTIVITY

Reflect on the ways in which Maria has provided a holistic case management intervention for this family and the benefits of this strategy as compared to one or two home visits only.

Evaluates the Impact of Public Health Nursing Interventions on Mental, Physical, Emotional, Social, Spiritual, and Environmental Health

As the intervention plan is being implemented, PHNs begin to evaluate the impact it is having on the target individual, family, community, or system. It is true that some outcomes might not be realized in the short term, yet PHNs need to pay careful attention to how the intervention is influencing aspects of health right away. Evaluating the impact of a PHN intervention can be complex. Generally, PHNs need to evaluate the intervention process, such as how it went, whether implementation was successful, and how future interventions could be improved. PHNs also need to focus on the impact of the intervention, as determined by the outcomes. Has the intervention contributed to health? How so? PHNs then return to the assessment strategies that identified the need for the intervention to reassess the situation. This return is a good way to determine whether changes have occurred and to complete a cycle of assessment, intervention, evaluation, and assessment, which can then lead to refined interventions.

Evidence Example: Evidence for Home Visits With Mothers and Children

One of the most exemplary studies evaluating the effectiveness of public health nursing interventions is a randomized controlled trial that measured outcomes of public health nursing visits to 743 mothers and children (Olds et al., 2007). Numerous aspects of health were evaluated over 9 years, including the economic, social, physical, and educational health of the mothers and the physical and educational health of the children. Importantly, children receiving the PHN home visits were less likely to die between birth and 9 years of age and more likely to report higher grade point averages and reading scores than those who did not receive PHN visits. Mothers who received home visits from PHNs were more likely to wait longer to become pregnant with their second child and to maintain longer relationships with their partners and reported less use of economic assistance (e.g., welfare assistance or food stamps) than mothers who did not receive home visits from PHNs. The findings from this study have informed national initiatives across the United States to implement PHN home-visiting programs for at-risk first-time mothers.

A qualitative approach can also be used to evaluate the effectiveness of the nursing process (see the following Evidence Example). In another example of qualitative evaluation, essays written by 62 clients who received PHN home visits in Alaska to help prevent child abuse and neglect were analyzed (DeMay, 2003). Some clients received "intense" services and about twice as many home visits as those assigned to receive "standard" home visit services. The evaluation, however, was not focused on whether one group showed greater benefits compared to the other but instead focused on the extent to which the essays about the PHN visits reflected the PHNs' perspectives about the visits. Interestingly, parents in both groups wrote in their essays about the trusting relationships developed with their PHNs and the importance of these positive relationships. It was noted that those receiving more visits (the intense group) wrote much longer essays than those in the other group, possibly reflecting the depth of relationship that can be built when more home visits are involved.

Evidence Example: PHN Home Visits to Elderly Clients

A qualitative approach was used to evaluate the impact of PHN home visits to elderly clients after they had been hospitalized (McKeown, 2007). In interviews, the older people shared that the PHNs helped meet many, but not all, of the needs they experienced following hospitalization (e.g., access to services, social aspects, home environment safety). In this study, it appears that only one home visit was provided, which certainly could be important in interpreting the findings specific to unmet needs. The study is helpful in that it shows the importance of evaluating PHN services to (a) identify what has been successful and (b) what is lacking or could be strengthened. It is very likely that with increased visits and support, these older adults would have shared different experiences in their interviews.

At the community level, a child-obesity surveillance program implemented in numerous Canadian public health clinics with more than 7,000 participants was evaluated (Flynn et al., 2005). In addition to such outcomes as rates of childhood obesity, parent satisfaction was evaluated because the authors of this study believed that one measure of the program's success was the extent to which the parents participating were content with their experience. PHNs administered the obesity surveillance program with families; among those who completed the evaluation survey about the program, more than 98% indicated being "very happy" or "happy" with the information received. The PHNs' confidence in conducting obesity screenings, providing education, and making referrals for follow-up was also assessed in questions posed to the PHNs who participated in the screening pilot project. This assessment is important, because the success of any nursing intervention depends in part not only on the nurses' abilities but also on their confidence in those abilities. Study results indicated that after participating in this screening program, the PHNs had increased confidence in their abilities to screen children accurately for weight and obesity risks and to provide parents with information they could use to improve their children's health.

An evaluation of services delivered via a public health nursing sexual health clinic also yielded valuable information about the PHNs' roles and successes. Surveys and semistructured interviews were conducted with 166 at-risk young people who had visited the clinic to learn their perspectives toward the services they received from the PHNs (Hayter, 2005). In the interviews, participants reported having confidence in the PHNs' ability to provide services in a confidential manner. Other abilities and attributes of the PHNs were assessed via the survey, and the majority of respondents indicated feeling comfortable talking with the PHNs (84%) and perceiving the PHNs as good listeners (more than 90%). These findings led to the conclusion that PHNs were successfully delivering sexual healthcare to at-risk, marginalized young people in a manner that was acceptable and welcoming to the youth. These data were important, because they informed program planning about how to staff and continue the sexual health clinic.

These types of evaluations, including not only the participants but also the PHNs delivering the interventions, require more time and economic resources, yet they yield more holistic information that can be useful in determining whether an intervention is effective and efficient. In today's world, interventions need to be cost-effective and efficient (e.g., with respect to staffing), or they will not be sustained over time. Evaluations that include data to justify the value and efficiency of an intervention are critical.

Time passes. Maria has not seen this family for a while since they have moved out of the county. She receives a phone call from the mother to update her on the family's situation, including that she and her boyfriend are expecting a baby. Maria asks how Marcus is doing with his asthma. His mother states that he has not had any episodes for 6 months and takes his medication every day. They discuss the development and successes of all the children. The mother calls again prior to the birth of her baby to tell Maria she is being induced the following day at a local hospital. Maria states that she might be able to stop by and see her and her new baby. The mother is very excited. Maria enters the hospital room and is greeted by the mother nursing her newborn. No concerns or crises arise during this visit. Maria leaves with tears in her eyes. This is the beginning of a new "family," and they will be residing in another county. Therefore, Maria has to accept that she can no longer serve this family she has become part of for the past 3 years. She reflects on the journey from that first flea-infested day to the sharing of this birth. Maria has addressed many physical, emotional, environmental, and spiritual issues with this family.

Ethical Considerations

PHNs must conduct assessment, planning, implementation, and evaluation in an ethical manner. PHNs should engage with individuals, communities, and systems in ways that demonstrate respect, a willingness to listen and learn, and a desire to come alongside rather than dictate or demand. The way in which an assessment is conducted directly informs the type of intervention that is developed and implemented; if the assessment focuses only on problems or risks, the intervention might not build on existing strengths or assets. This approach can lead to dependency rather than autonomy or capacity building. Instead, PHNs' assessments should be holistic, focused on strengths and weaknesses, assets, and risks. Interventions should not be dictated but collaboratively designed, with input from those who are receiving the intervention. This collaboration should enhance the potential that the intervention will be welcomed or adhered to, which will increase its likelihood of success. PHNs will find evaluation of the impact an intervention has made most useful when that evaluation is thorough and includes multiple sources of data. When PHNs take care to make sure that the public health nursing process is holistic and inclusive, they gather the ingredients for successful health promotion and disease prevention. And when ethical ideals are adhered to, PHNs are doing what is needed to yield healthy, sustainable outcomes. See Table 12.4 for an application of ethical perspectives to the holistic nursing process.

Table 12.4   Ethical Action in Holistic Assessment, Intervention, Planning, and Evaluation

Ethical perspective	Application
Rule ethics (principles)	• The goal of a holistic public health nursing process should be beneficence or the promotion of good (improvement in health status). • Encourage autonomy by ensuring that those being affected, including children, have input in determining interventions to improve health.
Virtue ethics (character)	• Be respectful when conducting an assessment and carrying out an intervention. • Be persistent in obtaining what is needed to successfully intervene based on what the assessment reveals. • Be patient when it takes time for an intervention to bear fruit or to be acceptable to those it is for (e.g., a family or a community).
Feminist ethics (reducing oppression)	• Ensure that assessment includes strengths and assets in addition to the risks, problems, or challenges. • Respect everyone. • Emphasize strengths and assets when developing an intervention. • Advocate for individuals and community groups that have less power. • Evaluate using qualitative and quantitative approaches that consider the broad ways in which an intervention has or has not been effective.

Key Points

- The process of assessment, planning, intervention, and evaluation is a cycle.

- Thorough assessment is critical to the success of the other nursing process phases.

- Assessment should include consideration of mental, physical, emotional, social, spiritual, and environmental assets and risks.

- Successful interventions build on strengths and are implemented with the collaboration and support of those being served.

- Evaluation of interventions should be planned before the intervention is initiated.

- Thorough evaluation should include qualitative and quantitative strategies.

- PHNs are uniquely positioned to collaborate with many different agencies in promoting the health and well-being of individuals/families, communities, and systems.

Learning Examples for Effective Assessment, Intervention, Planning, and Evaluation Strategies

You can find many examples of PHNs undertaking activities for individuals and communities that reflect obvious consideration of not only physical needs and concerns but also emotional, social, environmental, and spiritual needs and concerns. These examples should encourage you to consider the ways in which you can thoroughly and holistically promote the health and well-being of those you serve in public health settings. The following are learning examples for holistic assessment, planning, intervention, and evaluation.

Environmental Health

- Nursing students and students from an environmental education program collaborated to conduct walkthrough assessments of a local community.

- Student teams presented their assessment that integrated concepts of environmental health to their class and health policy representatives.

- Parish nurses and school nurses worked together to screen children in Catholic schools for vision problems, leading to quicker identification of problems and subsequent in-depth eye examinations (Hayes, Davis, & Miranda, 2006).

Bioterrorism Planning

- PHNs had a critical valuable role in the planning, implementation, and evaluation of bioterrorism drills and activities.

- PHNs facilitated important collaboration of diverse disciplines mutually concerned with the prevention of bioterrorism (Mondy, Cardenas, & Avila, 2003).

Reflective Practice

Conducting a blood pressure screening clinic in a church with a Spanish-speaking congregation takes careful and thoughtful planning. Parish nurses need to carefully conduct an assessment that considers the extent to which the congregation needs and is ready for screening activities. They also have to thoughtfully address many logistical aspects. Realizing that holistic assessment, planning, implementation, and evaluation processes are complex, consider how you might answer the following questions:

1. What might Maria need to consider in planning a health promotion activity in the neighborhood near the family she has been visiting?

    _____

    _____

2. Where might Maria go to find out whether the needs she is observing in one family are common to others in the neighborhood?

    _____

    _____

3. Who would be potentially valuable partners to Maria when she decides that a health promotion/nutrition screening fair might be of benefit to the neighborhood?

    _____

    _____

4. How will Maria know whether the health promotion fair has been successful?

    _____

    _____

5. What will Maria want to know following this health fair before she organizes another one?

    _____

    _____

6. How might Maria self-reflect on the process to realize the holistic nature of the screening and to encourage even more effective public health nursing in her future work?

    _____

    _____

7. Refer to the Cornerstones of Public Health in Chapter 1. Which of these Cornerstones supports efforts to be holistic in conducting PHN interventions or assessments?

_____

_____

 ## Application of Evidence

1. When PHNs conduct a neighborhood needs assessment, where will they find data, and whom might they want to speak with about the community?

2. To enhance the potential for the nutrition health fair to be successful, who are the people/agencies PHNs will want to partner with in planning, implementing, and evaluating the fair and its outcomes?

3. What are the differences in home safety checklists that PHNs might provide to families with young children, families with adolescents, or families with elderly members?

4. What are some qualitative and quantitative ways to assess the successes of public health nursing programs or interventions?

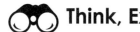 ## Think, Explore, Do

1. Why is assessment necessary before you intervene with a family?

2. Which data might you collect as part of an assessment of community violence?

3. How might you create a safety checklist so that it is attractive and accessible to families with a child who is hearing-impaired? What information would you include? Would the checklist be paper or electronic?

4. If you are planning a community health screening event, how will you publicize it so that you have a successful, well-attended event?

5. When might you use an interview to evaluate the success of a health screening event instead of surveys? (Hint: Consider education levels, the population being served, languages spoken, etc.)

6. The National Asthma Education and Prevention Program (NAEPP) has done some great work regarding addressing asthma in the school. Please visit its website and identify some priority strategies you might use to engage in asthma prevention efforts at the community and systems levels (not just the individual level).

7. Consider the ways in which the Adverse Child Experiences (ACE) initiative in Minnesota promotes holistic assessment and intervention. Select one of the nine ACEs and develop a holistic strategy that includes targets at the individual, community, and system levels. http://www.health.state.mn.us/divs/cfh/program/ace/content/document/pdf/acesum.pdf

References

Crisp, B. R., & Green Lister, P. (2004). Child protection and public health: Nurses' responsibilities. *Journal of Advanced Nursing, 47*(6), 656–663.

DeMay, D. A. (2003). The experience of being a client in an Alaska public health nursing home visitation program. *Public Health Nursing, 20*(3), 228–236.

Flynn, M. A., Hall, K., Noack, A., Clovechok, S., Enns, E., Pivnick, J., . . . Pryce, C. (2005). Promotion of healthy weights at preschool public health vaccination clinics in Calgary: An obesity surveillance program. *Canadian Journal of Public Health, 96*(6), 421–426.

Friedman, M. M., Bowden, V. R., & Jones, E. G. (2003). *Family nursing: Research, theory and practice*, 5th ed. Upper Saddle River, NJ: Prentice Hall.

Gerrity, P. (2010). And to think that it happened on 11th street: A nursing approach to community-based holistic care and health care reform. *Alternative Therapies in Health and Medicine, 16*(5), 62–67.

Hayden, D. (2011). Spirituality in end-of-life care: Attending the person on their journey. *British Journal of Community Nursing, 16*(11), 546–551.

Hayes, J. C., Davis, J. A., & Miranda, M. L. (2006). Incorporating a built environment module into an accelerated second-degree community health nursing course. *Public Health Nursing 23*(5), 442–452.

Hayter, M. (2005). Reaching marginalized young people through sexual health nursing outreach clinics: Evaluating service use and the views of service users. *Public Health Nursing, 22*(4), 339–346.

Kemp, L., Anderson, T., Travaglia, J., & Harris, E. (2005). Sustained nursing home visiting in early childhood: Exploring Australian nursing competencies. *Public Health Nursing, 22*(3), 254–259.

Kemper, A. R., Fant, K. E., & Clark, S. J. (2005). Informing parents about newborn screening. *Public Health Nursing, 22*(4), 332–338.

Labun, E. (1988). Spiritual care: An element in nursing care planning. *Journal of Advanced Nursing, 13*(3), 314–320.

McKeown, F. (2007). The experiences of older people on discharge from hospital following assessment by the public health nurse. *Journal of Clinical Nursing, 16*(3), 469–476.

McSherry, W., Cash, K., & Ross, L. (2004). Meaning of spirituality: Implications for nursing practice. *Journal of Clinical Nursing, 13*(8), 934–941.

Minnesota Department of Health (MDH). (2009). Early identification of young children with special health care needs. *Minnesota Department of Health Fact Sheet: Title V (MCH) Block Grant Children and Adolescents with Special Health Care Needs.* St. Paul, MN: Author.

Minnesota Department of Health (MDH). (2013a). *Adverse childhood experiences in Minnesota.* Retrieved from http://www.health.state.mn.us/divs/cfh/program/ace/content/document/pdf/acereport.pdf

Minnesota Department of Health (MDH). (2013b). *How-to: Community health assessment.* Retrieved from http://www.health.state.mn.us/divs/opi/pm/lphap/cha/howto.html

Mondy, C., Cardenas, D., & Avila, M. (2003). The role of an advanced practice public health nurse in bioterrorism preparedness. *Public Health Nursing, 20*(6), 422–431.

Olds, D. L., Kitzman, H., Hanks, C., Cole, R., Anson, E., Sidora-Arcoleo, K., . . . Bondy, J. (2007). Effects of nurse home visiting on maternal and child functioning: Age-9 follow-up of a randomized trial. *Pediatrics, 120*(4), 832–845.

Ricketts, S. A., Murray, E. K., & Schwalberg, R. (2005). Reducing low birthweight by resolving risks: Results from Colorado's Prenatal Plus Program. *American Journal of Public Health, 98*(11), 1952–1957.

Schim, S., Doorenbos, A., Benkert, R., & Miller, J. (2007). Culturally congruent care: Putting the puzzle together. *Journal of Transcultural Nursing, 18*(2), 103–110.

Schneiderman, J. U. (2006). Innovative pediatric nursing role: Public health nurses in child welfare. *Pediatric Nursing, 32*(4), 317–321.

Sittner, B., Hudson, D., & Defrain, J. (2007). Using the concept of family strengths to enhance nursing care. *MCN: American Journal of Maternal/Child Health Nursing, 32*(6), 353–357.

Somervell, A. M., Saylor, C., & Mao, C. L. (2005). Public health nurse interventions for women in a dependency drug court. *Public Health Nursing, 22*(1), 59–64.

Strass, P., & Billay, E. (2008). A public health nursing initiative to promote antenatal health. *Canadian Nurse, 104*(2), 29–33.

World Health Organization (WHO). (n.d.). *Environmental Health.* Retrieved from http://www.who.int/topics/environmental_health/en/

COMPETENCY #11

Demonstrates Leadership in Public Health Nursing With Communities, Systems, Individuals, and Families

Patricia M. Schoon and Marjorie A. Schaffer
with Bonnie Brueshoff

José is with the Elders at Home Program for his public health nursing clinical. He is assigned to Mr. and Mrs. Santos, a couple in their 70s struggling to manage their healthcare needs and stay in their home in an older inner-city neighborhood. Mrs. Santos provides primary assistance for her husband, who has advanced chronic obstructive pulmonary disease (COPD). After a recent hospitalization, Mr. Santos received home care services from a home care nurse, respiratory therapist, occupational therapist, and a home health aide. These services were reimbursed by Medicare because Mr. Santos met the criteria of potential for rehabilitation and progress toward independent living. All went well. Then a 60-day health assessment resulted in a determination that Mr. Santos was no longer eligible for home care services. He was referred to the county public health Elders at Home Program but has been resisting a home visit. José wonders, "I am just a student nurse. What can I do?" He sighs, "Well, it looks like my preceptor has handed me a challenge I can't avoid. Isn't there a chapter we are supposed to read on leadership in public health nursing?"

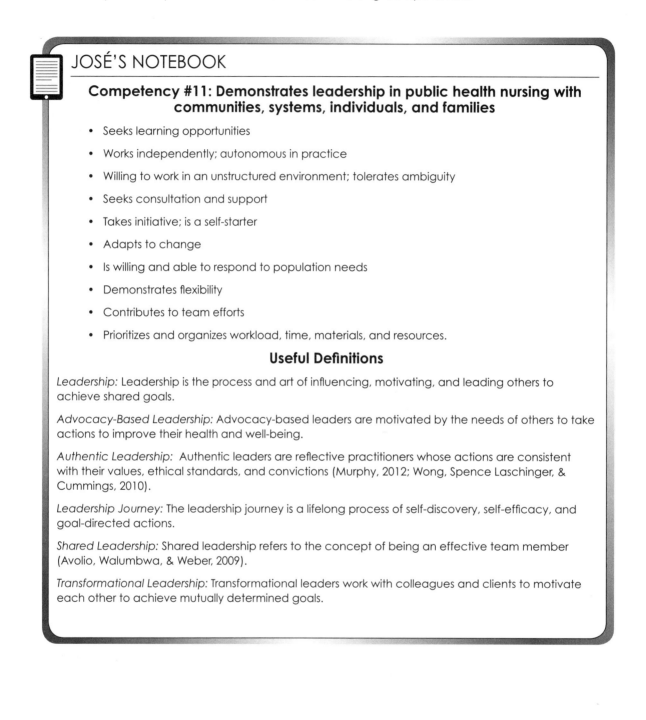

JOSÉ'S NOTEBOOK

Competency #11: Demonstrates leadership in public health nursing with communities, systems, individuals, and families

- Seeks learning opportunities

- Works independently; autonomous in practice

- Willing to work in an unstructured environment; tolerates ambiguity

- Seeks consultation and support

- Takes initiative; is a self-starter

- Adapts to change

- Is willing and able to respond to population needs

- Demonstrates flexibility

- Contributes to team efforts

- Prioritizes and organizes workload, time, materials, and resources.

Useful Definitions

Leadership: Leadership is the process and art of influencing, motivating, and leading others to achieve shared goals.

Advocacy-Based Leadership: Advocacy-based leaders are motivated by the needs of others to take actions to improve their health and well-being.

Authentic Leadership: Authentic leaders are reflective practitioners whose actions are consistent with their values, ethical standards, and convictions (Murphy, 2012; Wong, Spence Laschinger, & Cummings, 2010).

Leadership Journey: The leadership journey is a lifelong process of self-discovery, self-efficacy, and goal-directed actions.

Shared Leadership: Shared leadership refers to the concept of being an effective team member (Avolio, Walumbwa, & Weber, 2009).

Transformational Leadership: Transformational leaders work with colleagues and clients to motivate each other to achieve mutually determined goals.

What Does Leadership Mean in Public Health Nursing Practice?

Public health nurses (PHNs) spend their daily lives in the community and deal with social determinants of health and the impact of these determinants on health outcomes with individuals, families, populations, and communities. They know that they must go outside the healthcare system to promote and protect their clients' health. The use of leadership is crucial to the success of their efforts. PHNs carry out leadership at the individual/family, community, and systems levels, whether in the home, in the multidisciplinary public health team, in the community, or within diverse systems, such as government, healthcare organizations, schools, home-care agencies, prisons, faith-based communities, and homeless shelters. They employ many leadership strategies and interventions, such as collective social action, persuasion, influencing, role-modeling, coalition building, networking, social marketing, collaboration, passionate commitment, risk-taking, and personal bravery:

> Public health nurses practice at that intersection where societal attitudes, government policies, and people's lives meet. Such privilege creates a moral imperative not only to attend to the health needs of the public but also, like Nightingale, to work to change the societal conditions contributing to poor health. (Falk-Rafael, 2005, p. 219)

The Leadership Journey

Nurses are presented with leadership challenges throughout their careers. *Leadership challenges* are events or situations that require nurses to use critical thinking and ethical problem solving to arrive at equitable and effective solutions. These situations propel nurses along their leadership journey.

Nursing leadership begins with the nurse-patient relationship in clinical practice. You started your leadership journey as a nursing student the moment you identified an unmet patient need and advocated for your patient by working to influence other members of the care team to take actions to meet your patient's needs. In other words, you began to lead when you identified an unmet client need and took the lead in advocating for your client with others. In doing so, you demonstrated advocacy-based nursing leadership. The actions you took were based on your beliefs and values and reflected your own personal and professional way of being, the beginning of authentic leadership practice. You chose to enlist others to mutually achieve your goal to meet your patient's need, which was the beginning of transformational leadership. When you move beyond the nurse-client relationship and advocate within the healthcare system or community for changes in attitudes, beliefs, knowledge, actions, and resources that will help meet your client's needs, you are practicing leadership. You do not have to be in a formal position of authority, such as a supervisor or manager, to be a leader. Staff nurses usually work within healthcare teams and share the workload. Knowing how to work effectively within the healthcare team is referred to as shared leadership. The leadership journey is a lifelong process of self-discovery, self-efficacy, and goal-directed actions. Nursing students and professional nurses are on a lifelong journey as they develop their leadership potential, explore their authentic leadership styles, and identify their personal and professional reasons and motivations for taking leadership actions.

Authentic Leadership

Choosing to lead is a conscious choice to take action. The authentic leader moves from concerns about self to concerns about the other. Leadership is a journey from the "I" to the "We" (George & Sims, 2007). Leadership consciousness starts with an awareness and understanding of one's own values, beliefs, and convictions. Our self-awareness or consciousness leads us to develop our own personal and professional competencies. This consciousness then leads us to an awareness of the needs of others, thus creating a moral challenge and a call to action. When nurses respond to this call for action, they develop authentic personal and professional leadership styles and competencies. Figure 13.1 demonstrates how you will move along your leadership journey throughout your nursing career as you respond to transitional moments in your nursing practice. Which transition points do you think you might encounter during your leadership journey in public health nursing?

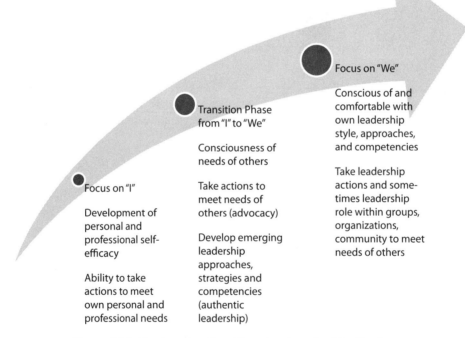

Figure 13.1. The Leadership—Ongoing Leadership Challenges
Source: Based on concepts from George & Sims, 2007

You have already developed some beginning leadership skills and practices in your previous nursing clinicals. These skills and practices are consistent with the situational challenges you have faced and your authentic sense of self. You may further develop your leadership style and skills as you progress through your public health clinical. This chapter provides guidance to help you understand the PHN's leadership styles and skills that you may use with each level of practice: individuals and families, communities, and systems.

The Leadership Journey: Reflections of a Public Health Nurse Leader

As you progress along your leadership journey, you may want to reflect on the situations, personal decisions, and role models or supporters who assisted you in developing your authentic leadership style and skills. In the following interview, a PHN leader describes her leadership journey and what she learned along the way (Brueshoff, 2013):

1. Tell a story about how your early experiences in public health nursing and the leadership challenges you confronted helped you along your leadership journey.

   My first job as a nurse was working in a PHN position in northern Minnesota. I had a generalized caseload of young families and elderly clients. One of my specific roles in the department was to provide follow-up for the Sudden Infant Death Syndrome (SIDS) cases in the county. As a novice PHN, I found my knowledge base about SIDS to be inadequate, which led me to request additional training available at the state level. Through the training, I made valuable connections with the Minnesota SIDS Center and accessed expertise from SIDS Center staff that provided me with resources for families and much-needed emotional support. Needless to say, I became better prepared to provide the support and assistance that benefited SIDS families during subsequent home visits. This experience early on in my career reinforced the importance of ongoing education and reaching out to access resources and expertise from other professionals. Later in my career, my experience working with SIDS families helped me mentor other PHNs who were working with SIDS cases and was a factor in my leadership journey as I was hired in a position as an apnea home monitoring coordinator.

2. Who were your role models and guides along the way?

   I was extremely fortunate to have the support and guidance from two public health directors who offered me opportunities for growth and challenged me to take on leadership roles. I consider both directors to be my role models and mentors. I also looked to the Minnesota Department of Health (MDH) PHN nurse consultants for guidance with my PHN practice and took every opportunity I could to volunteer for state work groups and committees. Through the encouragement that was given to me, I gained confidence and was motivated to advance my knowledge and skills. For example, I received the support to apply to serve on the MDH Maternal and Child Health (MCH) State Advisory Task Force. I was appointed to be a member of this task force, which gave me leadership experience in dealing with statewide policy and programs and expanded my professional network. I was given support to pursue the Robert Wood Johnson (RWJ) Executive Nurse Fellowship program that I completed.

3. What inspires you and keeps you fresh in your leadership vision and strategies?

   Both my practice experiences and professional development activities have kept me inspired including (1) experiencing the impact that public health has in helping us all be healthy, because the focus of public health is on prevention; (2) being able to be innovative in trying new approaches and using evidence-based practice; (3) reading leadership literature and articles; (4) networking with my colleagues; (5) mentoring new PHN staff; and (6) working to influence policies and decision-making on all levels—local, state, and national.

4. What are your three most important "lessons learned" about leadership in your public health nursing practice?

- To lead, you have to be willing to take risks and know it is OK to fail and learn from your mistakes—to learn how to "fail forward."

- Networking and lifelong learning are key. You can do more with others than by being solo. Join professional organizations and stretch yourself. Get involved. Never stop. Learning self-awareness is very important and will help you immensely! Ask for honest feedback from others so you can build on your strengths.

- Become politically savvy. Learn about policies and processes that affect public health. The ability to influence policy has a far-reaching influence on nursing!

–Bonnie Brueshoff, DNP, RN, PHN, Public Health Director and Robert Wood Johnson executive nurse fellow (2006–2009), Dakota County Public Health

Leading Through Relationships

PHNs always work with others, their clients, team members, intraprofessional colleagues, and various members of the community in striving to meet their goals of improving population health. Public health nursing leadership requires influencing others to achieve public health goals (Morrison, Jones, & Fuller, 1997).You are starting your public health nursing leadership journey at the individual/family level of practice, which is where entry-level PHNs often begin to develop their skills and understanding of their role. Table 13.1 outlines leadership styles that are congruent with public health nursing practice.

Table 13.1   Nursing Leadership Styles

Advocacy-based leadership: Advocacy-based leaders are motivated by the needs of others to take actions to improve their health and well-being. Advocacy-based leadership is based on the ethical principles of social justice. Advocacy-based leaders are risk takers who act with moral purpose and demonstrate moral courage when faced with perceived or actual opposition. (Refer to discussion of advocacy and moral courage in Chapter 10.)

Authentic leadership: Authentic leaders are reflective practitioners whose actions are consistent with their values, ethical standards, and convictions. They are true to themselves and know why they do what they do. Authentic leaders objectively consider all available information and the opinions of others, clearly and openly share their perspectives, are open and honest in their communication, and have an awareness of their own strengths and weaknesses. They are considered trustworthy and reliable (Murphy, 2012; Wong et al., 2010).

Shared leadership: Shared leadership refers to the concept of being an effective team member: sharing responsibilities, mutually organizing the team's work, maintaining team communication, taking the initiative to try a new approach if something is not working, supporting team members, providing positive feedback, and allocating resources equitably (Avolio et al., 2009). When leadership is shared, PHNs have more time and energy to care for their clients.

Transformational leadership: Transformational leadership is the process by which leaders and followers motivate each other to attain and achieve success (O'Neill, 2013, p. 179). Transformational leaders are advocates who motivate others by appealing to higher ideas and values, are flexible and adaptable, provide supportive environments, share responsibilities, and lead followers to sustain the greater good (Doody & Doody, 2012; Wolf, 2012).

ACTIVITY

Think about the leadership journey you have been on since becoming a nursing student. Are you able to identify when you began to focus more on your patients than yourself? Can you identify a transformative moment when you realized that it was morally necessary for you to advocate for your patients' unmet needs by enlisting the help of others? Reflect on your nursing actions to meet your patients' needs. Do any of the leadership styles in Table 13.1 fit your nursing actions?

Advocacy-Based Leadership

Advocacy-based leadership is foundational in public health nursing. Advocating for clients—whether those clients are individuals, families, populations, or communities—is part of the social justice mission of public health nursing. Although all nurses advocate for the unmet needs of their individual clients, PHNs have a responsibility to advocate for the health of the public, to care about what is causing the health disparities in their communities, and to take action to improve the health status of the affected individuals, families, populations, and communities. This means that PHNs need to be aware of emerging health needs and connect the patterns of health disparities they observe among their individual clients. Sometimes advocacy-based leadership is an unconscious response to an unmet healthcare need. Sometimes it is a conscious choice triggered by an ethical or moral call to action. The following example illustrates this form of leadership from the perspective of a public health nursing student from a school of nursing in the Henry Street Consortium.

Evidence Example: PHN Student Initiative Demonstrates Leadership and Improves Population Health

A student nurse completed her leadership clinical in an inner-city school with a 95% poverty rate among its students. She developed a dental screening program for third-graders as her leadership project. After screening all the children, she found that almost all of them had dental disease, such as decay, bleeding gums, abscesses, and missing or broken teeth. Almost none of them had received dental care in the last year, and few owned a toothbrush. Each child was given a toothbrush and toothpaste and taught how to brush his or her teeth. The PHN student then attempted to screen all the children in the elementary school, managing to screen about 90%. She prepared a report showing the need for dental care in almost all the children screened, sent home referrals to all the parents, and included information on local dental clinics that provided care for low-income patients. The principal used the report to obtain a grant to put a dental clinic in the school. Within a few years, dental clinics were established in elementary schools located in high-poverty neighborhoods throughout the school district.

—Senior Student Nurse

José returns to visit with Mr. and Mrs. Santos. Mrs. Santos is crying and wringing her hands. José asks Mrs. Santos whether she would be willing to see a mental health case worker. She refuses. He remembers that the local Latino Catholic church has a pastoral ministry home visiting program. He wonders whether Mrs. Santos would allow the pastoral minister to visit her. Mrs. Santos agrees to let José contact the church. José is pleased that he has thought outside the box. He is really stretching himself to try to find ways to help Mr. and Mrs. Santos and be an effective advocate.

Margaret, José's public health nursing preceptor, says to him, "I hope you like a challenge, because this couple has lots of them. You are going to have to think outside the box to keep Mr. and Mrs. Santos in their own home. You really are going to have to use all your communication, advocacy, and leadership skills to work successfully with this family."

José wonders, "Do I have any leadership skills? I thought those came later, after 5 to 10 years of practice."

 ACTIVITY
Which leadership challenges can you identify in this home visit? How might José meet these leadership challenges? Which leadership styles might José use in meeting each of these leadership challenges as he works with the Santos family and the interprofessional care team?

What Are Foundational Leadership Skills for Becoming a Public Health Nursing Leader?

PHNs are often confronted with the need to use their leadership skills in advocating for their clients. As someone new to public health nursing, you might find thinking about the skills needed for leadership in this field daunting. Remember that all good nursing leaders start at the beginning by becoming competent in their practice specialties; then, as they develop confidence as expert practitioners, they build a repertoire of leadership skills. The Henry Street Consortium has generated a set of leadership skills that beginning PHNs need to build their expertise through learning experiences and establishing a foundation for leadership in public health nursing. See Table 13.2.

Table 13.2   Essential Leadership Skills for Public Health Nurses

Skill	Strategies and considerations	Your leadership action
Seeks learning opportunities	• Determine goals for professional development. • Strive to see the "big picture" by attending to community and systems processes.	Match your interests and goals to learning opportunities.
Works independently; is autonomous in practice	• PHNs make many independent decisions based on established programs or protocols. • PHNs make decisions based on their own expertise within the framework of ethical and professional standards or practices.	Attend a PHN team meeting to observe how PHNs share experiences. Seek suggestions about evidence-based practice and tools to use for complex family situations.
Willing to work in an unstructured environment; tolerates ambiguity	• PHNs practice in settings where people live, learn, and work—the priorities in these settings are often not health or healthcare. • Sometimes the goals of others are not clear or consistent with the goals of PHNs. • PHNs learn to be in ambiguous situations while working to determine individual, family, and community goals. • PHNs suggest health-oriented goals but ultimately work within the structure of each setting to accomplish goals that are mutually determined or sometimes rejected.	Talk with your preceptors about the challenges they have confronted. Identify a clinical situation that was ambiguous. Analyze your feelings and how you dealt with the situation.
Seeks consultation and support	• It is essential to seek consultation and support in a practice area where role models are often not physically present. • PHNs use technology to access resources and expertise when additional information is needed.	By reflecting on your experiences with expert practitioners, you can validate your thinking and actions and learn about more effective approaches to your work.

continues

Table 13.2   Essential Leadership Skills for Public Health Nurses   (continued)

Skill	Strategies and considerations	Your leadership action
Takes initiative; is a self-starter	• PHNs are responsible for organizing their own schedules. • Many activities in public health nursing involve long-term planning, especially when building partnerships and coalitions that focus on community and systems changes.	As you are learning the skills needed for public health nursing practice, you can be proactive in identifying ways to prepare for clinical experiences. Do you need to do background reading? Do you need to identify specific objectives to guide your preparation? Which questions do you need to ask?
Adapts to change	• The settings where people live, work, and learn undergo constant changes. • Adapting to change is a constant in public health nursing practice.	As someone new to public health nursing, you need to change your frame of thinking to a public health model in contrast to the medical model (Competency #4, Chapter 6).
Is willing and able to respond to population needs	• Healthy People 2020 priorities are based on the most recently identified health goals for the United States (U.S. DHHS, n.d.). • PHNs and local health departments must adapt to these changes if they are to be relevant in the interventions selected to improve population health.	Review the health data and health disparities data for your community. Ask your preceptor how the public health or community agency is responding to those needs. Identify a priority that you would like to work on as a student or volunteer in your community.
Demonstrates flexibility	• Flexibility is required in situations where families or other professionals oppose change. • Sometimes being flexible means being patient and waiting while encouraging others to make a change.	Compare your plan for the day and reflect on what actually occurred. Analyze how you were flexible in adapting to changes in your plan.
Contributes to team efforts	• PHNs need to cultivate skills that make them effective team leaders and team players. • Listening, being open, valuing the contributions of others, and identifying a common vision and goals are all important when bringing others together to improve public health.	Many public health learning experiences include collaborating with your peers on a health promotion project for the community. Use this experience to work on your team-building skills. Take time to learn more about team members and different styles of working together.

| Prioritizes and organizes workload, time, materials, and resources | • Public health nursing can be overwhelming because so many areas exist in which nurses could spend time and energy for improving population health.

 • PHNs use technology (e.g., cell phones, digital calendars) to organize their workloads and manage their time. | Learning time-management skills at the beginning of your public health nursing experience can serve you well. Make a plan for what you need to do, gather the information you need, and seek needed resources. You can always modify your plan as you evaluate how well your plan is working. You can also share your plan with your preceptor or mentor, who can help you reflect on your organization and preparation for your learning experiences. |

Which of the skills in Table 13.2 might José demonstrate as he works with the Santos family? Give some examples.

Working in the community is challenging because of the diversity, uncertainty, and constant change you experience in an environment that is not within your control. As one student said, "The patients aren't lined up nicely in their beds all in a row down the hall." In home settings, children are running around, animals abound, and the sounds of the television and people coming and going are often disconcerting. Older or disabled adults might like their slippery throw rugs on the floor and might want to have their favorite snacks available even though they are not on their prescribed diets. You might find homes without heat in the winter and homes without refrigerators in the summer. Some people live alone, and others live with a myriad of relatives and friends. You never know what to expect when you knock on the door. But you need to be ready for both the expected and unexpected. The following student example demonstrates several leadership skills. Can you identify them?

> One student several years ago was in the process of changing a catheter for a paraplegic man when the man's cat jumped on the bed. What was the student to do? Her sterile field was about to be compromised. She was wearing her only pair of sterile gloves, and her equipment was laid out on the bed. She thought for a moment. Then, very calmly, she asked the man whether he would hold his cat while she changed his catheter. This student responded with flexibility, creativity, adaptability to a changing environment, and comfort with making decisions autonomously. As you develop the ability to practice nursing in the community, whether in a home, school, clinic, faith-based organization, or other type of community agency, you will be developing your leadership skill set.

What Are the Expected Leadership Competencies for Public Health Nursing?

Nursing leadership can be formal or informal. Nurses can demonstrate leadership at all levels of nursing practice from novice to expert and as staff nurses, clinical experts, nursing specialists, supervisors, managers, educators, or administrators. Leadership is a process, not a role. Much of the research on leadership in the literature looks at the leadership roles of managers; however, all nurses can utilize leadership styles and strategies. Leadership is an expected competency for PHNs, regardless of their position (ANA, 2013; Quad Council of Public Health Nursing Organizations, 2011). Table 13.3 provides an overview of the ANA leadership standard for public health nursing.

Table 13.3   Public Health Nursing Leadership Competencies

Standard 12: Leadership—The public health nurse demonstrates leadership in the professional practice setting and the profession

Competencies

The public health nurse:

- Oversees the nursing care given by others while retaining accountability for the quality of public health nursing care provided.
- Abides by the vision, the associated goals, and the plan to implement and measure progress of an individual, family, community, or population.
- Abides by organizational goals, including participating in emergency preparedness and response activities.
- Participates as a team member in developing organizational plans to implement programs and policies.
- Participates in teams to ensure compliance with organizational policies.
- Mentors colleagues in the acquisition of clinical knowledge, skills, abilities, and judgment.
- Treats colleagues with respect, trust, and dignity.
- Develops conflict-resolution skills.
- Contributes to the promotion of a culturally responsive work environment.
- Participates in professional organizations.
- Communicates effectively with the population.
- Seeks ways to advance nursing autonomy and accountability.
- Articulates nursing and public health knowledge and skills to the interdisciplinary team, administrators, educators, policy makers, and appropriate intersectoral partners.
- Participates in efforts to influence healthcare policy to increase access to care, improve quality of care provided, and ensure ethical and equitable provision of care.

Source: ANA, 2013

New PHNs need to be able to carry out entry-level leadership competencies. Initially, their leadership opportunities will be tied to their daily clinical practice with individuals and families. However, depending on the size and nature of the agency, they might soon become involved in leadership activities at the community and systems levels of practice. Some public health agencies include leadership development in their annual performance appraisals (Kalb et al., 2006). You might be expected to demonstrate the leadership skills you have developed after you have been in public health nursing for a year or so.

ACTIVITY

Think about the leadership competencies outlined in the ANA leadership standard for public health nursing (ANA, 2013). Which competencies have you identified in the PHNs you have observed in the community? Which competencies have you started to develop?

> *José makes a follow-up visit to Mr. and Mrs. Santos. Mrs. Santos is experiencing caregiver fatigue, and Mr. Santos is becoming less and less active. He loves to smoke even though he has a portable oxygen tank in his bedroom. The Santoses do not want nurses and social workers coming in and telling them what to do. They are afraid of strangers. José tells them he will make a joint visit with the social worker and introduce them to her. He is going to take the initiative to find the resources Mr. and Mrs. Santos need to live independently in their own home.*

Which public health nursing leadership skills has José demonstrated? Which ANA leadership competencies might he use in helping Mr. and Mrs. Santo live independently in their home?

Achieving the Work of the Organization

The day-to-day work of the public health or community health agency needs to be accomplished. This means two things: carrying out the organization's mission and goals and carrying out the organization's priority work. For staff nurses, that means managing their caseload of clients on a daily basis, setting priorities based on the changing needs of their clients, and being willing to take on tasks that need to be done. As you work with preceptors and expert nurses in the community, notice the leadership approaches and styles they use that meet the health needs of their clients as well as the needs of the organization.

Which nursing skills might you use to help achieve the mission and work of the public health/community health agency in which you are working? Refer to Table 13.2.

> *José makes a joint visit with the social worker. Mr. and Mrs. Santos are committed to living in this home that they have worked so hard to purchase and maintain. It is obvious that home maintenance is poor. Stacks of old papers litter the house, they lack working smoke detectors, and they have minimal food stored in the cupboards or refrigerator. The kitchen sink is not draining properly, and the washer and dryer are not working. The social worker offers to help the couple apply for assistance for home repairs and for Meals on Wheels. José is glad he can share the care needs with the social worker. He believes they will be more effective in helping Mr. and Mrs. Santos by working as a team.*

Which leadership skills is José demonstrating during this visit?

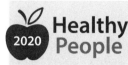

Healthy People 2020 Immunization Rates across the lifespan are highlighted in Healthy People 2020 Topics and Objectives. Click the National Snapshot tab under the topic "Immunizations" to find out the proportion of children in your state who have been immunized for measles, mumps, rubella, Hepatitis B, and pneumonia. Which vaccination rate is of most concern to you? Click the Interventions and Resources tab to find evidence-based information and recommendations for best practices for immunizations. Which intervention would you like to see implemented in your community to increase immunization rates? Which leadership strategies might you use to convince elected officials to fund this intervention to increase the immunization rate in your community?

Students can take the initiative to create their own leadership opportunities and share leadership with their peers. The following evidence example demonstrates that when students worked together to plan and organize their nursing care, their shared leadership actions enhanced their ability to provide patient-centered care.

Evidence Example: Shared Leadership Enhances Nursing Care in a Homeless Center

An example of how nursing students effectively practiced leadership occurred during a clinical at a homeless shelter. Public health nursing students conducted a monthly foot-care clinic from September through May each year. During a 3-hour clinic, six to eight students usually provided foot care to 20 to 45 clients. The instructor and homeless shelter staff oriented the students to the shelter and the foot-care clinic. Then the instructor turned the clinic over to the students to manage. The students determined how to arrange the clinic space, how to allocate the foot-care supplies, and who would carry out the different clinic roles (i.e., recruitment and registration of the clients; assigning the clients to different students for their foot care; keeping each workspace stocked with supplies; providing hospitality; documenting client assessments and services given; and following up with clients after they received care to make sure all their priority health needs were met). The instructor noticed that when she turned over the management of the clinic to the students, they were much more engaged and took more responsibility for the clinic and their clients. Every group of students organized its clinic a little differently. Each month, the shared responsibility, freedom to be creative and practice autonomously, and mutual contributions to team efforts always led to a successful clinic. Because of their ability to prioritize what needed to be done and organize their workload effectively, students managed to take the time to provide a therapeutic encounter with each client who visited the clinic. As one man said after he spent an hour with one of the students who listened patiently to his story, "This has been the best day of my life." (Schoon, 2013).

Which leadership styles and skills did these students demonstrate? How did they support the mission and work of the homeless shelter?

José makes a joint visit with the social worker. They talk to Mr. and Mrs. Santos about their health-care needs. Mr. Santos is on oxygen therapy. Mrs. Santos states that she knows her husband should stop smoking and that she turns off his oxygen when he does smoke. Mr. Santos cannot care for his personal needs. Mrs. Santos says that she is uncomfortable assisting him with hygiene and that he has not had a good bath or shower for several weeks. Mrs. Santos is becoming stressed and showing signs of depression. No one has contacted Mr. and Mrs. Santos about home maintenance. José decides he needs to prioritize their health needs. The social worker starts the application process for a home health aide to assist Mrs. Santos with Mr. Santos's personal needs. José is going to follow up on the home-maintenance referral and also work with Mr. Santos on a safe smoking program. He will focus on Mrs. Santos's stress and possible depression on the next visit. José is excited to share with his fellow students what he has learned about his own leadership abilities and how he has been able to work with Mr. and Mrs. Santos and the social worker to help the Santoses stay independent in their own home.

ACTIVITY

You can tell that José is becoming comfortable using leadership skills. Think about how you feel as you become comfortable working in the community and in people's homes. Do you share your successes with your classmates and give them helpful suggestions? If you do, are on your way to becoming an effective leader? Which leadership actions have you taken to facilitate the work of the public health nursing or community agency?

Organizational Culture and Leadership

The leadership and culture of the organization in which the PHN works determines the support available for effective public health nursing practice. The culture of support for achieving public health nursing practice goals must permeate the entire organization, as demonstrated in Figure 13.2. Nurses at all levels within the organization must take responsibility and leadership for carrying out the work of public health nursing practice.

ACTIVITY

Think about the organizational culture of the agency and the leadership styles of the PHN staff where you are completing your public health clinical. What if you were to apply for an entry-level PHN position here? What do you already know about the organizational culture and PHN leadership? Which questions would you ask to determine the type of support the organization provides to help you learn and accomplish expectations for practice? Which type of orientation is provided to newly hired PHNs? Would a preceptor or mentor be available to help you reflect on and guide your work? Do annual performance evaluations also focus on your development as a PHN?

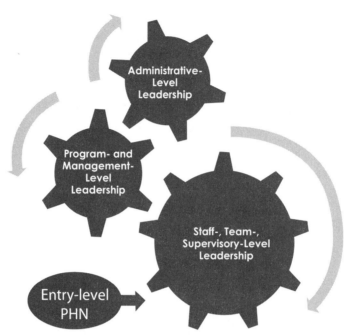

Figure 13.2. Organizational Culture of Support for Public Health Nursing Practice

Figure 13.2 illustrates how leadership needs to be part of the culture at all levels within a public health nursing agency. The following evidence example identifies the organizational attributes that support public health nursing leadership and practice.

Evidence Example: Organizational Attributes That Support Public Health Nursing Practice

A Canadian study (Meagher-Stewart et al., 2010; Underwood et al., 2009) identified effective leadership as an organizational attribute that supports public health nursing practice. The study analyzed survey data from more than 13,000 community nurses across Canada and data from 23 focus groups of PHNs and policy makers. The organizational factors that were identified as requisite for effective public health nursing practice included government policy that supports public health, supportive organizational culture, and good management practices. Visionary and empowering leadership that permeated the organization were identified as key factors that facilitated the PHNs' ability to practice their full scope of competencies. These organizational attributes and leadership qualities empowered and motivated staff to be effective in their roles. Researchers concluded that it was essential for leadership to respect, trust, and value public health for PHNs to be effective.

ACTIVITY

Which leadership qualities have you observed in your preceptor, nursing faculty, or expert public health nurses?

How do these leadership qualities contribute to effective public health nursing practice?

Which leadership qualities would you like to purposefully develop?

What are some strategies you could use to develop these leadership qualities?

José makes another visit to Mr. and Mrs. Santos. He notices that Mr. Santos is still smoking in the same room as his oxygen tank. José is concerned about the safety issues and the possible neglect of a vulnerable adult. He wants to honor the couple's independence and wishes but understands that his professional responsibility requires him to report the potential for harm to this vulnerable adult. José consults with Margaret, his preceptor. She says she will make a joint visit with José the next day to determine whether there is anything else they can do. During the visit the next day, José observes Margaret's approach to Mr. Santos. Margaret and Mr. and Mrs. Santos set up a smoking schedule for Mr. Santos that allows him to smoke while on the front porch. Mr. Santos will use his oxygen before and after each smoking session but not during it. José is impressed with Margaret's skill in working with Mr. Santos. He is going to use her technique during his next visit.

Which leadership styles and skills has Margaret demonstrated that José might use on his next visit?

Developing Leadership at the Community Level of Practice

As leaders, PHNs aim to be change agents to reduce the social conditions that contribute to poor health. Power to influence is gained through developing alliances (coalition building) with individuals and groups who have influence and power in the community. Florence Nightingale made alliances with politicians, journalists, philosophers, scientists, and influential thinkers and writers who contributed to her understanding of the public health issues of her time but also helped her bring about change for improving the health of populations (Falk-Rafael, 2005). PHNs need to move from behind the scenes to put forward strategies that can make a difference for the health of populations. This means increasing one's knowledge about the sociopolitical environment, increasing self-confidence, and developing political advocacy skills to bear witness to the effects of policy decisions on people's lives (Falk-Rafael, 2005; Mason, Backer, & Georges, 1991).

Taking the initiative to search for evidence to support nursing practice interventions also demonstrates nursing leadership. The following evidence example reports three leadership interventions that PHNs can use to bring childhood poverty, one of the major causes of health disparities in children, to the attention of the community and policy makers.

 Evidence Example: Bringing About Social Change to Reduce Child Poverty

Benita Cohen and Linda Reutter (2007) reviewed literature from Canada, the United States, and the United Kingdom as well as the professional standards and competencies for nursing practice in Canada. Based on their review, the authors recommend using Clare Blackburn's (1992) framework for working with families living in poverty. Blackburn conceptualizes three broad roles, which can be carried out at all levels of practice: (1) *monitoring*—collecting and analyzing information to determine the impact of poverty on families; (2) *alleviating and preventing*—helping families avoid, reduce, and counteract the impact of poverty; and (3) *bringing about social change*—working with organizations and the government to create policies that reduce or eliminate poverty.

PHNs can bring about social change through initiating public discussion on the effects of poverty and the contribution of policy decisions to creating poverty. Actions include putting poverty on the agenda of professional organizations and using the media to increase awareness. PHNs can use the data from their monitoring activities to inform other professionals, organizations, and the public about how poverty contributes to health disparities. Partnership skills for collective action (Competency #3, Chapter 5) are essential in bringing about change through advocacy action.

Although PHNs can identify and study the impact of social determinants of health, they cannot solve such problems as poverty, housing, unemployment, and unsafe environments. PHNs can, however, call attention to these problems and get them on the policy agenda and into the public discourse. PHNs can also study the causes and results of these health determinants and examine the effectiveness of social and collective responses to these problems. And they can help mobilize public will and coordinate actions of the public and private healthcare, education, and business sectors. Leading successful change in communities involves many different strategies (Hill, 2008; Nissen, Merrigan, & Kraft, 2005). Examples of such strategies are outlined in Table 13.4.

Table 13.4   Leadership Strategies for Successful Community Change

- Define the roles and responsibilities for stakeholders involved in leading the change.
- Seek input from all who will experience the change.
- Be present "at the table." "Interpersonal and political skills and personal presence are essential during periods of change" (Hill, 2008, p. 460).
- Look for traditional as well as nontraditional partners, including funding sources.
- Consider the big picture.
- Collaborate with others to create a positive vision of the future and choose strategies to work toward that vision.
- Remember that leadership is about relationships every day.
- Engage in self-examination and self-correction.
- Consistently integrate evidence-based approaches.
- Be hopeful but realistic when planning change.

Sources: Hill, 2008; Nissen, Merrigan, & Kraft, 2005

Working with the community as your client, just as working with individuals and families, requires a mutual egalitarian approach as you share data collection, problem solving, planning, and evaluation with community members. See Chapter 5 for examples of PHNs collaborating with communities and note in Chapter 3 how they work with community members in carrying out a community assessment. These approaches involve both shared and transformational leadership approaches.

Developing Entry-Level PHN Competencies as Part of the Leadership Journey

You might have noticed that José is practicing many of the public health nursing interventions described in Chapter 2 in his role as Mr. and Mrs. Santos's PHN. Leadership is integrated into many of the activities that PHNs and student nurses carry out. Table 13.5 has examples of leadership activities utilizing the Public Health Intervention Wheel (Dakota County Public Health, 2004). The intervention examples are suggested student learning activities outlined in a clinical menu of a public health agency.

Table 13.5 Entry-Level PHN Leadership Activities for Novice PHNs and Students

PHN interventions—Example

Advocacy
- Observing/participating in a town meeting designed to address or change a determinant of health
- Advocating for parenting classes at a conference center in an apartment complex (community level)

Policy development
- Working with schools/work sites to change vending and fund-raiser policies to include healthy food choices (systems level)

Policy enforcement
- Responding to concerns/complaints about smoking in restricted areas based on the Freedom to Breathe Act (community level)

Surveillance
- Attending or participating in immunization registry meetings (systems level)
- Locating unlicensed day care providers and providing teaching on home safety (individual level)

Coalition building
- Recruiting and inviting family day care providers to join the childhood-obesity prevention committee (community level)

Community organizing
- Participating in/helping plan youth programs, such as smoking or alcohol-use prevention (community level)
- Helping/coordinating a bioterrorism tabletop exercise (systems level)

continues

Table 13.5 Entry-Level PHN Leadership Activities for Novice PHNs and Students (continued)

PHN interventions—Example

Disease and health event investigation
- Following up on reports of pertussis cases; communicating with the state health department, clinics, and area schools about the outbreak and doing case investigation
- Meeting with clinics and hospitals regarding prenatal Hepatitis B program
- Working with veterinarians, meat packers, and hunting associations on chronic wasting disease (individual and systems levels)

Case management
- Participating in a Student Attendance Review Board (SARB) meeting within a school (systems level)

Collaboration
- Participating in meetings to observe the collaborative process, decision-making, and problem solving in groups (e.g., children's mental health, early childhood family education) (systems level)

Consultation
- Working with child day care centers, adult day care centers, and battered women's shelters to establish standards and criteria for prevention of infectious disease (systems level)

Social Marketing
- Designing messages and materials on "how to make a healthy home" that PHNs can use on home visits to help families deal with asthma (systems level)

Source: Brueshoff, 2010; Dakota County Public Health, 2004; Henry Street Consortium, 2004; MDH, 2001

What Are Leadership Expectations for Entry-Level Public Health Nurses?

Leadership needs change depending on the situations of the organization and the community. Different nurses also bring different leadership abilities to their work. Diverse styles of leadership are necessary to get the work of public health nursing accomplished. PHNs select leadership strategies and interventions based on what is most effective. Flexibility, a willingness and openness to develop new skills, and the courage to practice your new skills in the public arena are the key to your success in developing new leadership skills. Consider what a public health nursing director (Brueshoff, 2010) has to say about leadership and PHNs who are just starting out:

Based on the PHN population-based practice focus in public health, a new PHN needs to demonstrate clinical leadership for the work with individuals and families while also providing leadership at the community level. This leadership might be as a participant or a lead role on various committees such as a family service collaborative, early intervention, or other school teams. The PHN must also be a leader in doing community outreach and group education. The "client" in public health is often the community, and having skills to lead groups, coalitions, and committees is essential to achieve the goals of improving the health of the population.

–Bonnie Brueshoff, DNP, RN, PHN, Public Health Director and Robert Wood Johnson Executive Nurse Fellow (2006–2009), Dakota County Public Health

José has almost completed his public health nursing clinical. He is going to attend a Nurses Day on the Hill event at his state capitol. He wants to talk with his senator and representative about the need for funding programs to help people like Mr. and Mrs. Santos stay in their own homes. He asked Mr. and Mrs. Santos whether it would be okay with them if he shared their story. He knows that real-life stories are more effective than statistical data. José attended Nurses Day on the Hill and talked with his senator and representative. He was surprised at how receptive they were to him and that they treated him as an expert! More than 1,000 nurses were at the event. José was surprised that so many nurses and students took the time to attend. He felt proud to be part of such a large group that advocated for the health needs of the community. He realized that nursing requires more than just working a shift. If José is going to make a difference, he needs to advocate for his clients at both the systems and community levels of practice.

Participating in the Political Process

Professional nurses are expected to advocate for populations experiencing health disparities by using the political process. The role of a political advocate is embedded in the social contract that the profession of nursing has with society (Des Jardin, 2001). Nurses who have personal and professional senses of empowerment are able to work within and with their communities to improve population health through the political process (Carnegie & Kiger, 2009). PHNs are uniquely suited to participate in the political process, as they are confronted daily with the social determinants of health that often negatively affect their clients' health.

PHNs often participate in the Policy Development and Enforcement process, which requires an understanding of how the political process works and the critical points in moving forward. Taking the time to understand the policy-making process is essential if you want to advocate for vulnerable populations with your elected officials (e.g., legislators, mayor, city council, county commissioners, school board). After you understand how laws, regulations, and ordinances are made, you can be more confident about participating in the process (see Chapter 6). Your knowledge of healthcare and the health needs of your community makes you an expert in the eyes of elected officials. Developing a trusting relationship with your legislators can help you influence health policy development (Deschaine & Schaffer, 2003).

Nurses need to be involved in the political process from the electoral process to the legislative audit process (see Figure 13.3). José decides to review some basic civics on the political process and think about what he might do to advocate for older adults who need assistance to stay in their homes. See Table 13.6 for examples of what José could do.

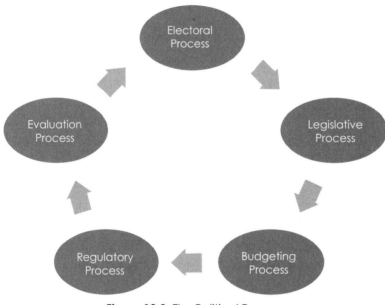

Figure 13.3. The Political Process

Table 13.6   Political Process—What Could José Do?

Electoral process Candidate selection, endorsement and support in the primary and general elections.	José can make phone calls, knock on doors, send mailings; he can also put up yard signs, donate money, and attend rallies and other campaign activities for candidates who support his political agenda for keeping older adults in their homes. He can participate in candidate screening through his local nurses' association.
Legislative process Writing, introducing, passing the bill, and enabling legislation for funding. Both houses of Congress (one or two at state level) must pass the bill, and the bill must then be signed by the governor.	José can contact his legislators about bills he wants them to support that provide funding for stay-at-home programs. He can write letters and emails or go to the Hill for a face-to-face meeting. He can attend hearings on the bill. Jose can also testify at conference hearings. He can write letters to the editor of the local newspaper, post blog entries, and call in to radio programs.

Budgeting process

The omnibus reconciliation bill at the end of each legislative session provides enabling funding. A government department is given "budget authority," or the right to implement the legislation and allocate the funding.

José can lobby for the bill's funding. He can find out which state agency has budget authority to enact and fund the legislation. He can provide testimony on the best way to fund programs and discuss who is going to benefit.

Regulatory process

The department with budget authority holds hearings to determine the rules and regulations that need to accompany the bill.

José can attend hearings about the rules and regulations that are going to enable the bill to be implemented and monitored for cost, quality, and access. He can ask to be put on an email list to receive notice of meetings and actions taken.

Evaluation process

There is generally a 2-year legislative budget cycle with a review of funded programs each biennium. A report may be generated by the agency with "budget authority" and/or by the Legislative Auditor's Office. Outcomes of program evaluation are a significant factor in determining whether the program is continued or renewed.

José can download a copy of the report and meet with his legislator's staff person, a staff member of the "budget authority" agency, or Legislative Auditors to discuss the evaluation. José can make recommendations for continuing or modifying the program to his legislator and/or appropriate legislative committee.

The American Public Health Association (APHA; 2010) has identified 10 key points of advocacy that might be helpful to you as you think about approaching your legislators (see Table 13.7). Which of these strategies would you feel comfortable using? Think about your authentic leadership style.

Table 13.7   Strategies for Working With Legislators

- Get to know legislators well—their districts and constituencies, voting records, personal schedules, opinions, expertise, and interests. Be sure to have a good understanding of the legislator and his/her concerns, priorities, and perspectives.

- Acquaint yourself with the staff members for the legislators, committees, and resource officials with whom you will be working. These people are essential sources of information and have significant influence in some instances in the development of policy.

- Identify fellow advocates and partners in the public health community to better understand the process, monitor legislation, and assess strengths and weaknesses. Finding common ground on an issue sometimes brings together strange bedfellows but makes for a stronger coalition.

- Identify the groups and other legislators with whom you may need to negotiate for changes in legislation. Do not dismiss anyone because of previous disagreements or because you lack a history of working together. Yesterday's opponent may be today's ally.

continues

Table 13.7 Strategies for Working with Legislators (continued)

- Foster and strengthen relationships with allies and work with legislators who are flexible and tend to keep an open mind. Don't allow anyone to consider you a bitter enemy because you disagree.

- Be honest, straightforward, and realistic when working with legislators and their staff. Don't make promises you cannot keep. Never lie or mislead a legislator about the importance of an issue, the opposition's position or strength, or other matters.

- Be polite, remember names, and thank those who help you—both in the legislature and in the public health advocacy community.

- Learn the legislative process and understand it well. Keep on top of the issues and be aware of controversial and contentious areas.

- Be brief, clear, accurate, persuasive, timely, persistent, grateful, and polite when presenting your position and communicating what you need/want from the legislator or staff member.

- Be sure to follow up with legislators and their staff. If you offer your assistance or promise to provide additional information, do so in a timely and professional manner. Be a reliable resource for them today and in the future.

Source: APHA, 2010

Ethical Considerations

In addition to considering the impact of decisions on the health of individuals, families, communities, and systems, public health nursing leaders must also consider how decisions affect PHNs and other public health staff. Nursing leaders can apply ethical perspectives to guide decisions that affect their teamwork and leadership activities (see Table 13.8).

> *José calls the social worker to report on how he and his preceptor have resolved the unsafe smoking situation with Mr. Santos. The social worker remains concerned and believes that Mr. Santos should be reported to county social services as a vulnerable adult. José believes that Mr. Santos should be allowed time to try the new approach. He advocates for the social worker to wait awhile to see how Mr. Santos does.*

ACTIVITY

Which ethical perspectives might José use in explaining this viewpoint to the social worker?

Table 13.8 Ethical Action in Public Health Nursing Leadership

Ethical perspective	Application
Rule ethics (principles)	• Make leadership decisions that promote good and prevent harm to families, communities, organizations, and public health workers. • Consider which leadership actions promote social justice in the community and among public health staff members. • Use advocacy-based leadership to improve population health at the individual/family and community levels of practice.
Virtue ethics (character)	• Be conscious of the needs of others, moving from the "I" to the "we" perspective. • Use your authentic leadership styles based on your beliefs, values, ethical standards, and convictions. • Be a leader who establishes caring relationships as a foundation for leadership actions. • Be a leader who values both the success of the organization and the well-being of public health staff members. • Value the contributions of all team members.
Feminist ethics (reducing oppression)	• Identify the moral and ethical leadership challenges related to population health and health disparities. • Be inclusive in the decision-making process within the community. Include all population groups that will receive services. • Use a team approach versus a hierarchical approach to prioritizing public health strategies. • Use a shared leadership approach to be an effective team member within the intraprofessional public health team and within the community. • Use a transformational leadership approach to empower communities to take charge of and manage their own healthcare needs.

Table based on work by Racher, 2007, and Volbrecht, 2002

Key Points

- Providing leadership at all three levels of public health nursing practice—individual/family, community, and system—is a professional expectation of nurses who work in public health.

- Students and professional nurses are on leadership journeys that will continue throughout their nursing careers. Leadership approaches that are particularly relevant to public health nursing practice include advocacy-based leadership, authentic leadership, shared leadership, and transformational leadership.

- Students and new graduates demonstrate entry-level leadership skills in public health by their ability to seek learning opportunities; work independently and autonomously; work in unstructured environments and tolerate ambiguity; contribute to team efforts; prioritize, organize, and complete assigned workloads; seek consultation and support; take initiative and be self-starters; be flexible and adapt to change; and respond to population needs.

- PHNs use many of the public health nursing interventions from the intervention wheel to carry out leadership activities.

- PHNs are able to be effective leaders when they are supported by an organizational culture that permeates all levels of the organization.

- PHNs are expected to advocate for improvement in population health and to reduce health disparities through navigating the political process.

- You will continue to develop your own unique leadership style and skill set in your public health nursing clinical and throughout your nursing career.

Learning Examples for Leadership

A concept called *glocal* means think global, act local. This is a good way to look at your leadership journey as a nursing student and when you begin your professional nursing practice. Select an issue you feel strongly about to start your leadership journey. Consider the following examples in which students chose to take leadership actions to resolve the leadership challenges confronting them. What might you do?

Action in Response to Suspicion of Child Abuse

A student nurse was carrying out health screening in an elementary school. She noticed that one young girl did not respond to questions, avoided eye contact, and flinched when she was touched. The student nurse conferred with her instructor and then took her concern about the child to the school principal.

Nurses Day on the Hill

Nursing students went to the state capitol to participate in an event sponsored by their state nurses association. Each student selected a health advocacy topic of interest, researched information about the topic, and prepared a 1-minute speech to present to a legislator that included a story about real people. Students visited with their elected representatives. They also participated in a rally in the capitol rotunda for safe patient care.

Infection Control Interventions With a Day Care

A team of student nurses was working with day care staffers to help them develop their disaster management plan. The students noticed that the day care had no infection control policies and procedures in place. They took their concerns to the day care director and proposed an intervention plan. The students then taught the staff members the basics of infection control and universal precautions. They also taught a hand-washing class to the preschoolers.

Groundwater Contamination in a Rural Community

Students working with a public health agency were asked to gather information about groundwater contamination by census track in a specific community. The students gathered the information and presented their results by creating a colorful map indicating different levels of groundwater contamination by census track. They also prepared a binder with the scientific data that supported the map and discussed the impact of the groundwater contamination on populations. The map and binder were prepared so well that county environmental health staff members used them both when testifying at the state legislature.

Reflective Practice

Think about the imperative that PHNs are expected to provide leadership to improve the health status of individuals, families, and communities. Think about how you might respond to an unexpected situation that might prompt you to take the *lead* in resolving a healthcare concern in the community. How might you respond to the leadership challenge in the following scenario?

> During a staff meeting, several PHNs in a health department shared their concerns about new moms dealing with postpartum depression and the lack of a postpartum depression support group in the county. Working with their supervisor, the PHNs discovered that a hospital bordering the county did have an active postpartum support group/program. Through several meetings and discussion of the needs that could be met and roles that each could provide, a partnership was established. The hospital agreed to provide staff with the expertise to facilitate the support group at no cost, and the PHNs were able to make space and child care available at no cost as well as do outreach and advertise this new program. Through these PHNs' leadership, the postpartum support group was established and continues to be successful in reaching

many new moms who benefit from the encouragement and support provided during the group meetings.

Consider the following questions:

- What was the leadership challenge in this situation?

  _____

  _____

- Which ethical principles might be used to resolve this leadership challenge?

  _____

  _____

- How did the PHNs demonstrate advocacy-based and authentic leadership?

  _____

  _____

- Which leadership skills did the PHNs demonstrate?

  _____

  _____

- Which levels of practice did PHNs use in planning and implementing nursing interventions?

  _____

  _____

 Application of Evidence

1. Which examples of public health nursing leadership have you observed at the individual, community, and systems levels in the agency where you have had your clinical experience?

2. Identify three leadership skills you have read about in this chapter that you have observed during your public health clinical.

3. Give an example of how a PHN has used advocacy-based leadership to improve the health of an individual/family or community during your public health nursing clinical.

4. Give an example of a PHN who has used authentic leadership to carry out the mission and the work of the public health agency.

Think, Explore, Do

1. How can you practice an advocacy-based leadership intervention? (For example, write a letter to the editor of your local newspaper about a public health issue in your community. Clearly state the problem, its causes, and make recommendations for what you would like to see happen.)

2. How could you use your authentic leadership style to work with a new immigrant family that knows nothing about the local healthcare system and needs to find a primary healthcare provider? Describe what you would do.

3. Think about your leadership journey during your public health nursing clinical. Identify a leadership challenge you experienced and how you met this challenge. How has this experience propelled you on your leadership journey?

4. Which leadership skills have you developed in your public health nursing clinical? Rate yourself according to the criteria listed in Table 13.9. What are your goals for further developing your leadership skills as you continue your leadership journey? How might you do this? Complete your learning goals and learning activities in Table 13.9.

Table 13.9   An Action Plan for Improving Your Entry-Level Leadership Skills in Public Health Nursing

Key for self-assessment: 1 = Always or usually; 2 = Sometimes; 3 = Rarely or never

Leadership behavior	Self-assessment			My learning goal and learning activities
Seeks learning opportunities	1	2	3	
Works independently; autonomous in practice	1	2	3	
Willing to work in an unstructured environment; tolerates ambiguity	1	2	3	
Seeks consultation and support	1	2	3	
Takes initiative; is a self-starter	1	2	3	
Adapts to change	1	2	3	
Is willing and able to respond to population needs	1	2	3	
Demonstrates flexibility	1	2	3	
Contributes to team efforts	1	2	3	
Prioritizes and organizes workload, time, materials, and resources	1	2	3	

Source: Adapted from Henry Street Consortium, 2003

References

American Nurses Association. (2013). *Public health nursing: Scope and standards of practice.* Silver Springs, MD: Nursesbooks.org.

American Public Health Association. (2010). *Top ten rules of advocacy.* Retrieved from http://www.apha.org

Avolio, B. J., Walumbwa, F. O., & Weber, T. J. (2009). Leadership: Current theories, research, and future directions. *Annual Review of Psychology, 60,* 421–449.

Blackburn, C. (1992). *Improving health and welfare work with families in poverty: A handbook.* Buckingham, UK: Open University Press.

Carnegie, E., & Kiger, A. (2009). Being and doing politics: An outdated model or 21st century reality? *Journal of Advanced Nursing, 65*(9), 1976–1984. doi:10.1111/j.1365-2648.2009.05084.x

Cohen, B. E., & Reutter, L. (2007). Development of the role of public health nurses in addressing child and family poverty: A framework for action. *Journal of Advanced Nursing, 60*(1), 96–107.

Dakota County Public Health (DCPH). (2004). *Dakota County Clinical Menu, modified from Henry Street Consortium Clinical Menu.* West St. Paul, MN: DCPH.

Deschaine, J., & Schaffer, M. (2003). Strengthening the role of public health nurse leaders in policy development. *Policy, Politics, and Nursing Practice, 4*(4), 266–274.

Des Jardin, K. (2001). Political involvement in nursing—Politics, ethics, and strategic action. *AORN Journal, 74*(5), 614–622.

Doody, O., & Doody, C. M. (2012). Transformational leadership in nursing practice. *British Journal of Nursing, (21)*20, 1212–1218.

Falk-Rafael, A. (2005). Speaking truth to power: Nursing's legacy and moral imperative. *Advances in Nursing Science, 28*(3), 212–223.

George, B., & Sims, P. (2007). *True north: Discover your authentic leadership.* Hoboken, NJ: Jossey-Bass/Wiley.

Henry Street Consortium. (2003). *Population-based public health nursing competencies.* St. Paul, MN: Author. Retrieved from http://www.health.state.mn.us/divs/opi/cd/phn/henrystreet/docs/0303henryst_corecomp.pdf

Henry Street Consortium. (2004). *The Henry Street Consortium Clinical Menu.* St. Paul, MN: HSC. Retrieved from http://www.health.state.mn.us/divs/opi/cd/phn/henrystreet/

Hill, K. S. (2008). Leading change: The creativity of a public health nurse leader. *Journal of Nursing Administration, 38*(11), 459–460.

Kalb, K. B., Cherry, N. M., Kauzloric, J., Brender, A., Green, K., Miyagawa, L. . . . & Shinoda-Mettler, A. (2006). A competency-based approach to public health nursing performance appraisal. *Public Health Nursing, 29*(3), 115–138.

Mason, D. J., Backer, B. A., & Georges, C. A. (1991). Toward a feminist model for the political empowerment of nurses. *Image Journal of Nursing Scholarship, 23*(2), 72–77.

Meagher-Stewart, D., Underwood, J., MacDonald, M., Schoenfeld, B., Blythe, J., Knibbs, K., . . . Crea, M. (2010). Organizational attributes that assure optimal utilization of public health nurses. *Public Health Nursing, 27*(5), 433–441.

Minnesota Department of Health. (2001). *Public health interventions—Applications for public health nursing practice.* St. Paul, MN: Author. Retrieved from http://www.health.state.mn.us/divs/opi/cd/phn/wheel.html

Morrison, R. S., Jones, L., & Fuller, B. (1997). The relation between leadership style and empowerment on job satisfaction of nurses. *Journal of Nursing Administration, 27*(5), 27–34.

Murphy, L. G. (2012). Authentic leadership—Becoming and remaining an authentic nurse leader. *Journal of Nursing Administration, 42*(11), 507–512.

Nissen, L. B., Merrigan, D. M., & Kraft, M. K. (2005). Moving mountains together: Strategic community leadership and systems change. *Child Welfare, 84*(2), 123–140.

O'Neill, J. A. (2013). Advancing the nursing profession begins with leadership. *Journal of Nursing Administration,43*(4), 179–181.

Quad Council of Public Health Nursing Organizations. (2011). *Quad Council Competencies for Public Health Nurses.* Retrieved from http://www.achne.org/files/Quad%20Council/QuadCouncilCompetenciesforPublicHealthNurses.pdf

Racher, F. (2007). The evolution of ethics for community practice. *Journal of Community Health Nursing, 24*(1), 65–76.

Schoon, P. (2013). *Shared leadership enhances nursing care in homeless shelter.* Unpublished manuscript.

Underwood, J. M., Mowat, D. L., Meagher-Stewart, D. M., Deber, R. B., Baumann, A. O., MacDonald, M. B., . . . Munroe, V. J. (2009). Building community and public health nursing capacity: A synthesis report of the national community health nursing study. *Canadian Journal of Public Health, 100*(5), I-1–I-11.

U.S. Department of Health and Human Services. (n.d.). *Healthy People 2020—About Healthy People.* Retrieved from http://www.healthypeople.gov/hp2020

Volbrecht, R. M. (2002). *Nursing ethics: Communities in dialogue.* Upper Saddle River, NJ: Pearson Prentice Hall.

Wolf, G. A. (2012). Transformational leadership: The art of advocacy and influence. *Journal of Nursing Administration, 42*(6), 309–310.

Wong, C. A, Spence Laschinger, H. K., & Cummings, G. G. (2010). Authentic leadership and nurses' voice behavior and perceptions of care equity. *Journal of Nursing Management, 18,* 889–900.

Marjorie A. Schaffer
with Patricia M. Schoon

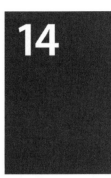

This is the beginning of your story as a public health nurse (PHN). The chapters in this book have given you a foundation in the Henry Street Consortium entry-level population-based public health nursing competencies, which emphasize the knowledge, skills, and attitudes needed to be an effective PHN. What are your next steps for developing your expertise in public health nursing?

What Do You Need to Know?

When PHNs and educators created the Henry Street Consortium competencies, they also generated a basic public health nursing knowledge base to serve as a foundation for public health nursing practice. In smaller local health departments, PHNs need a broader knowledge base so that they are competent to provide services in many areas of public health. In larger public health agencies, PHNs might need more in-depth knowledge and expertise in specific areas of public health, such as following up on a population with drug-resistant tuberculosis or working with schools and community agencies to prevent teen pregnancy. Keep in mind that PHNs also work in many organizations other than official public health agencies, such as home-visiting nurse associations, schools, corporations that include occupational health positions, and non-profit organizations that value and need the expertise of PHNs. Following is a list of basic public health nursing knowledge areas for population-based practice:

- Antepartum/postpartum

- Chemical health issues and behaviors

- Chronic disease prevention and management

- Death and dying

- Disaster and bioterrorism response

- Disease prevention and control

- Environmental health and safety

- Family development
- Family planning
- Health determinants
- Health informatics
- Health promotion for all ages
- Human growth and development
- Human sexuality
- Immunizations across the lifespan

- Injury prevention
- Medication administration/management
- Mental health
- Nutrition
- Parenting
- Social and market justice
- Technical nursing skills
- Violence prevention

Many nursing students worry about being knowledgeable in medication administration and technical nursing skills as they seek their first employment as a nurse. Nurses new to public health nursing might feel similarly less prepared in public health knowledge areas that are essential to successful public health nursing practice. Look carefully at your position description to determine whether you have an adequate knowledge base and skill set to perform the job responsibilities. Seek a mentor and establish a plan for strengthening your knowledge base and skill set.

ACTIVITY

Think about the basic knowledge base required for effective public health nursing practice related to the specific population health practice area of interest to you.

Analyze your strengths in basic public health nursing knowledge in that population health area.

Which knowledge areas do you need to strengthen? Consider your intended area of practice. If you are in a new public health nursing position, analyze the knowledge base you need for effective public health nursing practice in your setting and focus area.

Which strategies can you use to strengthen needed knowledge areas?

Who Do You Need to Be?

Henry Street Consortium members also identified personal characteristics that contribute to effective public health nursing practice. The following characteristics are virtues that can enhance your ability to be successful and committed to public health nursing:

- Adaptability
- Caring
- Compassion

- Confidence
- Courage
- Creativity

- Flexibility

- Hard work

- Humor

- Independence

- Leadership qualities

- Lifelong learning attitude

- Passion

- Persistence

- Positive attitude

- Resourcefulness

- Risk taking

- Self-care

 ## ACTIVITY

Consider the following questions as you review the table of personal characteristics/virtues that enhance your public health nursing practice.

Why are these characteristics important for effective public health nursing practice?

Which of these characteristics have you observed in practicing PHNs? Give a specific example of how you see the characteristic exemplified in the practice of the expert PHN.

How do you see these characteristics contributing to the accomplishment of the competencies (see Table 14.1 for competencies)?

How do you think your personal characteristics/virtues match with the kind of PHN you would like to be?

How Can You Use the Public Health Nursing Knowledge and Skills in Other Nursing Practice Settings?

As many of you will start your professional nursing career in an area other than public health nursing, think about how you can apply your public health nursing knowledge and competencies to your chosen area of practice. PHNs believe that public health nursing concepts and skills can be applied to all specialty areas in nursing practice. See Table 14.1 for reflection questions and examples related to each of the competencies.

Table 14.1 Reflection on Application of Public Health Nursing Competencies to Other Care Settings

Competency	Reflection question	Examples
1. Applies the public health nursing process to communities, systems, individuals, and families	How does thinking about an individual patient as part of a population contribute to your choosing nursing interventions for that patient?	Your patient is a frail elderly person who lives alone. What do you know about the health risks for this population? Which assessment data would you need to collect about this patient as part of your discharge planning process?
2. Utilizes basic epidemiological principles (the incidence, distribution, and control of disease in a population) in public health nursing practice	In the hospital setting, how can you use epidemiology to help you understand your patient's illness?	Your patient has been diagnosed with *Clostridium Difficile* infection, a common hospital-acquired infection. Which infection control practices would you need to institute? How would you prevent the spread of this infection to other patients on your unit?
3. Utilizes collaboration to achieve public health goals	How many different professionals and ancillary staff do you collaborate with in an acute care setting? How can you collaborate with them effectively?	A child with a traumatic brain injury has been admitted to your pediatric intensive care unit. You are the admitting nurse. Which other members of the interprofessional care team should you alert about the arrival of this patient?
4. Works within the responsibility and authority of the governmental public health system	Which governmental policies influence how care is delivered in hospitals?	An uninsured patient comes to the Emergency Department (ED) complaining of an earache that could probably be managed at the outpatient clinic. Based on the "duty to treat" mandate in the Emergency Medical Treatment and Active Labor Act (EMTALA), can you send the patient to the outpatient clinic rather than treat him in the ED?
5. Practices public health nursing within the auspices of the Nurse Practice Act	What are the independent actions covered by the Nurse Practice Act that you provide in nursing care in acute care settings?	A new mother on the postpartum unit is having difficulty getting her newborn to latch on during breastfeeding. Is it within your legal scope of practice to refer the patient to the lactation consultant?

6. Effectively communicates with communities, systems, individuals, families, and colleagues

What have you learned about effective communication in acute care settings?

A dying patient wants to be discharged to hospice, but her daughter wants her to stay in the hospital to try one more treatment approach. How might you approach the daughter to discuss her mother's wishes? Which other members of the care team might you want to enlist in working with this mother and daughter?

7. Establishes and maintains caring relationships with communities, systems, individuals, and families

How do the hospital environment, staff, and policies contribute to patient perceptions of caring?

You are teaching a non-English-speaking patient about her newly diagnosed diabetes. A family member is acting as a translator, but you are concerned that the patient is not receiving accurate information, and the patient is very anxious. What are your hospital policies about patients' relatives translating medical information? Which translation resources are available to you and your patient?

8. Shows evidence of commitment to social justice, the greater good, and the public health principles

How are hospital policies consistent or inconsistent with social justice?

A patient on your Behavioral Health Unit is being discharged. You believe that the patient is still a danger to herself and others. The patient's insurance will not pay for additional hospital days, and your hospital policy is to discharge patients when their insurance no longer certifies them for acute care hospitalization. Do any other hospital policies or laws allow an extended stay for this patient?

9. Demonstrates nonjudgmental and unconditional acceptance of people different from self

How are cultural differences and needs addressed in the acute care setting?

A Native American patient would like a native healer to conduct a smudging ceremony, which involves burning sage in his hospital room. Hospital rules do not allow any fires in hospital rooms. Which culturally sensitive interventions might you employ to meet this patient's needs?

continues

Table 14.1   Reflection on Application of Public Health Nursing Competencies to Other Care Settings   (continued)

Competency	Reflection question	Examples
10. Incorporates mental, physical, emotional, social, spiritual, and environmental aspects of health into assessment, planning, implementation, and evaluation	How does nursing care address the whole person in the acute care setting?	You are caring for an elderly male patient who has a terminal illness. He wants to share stories about his life with you. You realize that he is trying to complete the developmental task of his life review. However, you have four patients to care for and very little time to spend with this patient. How might you respond to this patient's needs?
11. Demonstrates leadership in public health nursing with communities, systems, individuals, and families	What does it mean to be an authentic leader in an acute care setting? Which actions might you take to advocate for your patients that are consistent with your beliefs, values, and convictions?	You are caring for a patient who has had a recent surgical procedure. The patient is in extreme pain, and the pain medication prescribed is not effective. The patient's physician is not comfortable increasing the patient's medication, as she knows that the patient is addicted to oxycodone. Which patient advocacy actions might you take in this situation?

Also, many of the public health interventions are applicable in acute care settings. When public health nursing students were asked how they used the public health interventions in other practice settings, they suggested the activities in Table 14.2. Think about how these activities are consistent with each intervention.

Table 14.2   Use of the Public Health Intervention Wheel in Other Settings

Intervention	Specific activities
Surveillance	Identify nosocomial infections (infections acquired in healthcare settings).
Disease and health event investigation	Determine contributing factors related to nosocomial infections.
Outreach	Offer a flu shot day or week for employees.

Screening	Provide mammograms and lab tests during yearly physical checkup; screen at-risk individuals for falls in hospital setting.
Referral and follow-up	Refer to home care, chaplain, or social services.
Case management	As a primary nurse, coordinate care for a hospitalized patient.
Delegated functions	Delegate certain tasks to certified nursing assistants (CNAs).
Health teaching	Provide discharge teaching, breastfeeding instruction, or teaching about "back to sleep" techniques.
Counseling	Offer breastfeeding support; conduct support groups on mental health units.
Consultation	Consult as a lactation expert; consult with family and care teams about palliative care.
Collaboration	Collaborate with the care team (surgeon, physician, nurse, aide, family).
Coalition building	Create a coalition of public television and medical society to promote advanced directives.
Community organizing	Promote a wellness initiative in a hospital or clinic setting.
Advocacy	Provide patient advocates in acute and clinic settings.
Social marketing	Advertise the availability of specialized units; publish data about outcomes indicating that quality care is provided.
Policy development and enforcement	Mandate the reporting of suspected child abuse for hospitalized children; establish no-smoking policy for health campus.

Evidence Example: What PHNs Say About Their Practice

Keller, Schaffer, and Reckinger (2013) explored PHN perceptions on how their activities contributed to health and well-being in the communities they served. The sample included 49 PHNs across the United States. PHN responses to a question on the activities that had the greatest impact on community health were grouped into four categories: (1) child immunization; (2) communicable disease surveillance, education, and investigation; (3) maternal and child health—early intervention, school readiness, prenatal and parenting education, case management of high-risk families, and growth and development follow-up; and (4) linking people to resources.

When PHNs were asked about the greatest impact on the community if there were no public health nursing services, five categories revealed their perceptions about potential negative effects on the community (see Table 14.3).

Table 14.3 PHNs Perceptions of the Impact of No Public Health Nursing Services on the Community

Category	PHN comments
Occurrence of disease and health problems	"I believe more children would be placed in increasingly violent or dangerous environments."
Lack of prevention accompanied by declining health in the community	"The biggest impact on the health of the community would be a much less healthy society."
Less care for vulnerable populations	"The most vulnerable among us would suffer immeasurably." "The poor and vulnerable would go without primary/preventive care and would flood our emergency departments." "Mentally ill and disabled clients that do not have health insurance would be wandering with nowhere to be treated."
Negative effects on public health infrastructure	"The high-risk individuals that are uninsured or underinsured would fall through the cracks of the system and would not have any resources for healthcare on any level, with the exception of the already overused and misused emergency room for their healthcare."
Negative effects on local health department programs	"The impact would be devastating. While all aspects of public health are important, it is the nurse who pulls all the little pieces together. It is the nurse who looks at the big picture to ensure services are being received."

The key message from this evidence about the work of public health nurses is that PHNs are essential contributors to community health and well-being. PHNs must continue to provide evidence about the outcomes of their work and become "visible" to policymakers who make decisions about public health funding. This means PHNs must advocate for themselves and their accomplishments as well as for services for the populations they serve. As citizens of communities, PHNs also have a civic responsibility to contribute to community well-being.

What Can You Learn From the Stories of Nursing Students?

We can also learn about public health nursing strategies from the stories of nursing students. The student stories represent the process and experiences encountered in becoming a PHN.

As you reflect on the meaning of the stories, think about how you are learning to be a PHN. Use the following questions to guide your reflections about the three student stories:

1. Which competencies is the student working on developing?

2. Which public health interventions are the student and preceptor using in this story?

3. Which public health nursing Cornerstones is the student expressing?

4. Which personal characteristics would it be helpful to have or develop to carry out this public health nursing practice example?

Student Story #1

School children comprise a population at high risk for infection and transmitting infectious organisms. In terms of epidemiology, the "chain of infection" is the process by which pathogens are transmitted from the environment to a host, invade the host, and cause infection. Breaking the chain of infection at any point prevents the spread of infection. Hand-washing is the most effective mechanism to break the chain and prevent the spread of infection. Two of my classmates and I taught three sessions on hand-washing to first graders. A curriculum and resource program had provided us with a hand-washing kit that consisted of a 3-minute video of a young boy explaining and demonstrating how to correctly wash one's hands to remove as many germs as possible, several bottles of "GloGerm Potion" that makes invisible germs glow a bright white under a black light, a black light, and a bunch of "Germbusters!" stickers.

As each session began, we did a few minutes' worth of very basic health teaching about how germs can cause illness; are everywhere, especially on our hands; and by washing our hands well and often, we can prevent the spread of germs and stay healthy. After our short presentation, we helped the children practice correct hand-washing techniques with the GloGerm product. This gave me a nice chance to do some one-on-one teaching and interact with a few children who were somewhat timid or shy and see them respond positively and come out of their shell. The kids absolutely loved the presentation and our "magic potion"!

This experience shows growth in my ability to communicate effectively and work with others to complete a task. Good communication and organization were required between me and my classmates to work out our own teaching time to learn about the hand-washing kit, pick up and return the kit, and put together a good presentation. It was also necessary to communicate with first-graders and to understand child development to teach health concepts at their developmental level and not speak over their heads. I believe any one of us could have done the job alone, but it was much more enjoyable to share the work and be a part of a team than to do it alone. Being a team player is something I, a loner by nature, need to work on. I learned that I am likable and competent, work well with others, and really enjoy it, and I showed that I am responsible by carrying my share of this clinical assignment. This teaching experience was FUN and gave me more confidence in my nursing knowledge and teaching skills. In looking back, I see that I have become more spontaneous and flexible and can laugh more as I spend more time in real-world settings as opposed to the nursing lab or classroom. This experience of working with others and the necessity of good communication were most useful to me and will help me continue improving in those areas. This teaching experience will serve as a positive example in times when I feel less confident in my abilities.

Source: Competency Portfolio, Senior Nursing Student

Student Story #2

My preceptor and I went out to a home to carry out a developmental assessment on a 2-year-old suspected of being developmentally delayed. My preceptor had a very friendly, informal, yet professional demeanor, which I believe is a very beneficial and important asset to have and develop; she explained what the assessment consisted of and the actions that would ensue following the assessment as well as the other areas of specialty services that might be involved. During the assessment, my preceptor was very warm and casual, but one could see that she was observing our young client very carefully. She observed him in a way that was not distressing to the mother. Afterward, my preceptor and I discussed the results and the process she uses when collecting and processing data within the realm of public health nursing. She stated that working within public health really exposes one in a community. For example, it is not uncommon to run into clients at the grocery store or in various other establishments around the area, and one has to face the questions, "Do I say hello? Do I ask how things are going? Do they recognize me?" I asked her how she deals with these simple, yet complex questions. She remarked that a nurse needs to be very sensitive and prepared for these issues: "We are in their lives and homes and must be respectful." She stated that she leaves it up to the clients to make the initial contact and allows them to lead the direction of the conversation. She also made it clear how important confidentiality is, because at times a PHN visits one family member and the other members are unaware, so even confidentiality within families is instituted and mandated by HIPAA [the Health Insurance Portability and Accountability Act].

I became more aware of the importance of having guidelines, such as the Nurse Practice Act, to help us provide effective and competent care. My preceptor was an excellent example and resource to whom I can look back and reflect when I begin my career as a nurse. The Nurse Practice Act encompasses nurses in all fields; however, the means by which it is carried out is customized to each specialty field. For example, independent nursing functions, in reference to public health nursing, differ from delegated medical functions that nurses carry out in hospitals. Independent functions consist of educating, teaching, and providing information to clients and not performing skilled nursing care, such as caring for wounds or giving injections that would be done in the hospital. Also, boundaries are harder to manage in public health nursing than within the hospital. It is the client who "runs" the show and is in charge, not the nurse; one must be extra cautious when exchanging information in the field. I feel I will be more adequately prepared and aware of when and how to set boundaries and how to deal with a situation where I might not want to reveal as much to clients as they might want or expect.

Source: Competency Portfolio, Senior Nursing Student

Student Story #3

I worked with my preceptor in a breast and cervical cancer screening program. Part of the screening consisted of checking total (fasting) cholesterol and blood glucose levels. I did a finger stick to draw up a drop of blood into a little plastic case that fit into a machine that would give us the cholesterol and glucose results in about 5 minutes. After we had the results, I entered the data into a computer program created by the Centers for Disease Control and Prevention (CDC) that analyzes and creates a bar graph and written description of the results that are very easy for the average nonmedical person to understand and learn from. It also generates a "Diagnostic Referral" form if any test result is too high. This form can then be faxed to a healthcare provider immediately, with no other data needing to be added. When I had printed out the report, I went over it in great detail with my client, asking her to stop me if she needed additional clarification or had any other questions. She was able to verbalize a general understanding of her results. The computer program had created a referral form for her to be evaluated by a physician because of high cholesterol, and she requested that my preceptor set up an appointment for her. My preceptor will follow up with the woman in 2 weeks to find out whether she has kept the doctor appointment and whether she wants to participate in the lifestyle interventions and counseling services that are also offered at the clinic.

I learned how to use new-to-me technology in both the blood testing and data entry experiences, and I learned so much about the community resources available for this (my) age group. More important to my nursing practice was the review of cholesterol and glucose normal values and the opportunity to do some teaching with my client, in which I had to use good communication and listening skills to facilitate her learning. I noticed afterward that I had picked up some of my preceptor's mannerisms in talking with clients—nonverbal communication skills, such as leaning forward toward the client. I also learned that I often get in a rush when I am talking about something I understand but the person I am talking to does not and that I need to slow down. I have become more aware of my interpersonal behaviors, and this will help make me a better nurse in the future.

Source: Competency Portfolio, Senior Nursing Student

Expert PHNs also have stories about their practice that illustrate how they accomplish public health nursing interventions (Minnesota Department of Health, 2006).

Transition From Student to Public Health Nursing Practice

You may feel overwhelmed by how much there is to know about public health nursing. How can a new graduate be a successful PHN? Molly Hoff, who recently began her public health nursing practice, reflects on the experience of becoming a PHN:

Question: What support helped you to make a transition to your new position?

Answer: The biggest support I had transitioning to PHN practice was other nurses and social workers in my orientation. Some of them were more experienced than me, and it was great to draw on that knowledge. With little experience, it was nice to be able to relate and lean on them for support.

Question: What knowledge areas and skills did you find you needed for public health nursing practice?

Answer: Far and above, you need to have great critical thinking skills—before anything else, you need that. I was taught this very well in school, but it got rusty in some of my clinical practice, which was less autonomous than this position. You need to be able to think through, around, and over a myriad of issues that are constantly coming up with our clients. Another skill needed is active listening/motivational interviewing—this is the crux of our contact with the clients and unless they feel supported and that they are not being judged, we will not be able to do our jobs. Having a base in holistic treatment doesn't hurt either, knowing how to look at the person as a complete being and not the sum of their diagnoses.

Question: What is especially rewarding to you about public health nursing practice?

Answer: Public health practice is great because it is helping people live their lives to the fullest possible degree. Going into the hospital is an event; what we do is everything after and before that—the person's everyday life.

Question: What advice do you have for a new PHN?

Answer: Learn as much as possible about health and wellness, because you never know what will come in handy or help you in your job.

Reflections on Being a Public Health Nurse

Expert PHNs explained why they practice public health nursing and what they find rewarding in practice. Their comments capture the essence of what is important to PHNs and what inspires them to do their work:

"Being a public health nurse is an honor and a privilege. You are constantly doing work important to the public 'common good.' You constantly give back each and every day. It is an amazing privilege to be allowed such an important place in others' lives." —Karen

"Being a public health nurse fits best with my philosophy—giving people the resources and supports they need to make good decisions that maximize their health, safety, and independence." —Chris

"Being a public health nurse includes looking beyond the obvious and looking for what is happening in the client situation that we do not yet know. Making genuine connections and building caring relationships undergirds public health. A public health nurse is both a nurse investigator and caregiver, blending holistic inquiry with thoughtful interventions that can make a real difference in people's everyday lives by impacting health and imparting hope." —Renee

"Public health nursing involves healthcare of an entire community. I personally thrive in a work environment where all aspects of nursing care might be required on any given day. A public health nurse needs to be flexible in the work day, because priorities can be continually changing." —BJ

"Public health nursing is rewarding when I help improve the health of the community while assisting individuals with taking action to optimize their own health." —Bruce

"I enjoy working with different cultures—learning about their traditions, beliefs, and how frequently there is a commonality to all people, regardless of which country they were born in or their economic status." —Mary

"I know that each family I visit will find their path a little easier and more focused because of me. As a public health nurse, I need to be flexible, nonjudgmental, caring, and empathetic, but I also need to keep myself distanced enough to see the big picture and to help my clients look at options and goals for their health and their lives. I am a public health nurse because I want to make a difference." —Barb

"Being in the community is so rewarding—I work with people of all ages and backgrounds and establish partnerships to carry out the public health mission to reach those in need. Being a public health nurse means being a voice for prevention and early intervention, being a voice for making healthy choices, and being an advocate to help people to be healthy. For me, public health nursing is fulfilling, rewarding, challenging, and is my passion. It is a true calling and a blessing to be a public health nurse." —Bonnie

References

Keller, L. O., Schaffer, M. A., & Reckinger, D. (2013). Visibility for public health nursing. Unpublished paper.

Minnesota Department of Health. (2006). Wheel of public health interventions: A collection of "Getting Behind the Wheel" stories, 2000–2006. Office of Public Health Practice. Retrieved from http://www.health.state.mn.us/divs/opi/cd/phn/docs/0606wheel_stories.pdf

APPENDIXES   III

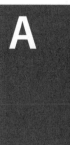

Chapter 1

American Nurses Association. (2003). *Nursing's social policy statement, 2nd ed.* Silver Spring, MD: Nursesbooks.org.

American Nurses Association. (2013). *Public health nursing: Scope and standards of practice.* Silver Spring, MD: Nursesbooks.org.

American Public Health Association, Public Health Nursing Section. (1996). *Definition and role of public health nursing.* Washington, DC: Author. Retrieved from http://www.apha.org/membergroups/sections/aphasections/phn/about/defbackground.htm

Clark, M. J. (2008). *Community health nursing.* Upper Saddle River, NJ: Pearson.

Core Public Health Functions Steering Committee. (1995). *Public health in America: Core functions and essential services of public health.* Adopted 1994. Retrieved from http://www.health.gov/phfunctions/public.htm

Dreher, M., Shapiro, D., & Asselin, M. (2006). *Healthy places, healthy people: A handbook for culturally competent community nursing practice.* Indianapolis, IN: Sigma Theta Tau International.

Education Committee of the Association of Community Health Nurse Educators. (2010). Essentials of baccalaureate nursing education for entry-level community/public health nursing. *Public Health Nursing, 27*(4), 371–382. doi:10.1111/j.1525-1446.2010.00867.x

Essential Public Health Services Work Group of the Core Public Health Functions Steering Committee Membership: American Public Health Association; Association of Schools of Public Health; Association of State and Territorial Health Officials; Centers for Disease Control and Prevention; Environmental Council of the States; Food and Drug Administration; Health Resources and Services Administration; Indian Health Service; Institute of Medicine; National Academy of Sciences; National Association of County and City Health Officials; National Association of State Alcohol and Drug Abuse Directors; National Association of State Mental Health Program Directors; National Institutes of Health; Office of the Assistant Secretary for Health; Public Health Foundation; Substance Abuse and Mental Health Services Administration; U.S. Public Health Service Agency for Health Care Policy and Research. (1994). *Public health core functions and essential services.* Retrieved from http://www.cdc.gov/nphpsp/essentialservices.html

Friedman, M., Bowden, V., & Jones, E. (2003). *Family nursing: Research, theory, and practice, 5th ed.* Upper Saddle River, NJ: Prentice Hall.

Henry Street Consortium. (2003). *Population-based public health nursing competencies.* St. Paul, MN: Author. Retrieved from http://www.health.state.mn.us/divs/opi/cd/phn/henrystreet/docs/0303henryst_corecomp.pdf

Institute of Medicine. (1988). *The future of public health.* Washington, D.C.: National Academy Press.

Institute of Medicine. (2011). *The future of nursing—Leading change, advancing health.* Washington, D.C.: National Academy Press.

International Council of Nurses. (2007). *Vision for the future of nursing.* Retrieved from http://www.icn.ch/about-icn/icns-vision-for-the-future-of-nursing/

Keller, L. O., Strohschein, S., & Schaffer, M. A. (2011). The cornerstones of public health nursing. *Public Health Nursing, 28*(3), 249–260. doi:10.1111/j.1525-1446.2010.00923.x

Marmot, M., & Wilkinson, R. G. (1999). *Social determinants of health.* Oxford, UK: Oxford University Press.

Minnesota Department of Health, Center for Public Health Nursing. (2003). *Definition of population-based practice.* Retrieved from http://www.health.state.mn.us/divs/opi/cd/phn/docs/0303phn_pop-basedpractice.pdf

Minnesota Department of Health, Center for Public Health Nursing. (2007). *Cornerstones of Public Health Nursing.* Adapted from original by Center for Public Health Nursing, 2004. St. Paul: Author. Retrieved from http://www.health.state.mn.us/divs/opi/cd/phn/docs/0710phn_cornerstones.pdf

Minnesota Department of Health, Division of Community Health Services, Public Health Nursing Section. (2001). *Public health interventions: Applications for public health nursing practice.* St. Paul, MN: Author. Retrieved from http://www.health.state.mn.us/divs/opi/cd/phn/docs/0301wheel_manual.pdf

Minnesota Department of Health, Public Health Nursing Section. (2000). *Public health nursing practice for the 21st century: Competency development in population-based practice.* National Satellite Learning Conference. St. Paul, MN: Author. Retrieved from http://www.health.state.mn.us/divs/opi/cd/phn/docs/0001phnpractice_learningguide.pdf

National Center for Health Statistics. (2012). *Healthy People 2010, final review.* Hyattsville, NY: U.S. DHHS. Retrieved from http://www.cdc.gov/nchs/data/hpdata2010/hp2010_final_review.pdf

Quad Council of Public Health Nursing Organizations. (2011). *Public health nursing competencies.* Retrieved from http://www.phf.org/resourcestools/Pages/Public_Health_Nursing_Competencies.aspx

Robert Wood Johnson Foundation. (2013). *Forum on the future of public health nursing, February 8, 2012—Proceedings and feedback: Summary report.* Retrieved from http://www.rwjf.org/content/dam/farm/reports/reports/2012/rwjf404144

Schaffer, M. A., Cross, S., Olson, L. O., Nelson, P., Schoon, P. M., & Henton, P. (2011). The Henry Street Consortium population-based competencies for educating public health nursing students. *Public Health Nursing, 28*(1), 78–90. doi:10.1111/j.1525-1446.2010.00900.x

Stanhope, M., & Lancaster, J. (2008). *Public health nursing: Population-centered health care in the community, 7th ed.* St. Louis, MO: Mosby.

U.S. Department of Health and Human Services. (n.d.). *Healthy People 2020: About Healthy People 2020: Leading health indicators.* Retrieved from http://healthypeople.gov/2020/default.aspx

U.S. Department of Health and Human Services. (2010). *Public health functions project: Public health in America statement.* Retrieved from http://www.health.gov/phfunctions

World Health Organization. (n.d.). *Public health.* Retrieved from http://www.who.int/trade/glossary/story076/en/

World Health Organization. (2013). *What are social determinants of health?* Retrieved from http://www.who.int/social_determinants/sdh_definition/en/index.html

Zahner, S. J., & Block, D. E. (2006). The road to population health: Using Healthy People 2010 in nursing education. *Journal of Nursing Education, 45*(3), 105–108.

Chapter 2

American Nurses Association. (2013). *Public health nursing: Scope and standards of practice.* Silver Spring, MD: Nursesbooks.org.

Armstrong, K. L., Fraser, J. A., Dadds, M. R., & Morris J. (1999). A randomized, controlled trial of nurse home visiting to vulnerable families with newborns. *Journal of Paediatrics and Child Health, 35*(3), 237–244.

Atkins, R. B., Williams, J. R., Silenas, R., & Edwards, J. C. (2005). The role of PHNs in bioterrorism preparedness. *Disaster Management Response, 3*(4), 98–105.

Brownson, R. C., Baker, E. A., Leet, T. L., & Gillespie, K. N. (Eds.). (2002). *Evidence-based public health.* New York, NY: Oxford University Press.

Caldera, D., Burrell, L., Rodriguez, K., Crowne, S. S., Rohde, C., & Duggan, A. (2007). Impact of a statewide home visiting program on parenting and on child health and development. *Child Abuse & Neglect, 31*(8), 829–852. doi:10.1016/j.chiabu.2007.02.008

Centers for Disease Control and Prevention. (n.d.). *Vaccines and immunizations.* Retrieved from http://www.cdc.gov/vaccines/

Corrarino, J. E. (2000). *Lessons learned: Successful strategies to implement a perinatal hepatitis B program.* Centers for Disease Control and Prevention Annual Hepatitis B Conference. San Diego, CA.

Corrarino, J. E., & Little, A. (2006). *Breathing easy: A public health nursing/community coalition success story.* American Public Health Association. 128th Annual Meeting. Boston, MA.

Corrarino, J. E., Walsh, P. J., & Nadel, E. (2001). Does teaching scald burn prevention to families of young children make a difference? A pilot study. *Journal of Pediatric Nursing, 16*(4), 256–262.

Corrarino, J. E., Williams, C., Campbell, W. S., 3rd, Amrhein, E., LoPiano, L., & Kalachik, D. (2000). Linking substance-abusing pregnant women to drug treatment services: A pilot program. *Journal of Obstetric, Gynecologic, and Neonatal Nurses, 29*(4), 369–376.

Dearholt, S. L., & Dang, D. (2012). *Johns Hopkins nursing evidence-based practice: Model and guidelines, 2nd ed.* Indianapolis, IN: Sigma Theta Tau International.

Eckenrode, J., GanzeI, B., Henderson, C. R., Jr., Smith, E., Olds, D. L., Powers, J., . . . Sidora, K. (2000). Preventing child abuse and neglect with a program of nurse home visitation: The limiting effects of domestic violence. *JAMA, 284*(11), 1385–1391.

Fetrick, A., Christensen, M., & Mitchell, C. (2003). Does public health nurse home visitation make a difference in the health outcomes of pregnant clients and their offspring? *Public Health Nursing, 20*(3), 184–189.

Fineout-Overholt, E., Melnyk, B. M., Stillwell, S., & Williamson, K. (2010). Critical appraisal of the evidence: Part I. *American Journal of Nursing, 110*(7), 47–52.

Hedberg, I. G. (2013). Barriers to breastfeeding in the WIC population. *American Journal of Maternal Child Health Nursing, 38*(4), 244–249. doi:10.1097/NMC.0b013e3182836ca2

Home Visiting Evidence of Effectiveness. (n.d.). *Healthy Families America: Evidence of program model effectiveness.* Retrieved from http://homvee.acf.hhs.gov/document.aspx?sid=10&rid=1&mid=1

Hopp, L., & Rittenmeyer, L. (2012). *Introduction to evidence-based practice: A practical guide for nursing.* Philadelphia, PA: F. A. Davis.

Izzo, C. V., Eckenrode, J. J., Smith, E. G., Henderson, C. R., Cole, R., Kitzman, H., & Olds, D. L. (2005). Reducing the impact of uncontrollable stressful life events through a program of nurse home visitation for new parents. *Prevention Science, 6*(4), 269–274.

Kang, N., Song, Y., Hyun, T. H., & Kim, K. (2005). Evaluation of the breastfeeding intervention program in a Korean community health center. *International Journal of Nursing, 42,* 409–413. doi:10.1016/j.ijnurstu.2004.08.003

Kearney, M. H., York, R., & Deatrick, J. A. (2000). Effects of home visits to vulnerable young families. *Journal of Nursing Scholarship, 32*(4), 369–376.

Kelaher, M., Dunt, D., Feldman, P., Nolan, A., & Raban, B. (2009). The effect of an area-based intervention on breastfeeding rates in Victoria, Australia. *Health Policy, 90,* 89–93.

Keller, L. O., & Strohschein, S. (2009, April). *E_2 evidence exchange: Your public health nursing e-source.* Public Health Nursing Faculty Conference. Otsego, MN.

Keller, L., Strohschein, S., Lia-Hoagberg, B., & Schaffer, M. (1998). Population-based public health nursing interventions: A model for practice. *Public Health Nursing, 15*(3), 207–215.

Keller, L., Strohschein, S., Lia-Hoagberg, B., & Schaffer, M. (2004). Population-based public health interventions: Practice-based and evidence-supported. *Public Health Nursing, 21*(5), 453–468.

Kitzman, H. J., Olds, D. L., Cole, R. E., Hanks, C. A., Anson, E. A., Arcoleo, K. J., . . . Holmberg, J. R. (2010). Enduring effects of prenatal and infancy home visiting by nurses on children: follow-up of a randomized trial among children at age 12 years. *Archives of Pediatrics & Adolescent Medicine, 164*(5): 412–418. doi:10.1001/archpediatrics.2010.76.

Lanigan, C. (2013). *Case Study: MVNA Evidence-Based Practice in Maternal/Child Health Home Visiting.* Unpublished manuscript for MVNA, Minneapolis, MN.

MacNeil, J., Lobato, M., & Moore, M. (2005). An unanswered health disparity: Tuberculosis among correctional inmates, 1993 through 2003. *American Journal of Public Health, 95*(10), 1800–1805.

Margolis, P. A., Lannon, C. M., Stevens, R., Harlan, C., Bordley, W. C., Carey, T., . . . Earp, J. L. (1996). Linking clinical and public health approaches to improve access to healthcare for socially disadvantaged mothers and children. A feasibility study. *Archives of Pediatric & Adolescent Medicine, 150*(8), 815–821.

Martin, K. S. (2005). *The Omaha System: A key to practice, documentation, and information management, 2nd ed.* Omaha, NE: Health Connections Press.

Melnyk, B. M., & Fineout-Overholt, E. (Eds.). (2005). *Evidence-based practice in nursing and healthcare: A guide to best practice, 1st ed.* Philadelphia, PA: Lippincott Williams and Wilkins.

Milbank Memorial Fund. (1998). *Partners in community health: Working together for a healthy New York.* New York, NY: Milbank Memorial Fund.

Minnesota Department of Health, Center for Public Health Nursing. (2001). *Public health interventions.* St. Paul, MN: Author. Retrieved from http://www.health.state.mn.us/divs/cfh/ophp/resources/docs/wheelbw.pdf

Minnesota Department of Health, Center for Public Health Nursing. (2003). *The nursing process applied to population-based public health nursing practice.* St. Paul, MN: Author. Retrieved from http://www.health.state.mn.us/divs/cfh/ophp/resources/docs/nursing_process.pdf

Monsen, K., & Keller, L. O. (2002). A population-based approach to pediculosis management. *Public Health Nursing, 19*(3), 201–208.

Newhouse, R. P., Dearholt, S. L., Poe, S. P., Pugh, L. C., & White, K. M. (2007). *Johns Hopkins evidence-based practice model and guidelines.* Indianapolis, IN: Sigma Theta Tau International.

Olds D. L., Kitzman, H. J., Cole, R. E., Hanks, C. A., Arcoleo, K. J., Anson, E. A., . . . Stevenson, A. J. (2010). Enduring effects of prenatal and infancy home visiting by nurses on maternal life course and government spending: Follow-up of a randomized trial among children at age 12 years. *Archives of Pediatrics & Adolescent Medicine, 164*(5): 419–424. doi:10.1001/archpediatrics.2010.49

Olds, D. L., Kitzman, H., Cole, R., Robinson, J., Sidora, K., Luckey, D. W., . . . Holmberg, J. (2004). Effects of nurse home-visiting on maternal life course and child development: Age 6 follow-up results of a randomized trial. *Pediatrics, 114*(6), 1550–1559.

Olds, D., Kitzman, H., Hanks, C., Cole, R., Anson, E., Sidora-Arcoleo, K., . . . Bondy, J. (2007). Effects of nurse home visiting on maternal and child functioning: Age 9 follow-up of a randomized trial. *Pediatrics, 120,* e832–e845, 2006–2111.

Olds, D. L., Robinson, J., O'Brien, R., Luckey, D. W., Pettitt, L. M., Henderson, C. R., Jr., . . . Talmi, A. (2002). Home visiting by paraprofessionals and by nurses: A randomized, controlled trial. *Pediatrics, 110*(3), 486–496.

Padget, S. M., Bekemeirer, B., & Berkowitz, B. (2004). Collaborative partnerships at the state level: Promoting systems changes in public health infrastructure. *Journal of Public Health Management Practice, 10*(3), 251–257.

Poe, S. S., & White, K. K. (2010). *Johns Hopkins nursing evidence-based practice: Implementation and translation.* Indianapolis, IN: Sigma Theta Tau International.

Porter-O'Grady, T. (1984). *Shared governance for nursing: A creative approach to professional accountability.* Rockville, MD: Aspen Systems Corporation.

Quad Council of Public Health Nursing Organizations. (2007, February). The public health nursing shortage: A threat to the public's health. Endorsed by the Quad Council of Public Health Nursing Organizations, American Nurses Association, Congress on Nursing Practice & Economics.

Renfrew, M. J., Dyson, L., Herbert, B., McFadden, A., McCormick, F., Thomas, J., & Spiby, H. (2008). Developing evidence-based recommendations in public health—Incorporating the views of practitioners, service users, and user representatives. *Health Expectations, 11,* 3–15. doi:10.1111/j.1369-7625.2007.00471.x

Schaffer, M. A., Goodhue, A., Stennes, K., & Lanigan, C. (2012). Evaluation of a public health nurse visiting program for pregnant and parenting teens. *Public Health Nursing, 29*(3), 218–231. doi:10.1111/j.1525-1446.2011.01005.x

Schaffer, M. A., Sandau, K. E., & Diedrick, L. (2012). Evidence-based practice models for organizational change: Overview and practice applications. *Journal of Advanced Nursing, 69*(5),1197–1209. doi:10.1111/j.1365-2648.2012.06122.x

Stillwell, S. B., Fineout-Overholt, E., Melnyk, B. M., & Williamson, K. M. (2010). Evidence-based practice: Step by step. *American Journal of Nursing, 110*(5), 41–47.

Tembreull, C., & Schaffer, M. (2005). The intervention of outreach: Best practices. *Public Health Nursing 22*(4), 347–353.

Vari, P., Vogeltanz-Holm, N., Olsen, G., Anderson, C., Holm, J., Peterson, H., & Henly, S. (2013). Community breastfeeding attitudes and beliefs. *Healthcare for Women International, 34*(7), 592–606. doi:10.1080/07399332.2012.655391

Walsh, N. (2010). Dissemination of evidence into practice: Opportunities and threats. *Primary Healthcare, 20*(3), 26–30.

Yousey, Y., Leake, J., Wdowik, M., & Janken, J. (2007). Education in a homeless shelter to improve the nutrition of young children. *Public Health Nursing, 24*(3), 249–255.

Chapter 3

Ailinger, R. L., Molloy, S. B., & Sacasa, E. R. (2009). Community health nursing student experience in Nicaragua. *Journal of Community Health Nursing, 26,* 47–53. doi:10.1080/07370010902805072

Alkon, A., To, K., Mackie, J. F., Wolff, M., & Bernzweig, J. (2009). Health and safety needs in early care and education programs: What do directors, child health records, and national standards tell us? *Public Health Nursing, 27*(1), 3–16. doi:10.1111/j.1525-1446.2009.00821.x

American Nurses Association. (2013). *Public health nursing: Scope and standards of practice.* Silver Spring, MD: Nursesbooks.org.

Centers for Disease Control and Prevention. (2010a). *Definition of public health informatics.* National Center for Public Health Informatics. Retrieved from http://www.cdc.gov/ncphi/about.html

Centers for Disease Control and Prevention. (2010b). *CDC's Advisory Committee on Immunization Practices (ACIP) recommends universal annual influenza vaccination.* Retrieved from http://www.cdc.gov/media/pressrel/2010/r100224.htm

Clark, M. J. (2008). *Community health nursing.* Upper Saddle River, NJ: Pearson/Prentice Hall.

Cross, S. (2010). *Public health teen parent program.* Unpublished manuscript from Ramsey County Public Health. St. Paul, MN.

Dreher, M. C., Skemp, L. E., & Asselin, M. (2006). *Healthy places—Healthy people.* Indianapolis, IN: Sigma Theta Tau International.

Eide, P. J., Hahn, L., Bayne, T., Allen, C. B., & Swain, D. (2006). The population-focused analysis project for teaching community health. *Nursing Education Perspectives, 27*(1), 22–27.

Eriksson, I., & Nilsson, K. (2008). Preconditions needed for establishing a trusting relationship during health counseling: An interview study. *Journal of Clinical Nursing, 17*(17), 2352–2359.

Gardner, A. (2010). Therapeutic friendliness and the development of therapeutic leverage by mental health nurses in community rehabilitation settings. *Contemporary Nurse, 34*(2), 140–148.

Hargate, C. (2013). *Windshield survey.* Unpublished manuscript from Bethel University. St. Paul, MN.

Hunt, R. (2013). *Introduction to community-based nursing.* Philadelphia, PA: Wolters Kluwer Health/Lippincott Williams and Williams.

Jansson, A., Petersson, K., & Uden, G. (2001). Nurses' first encounters with parents of new-born children: Public health nurses' views of a good meeting. *Journal of Clinical Nursing, 10,* 140–151.

Kaakinen, J. R., Gedaly-Duff, V., Coehlo, D. P., & Hanson, S. M. H. (2010). *Family health care nursing: Theory, practice and research, 4th ed.* Philadelphia: F. A. Davis.

Keller, L. O., Strohschein, S., Lia-Hoagberg, B., & Schaffer, M. A. (2004). Population-based public health interventions. *Public Health Nursing, 21*(5), 453–468.

Kelly, P. J. (2005). Practical suggestions for community interventions using participatory action research. *Public Health Nursing, 22*(1), 65–73.

Kleinfehn-Wald, N. (2010). *Determining population needs in a rural/suburban county.* Unpublished manuscript from Scott County Public Health. Shakopee, MN.

Lanigan, C. (2010). *In-home influenza immunizations.* Unpublished manuscript from Minnesota Visiting Nurse Association. Minneapolis, MN.

Mansfield, R., & Meyer, C. L. (2007). Making a difference with combined community assessment and change projects. *Journal of Nursing Education, 46*(3), 132–134.

Martin, K. S. (2005). *The Omaha System: A key to practice, documentation, and information management, 2nd ed.* Omaha, NE: Health Connections Press.

Martin, K. S., Monsen, K. A., & Bowles, K. H. (2011). The Omaha System and meaningful use: Applications for practice, education, and research. *CIN: Computers, Informatics, Nursing, 29*(1), 52–58. doi:10.1097/NCN.0b013e3181f9ddc6

McCann, T. V., & Baker, H. (2001). Mutual relating: Developing interpersonal relationships in the community. *Journal of Advanced Nursing, 34*(4), 530–537.

McNaughton, D. B. (2005). A naturalistic test of Peplau's theory in home visiting. *Public Health Nursing, 22*(5), 429–438.

Meagher-Stewart, D., Edwards, N., Aston, M., & Young, L. (2009). Population health surveillance practice of public health nurses. *Public Health Nursing, 26*(6), 553–560. doi:10.1111/j.1525-1446.2009.00814.x

Minnesota Department of Health. (n.d.). *How to: Community health assessment.* Retrieved from http://www.health.state.mn.us/divs/opi/pm/lphap/cha/howto.html

Minnesota Department of Health. (2001). *Public health interventions—Application for public health nursing practice.* St. Paul, MN: Author.

Minnesota Department of Health, Center for Public Health Nursing Practice. (2003). *The nursing process applied to population-based public health nursing practice.* Retrieved from http://www.health.state.mn.us/divs/opi/cd/phn/docs/0303phn_processapplication.pdf

Minnesota Department of Health, Office of Public Health Practice. (2006). *A collection of "Getting Behind the Wheel Stories" 2000–2006.* Retrieved from http://www.health.state.mn.us/divs/opi/cd/phn/docs/0606wheel_stories.pdf

Monsen, K. A., Fitzsimmons, L. L., Lescenski, B. A., Lytton, A. B., Schwichtenberg, L. D., & Martin, K. S. (2006). A public health nursing informatics data-and-practice quality project. *CIN: Computers, Informatics, Nursing, 24*(3), 152–158.

Monsen, K. A., Fulkerson, J. A., Lytton, A. B., Taft, L. L., Schwichtenberg, L. D., & Martin, K. S. (2010). Comparing maternal child health problems and outcomes across public health nursing agencies. *Maternal and Child Health Journal, 14*(3), 412–421. doi:10.1007/s10995-009-0479-9

Omaha System. (2010). *Omaha System website.* Retrieved from http://www.omahasystem.org

Otterness, N., Gehrke, P., & Sener, I. M. (2007). Partnerships between nursing education and faith communities: Benefits and challenges. *Journal of Nursing Education, 46*(1), 39–44.

Parris, K. M., Place, P. J., Orellana, E., Calder, J., Jackson, K., Karolys, A, . . . Smith, D. (1999). Integrating nursing diagnoses, interventions, and outcomes in public health nursing practice. *Nursing Diagnosis, 10*(2), 49–56.

Racher, F. (2007). The evolution of ethics for community practice. *Journal of Community Health Nursing, 24*(1), 65–76.

Reinberg, S. (2010). *U.S. government sets new health goals for 2020.* Retrieved from http://consumer.healthday.com/Article.asp?AID=646932

Schaffer, M. A., Jost, R., Peterson, B. J., & Lair, M. (2008). Pregnancy-free club: A strategy to prevent repeat adolescent pregnancy. *Public Health Nursing, 25*(4), 304–311. doi:10.1111/j.1525-1446.2008.00710.x

Schoon, P. (2010). *Elementary school health assessment.* Unpublished manuscript.

Schoon, P. M., Champlin, B., & Hunt, R. (2012). Developing a sustainable foot care clinic in a homeless shelter within an academic-community partnership through curricular integration and faculty engagement. *Journal of Nursing Education, 51*(12), 714–718. doi:10.3928/01484834-20121112-02

Scroggins, L. M. (2008). The developmental processes for NANDA international nursing diagnoses. *International Journal of Nursing Terminologies and Classifications, 19*(2), 57–64.

Truglio-Londrigan, M., & Lewenson, S. B. (2013). *Public health nursing: Practicing population-based care.* Sudbury, MA: Jones and Bartlett.

U.S. Department of Health and Human Services. (2010). *Introducing Healthy People 2020.* Retrieved from http://www.healthypeople.gov/2020/about/default.aspx

Volbrecht, R. M. (2002). *Nursing ethics: Communities in dialogue.* Upper Saddle River, NJ: Pearson/Prentice Hall.

Chapter 4

Alfred, R. (2009). *Sept. 8, 1854: Pump shutdown stops London cholera outbreak.* Retrieved from http://www.wired.com/thisdayintech/2009/09/0908london-cholera-pump

Aschengrau, A., & Seage, G. R. (2008). *Essentials of epidemiology in public health, 2nd ed.* Sudbury, MA: Jones and Bartlett.

Centers for Disease Control and Prevention (CDC). (2001). Updated guidelines for evaluating public health surveillance systems: Recommendations from the Guidelines Working Group. *MMWR, 50*(RR13), 1–35. Retrieved from http://www.cdc.gov/mmwr/preview/mmwrhtml/rr5013a1.htm

Centers for Disease Control and Prevention (CDC). (2013). *Pertussis outbreak trends.* Retrieved from http://www.cdc.gov/pertussis/outbreaks/trends.html

Centers for Disease Control and Prevention (CDC). (2013). *Reported cases of Lyme disease—United States, 2011.* Retrieved from http://www.cdc.gov/lyme/stats/maps/map2011.html

Clark, M. (2008). *Community health nursing: Advocacy for population health, 5th ed.* Upper Saddle River, NJ: Pearson Education.

County Health Rankings and Roadmaps: Health Outcomes in Minnesota. (2012). University of Wisconsin Population Health Institute. Retrieved from http://www.countyhealthrankings.org/app/minnesota/2012/rankings/outcomes/overall

Earl, C. (2009). Medical history and epidemiology: Their contribution to the development of public health nursing. *Nursing Outlook, 57*(5), 257–265.

Friis, R. H., & Sellers, T. A. (1999). *Epidemiology for public health practice, 2nd ed.* Gaithersburg, MD: Aspen.

Guadarrama-Celaya, F., Otero-Ojeda, G. A., Pliego-Rivero, F. B., Porcayo-Mercado, M., Ricardo-Garcell, J., & Perez-Abalo, M. C. (2012). Screening of neurodevelopmental delays in four communities of Mexico and Cuba. *Public Health Nursing, 29*(2), 105–115.

Klopf, L. (1998). Tuberculosis control in the New York State Department of Correctional Services: A case management approach. *American Journal of Infection Control, 26*(5), 534–538.

Krieger, N. (1997). Epidemiology and the web of causation: Has anyone seen the spider? *Social Science and Medicine, 39*(7), 887–903.

Krieger, N. (2001a). A glossary for social epidemiology. *Journal of Epidemiology and Community Health, 55*(10), 693–700.

Krieger, N. (2001b). Theories for social epidemiology in the 21st century: An ecosocial perspective. *International Journal of Epidemiology, 30*(4), 668–677.

Kuh, D., Ben-Shlomo, Y., Lynch, J., Hallqvist, J., & Power, C. (2003). Life course epidemiology. *Journal of Epidemiology and Community Health, 57*(10), 778–783.

Le, C. T. (2001). *Health and numbers: A problem-based introduction to biostatistics, 2nd ed.* New York, NY: Wiley-Liss.

Lind, C., & Smith, D. (2008). Analyzing the state of community health nursing: Advancing from deficit to strengths-based practice using appreciative inquiry. *Advances in Nursing Science, 31*(1), 28–41.

Merrill, R. M., & Timmreck, T. C. (2006). *Introduction to epidemiology, 4th ed.* Sudbury, MA: Jones and Bartlett.

Minnesota Department of Health (MDH). (2013). *Reported cases of Lyme disease in Minnesota by year, 1986–2012.* Retrieved from http://www.health.state.mn.us/divs/idepc/diseases/lyme/casesyear.html

Missouri Department of Health and Senior Services (MDHSS). (2010). *Geographic Information Systems (GIS) and maps.* Retrieved from http://www.dhss.mo.gov/GIS/

Pew Hispanic Center. (2006). *Population pyramids by ethnicity, 2005.* Cited in Hakimzadeh, S. (2006). 41.9 million and counting: A statistical view of Hispanics at mid-decade. Retrieved from http://pewresearch.org/pubs/251/419-million-and-counting

Richter, M. (2010). It does take two to tango! On the need for theory in research on the social determinants of health. *International Journal of Public Health, 55,* 457–458.

Stein, Z., Susser, M., Saenger, G., & Marolla, F. (1975). *Famine and human development: The Dutch hunger winter of 1944–45.* New York, NY: Oxford University Press.

University of California, Los Angeles (UCLA). (2010). *John Snow.* Retrieved from http://www.ph.ucla.edu/epi/snow.html

Valanis, B. (1999). *Epidemiology in health care, 3rd ed.* Stamford, CT: Appleton and Lange.

World Health Organization (WHO). (2012). *World: Estimated tuberculosis (TB) incidence rates, 2011 (as of 5 Nov 2012).* Retrieved from http://reliefweb.int/map/world/world-estimated-tuberculosis-tb-incidence-rates2011-5-nov-2012

Chapter 5

American Nurses Association. (2013). *Scope and standards of public health nursing practice.* Silver Springs, MD: Nursebooks.org.

Aston, M., Meagher-Stewart, D., Edwards, N., & Young, L. M. (2009). Public health nurses' primary health care practice: Strategies for fostering citizen participation. *Journal of Community Health Nursing, 26,* 24–34.

Baker, I. R., Dennison, B. A., Boyer, P. S., Sellers, K. F., Russo, T. J., & Sherwood, N. A. (2007). An asset-based community initiative to reduce television viewing in New York state. *Preventive Medicine, 44*(5), 437–441.

Bazarman, M. H. (Ed.). (2005). *Negotiating, decision making and conflict management.* Cheltenam, UK: Edward Elgar Publishing United.

Bonin, E., Brehove, T., Kline, S., Misgen, M., Post, P., Strehlow, A. J., & Yungman, J. (2010). *Adapting your practice: General recommendations for the care of homeless patients.* Nashville, TN: Health Care for the Homeless Clinicians' Network, National Health Care for the Homeless Council, Inc.

Bredesen, J. A. (2012). *A comparison of recommended practice guidelines for health care of the homeless and the current health status of homeless families in St. Paul, Minnesota, as assessed through the use of Photo-Voice methodology.* Doctor of Nursing Practice Project.

Carter, M. R., Kelly, R. K., Montgomery, M., & Cheshire, M. (2013). An innovative approach to health promotion experiences in community health nursing: A university collaborative partnership. *Journal of Nursing Education, 52*(2), 108–111. doi:10.3928/01484834-20130121-04

Chaudry, R. V., Polivka, B. J., & Kennedy, C. W. (2000). Public health nursing director's perceptions regarding interagency collaboration with community mental health agencies. *Public Health Nursing, 17*(2), 75–84.

Clatworthy, W. (1999). Community care: Collaborative working. *Journal of Community Nursing, 13*(4), 4.

Community Tool Box. (2001). Identifying community assets and resources. Retrieved from http://ctb. ku.edu/en/tablecontents/sub_section_main_1043.aspx

Crist, J. D., & Escandon-Dominguez, S. (2003). Identifying and recruiting Mexican American partners and sustaining community partnerships. *Journal of Transcultural Nursing, 14*(3), 266–271.

D'Amour, D., Ferrada-Videla, M., Rodriguez, L., & Beaulieu, M. (2005). The conceptual basis for interprofessional collaboration: Core concepts and theoretical frameworks. *Journal of Interprofessional Care,* Suppl. 1, 116–131.

Fawcett, S. B., Francisco, V. T., Paine-Andrews, A., & Schultz, J. A. (2000). A model memorandum of collaboration: A proposal. *Public Health Reports, 155*(2–3), 174–190.

Findley, S. A., Irigoyen, M., See, D., Sanchez, M., Chen, S., Sternfels, P., & Caesar, A. (2003). Community-provider partnerships reduce immunization disparities: Field report from northern Manhattan. *American Journal of Public Health, 93*(7), 1041–1044.

Foss, G. F., Bonaiuto, M. M., Johnson, Z. S., & Moreland, D. M. (2003). Using Polivka's model to create a service-learning partnership. *Journal of School Health, 73*(8), 305–310.

Franklin, L., Exline, J., & Stringer, K. (2002). Using coalition and community-based partnerships to improve immunization rates in Mississippi: A case study. *Texas Journal of Rural Health, 20*(3), 31–37.

Fuller, T., Guy, D., & Pletsch, C. (2002). Canadian Rural Partnership asset mapping: A handbook. Canadian Rural Partnership: Canada. Retrieved from http://www.planningtoolexchange.org/browse/results/asset%20mapping%20handbook

Gamm, L. D. (1998). Advancing community health through community health partnerships. *Journal of Healthcare Management, 43*(1), 51–67.

Goldman, K. D., & Schmalz, K. J. (2005). "Accentuate the positive!" Using an asset-mapping tool as part of a community-health needs assessment. *Health Promotion Practice, 6,* 125–128.

Goodhart, W., Hsu, J., Baek, J. H., Coleman, A. L., Maresca, F. M., & Miller, M. B. (2006). A view through a different lens: PhotoVoice as a tool for student advocacy. *Journal of American College Health, 55*(1), 53–56.

Grant, R. W., & Finnocchio, L. J. (1995). *Interdisciplinary collaborative teams in primary care: A model curriculum and resource guide.* San Francisco, CA: Pew Health Professions Commission.

Henneman, E. A., Lee, J. L., & Cohen, J. I. (1995). Collaboration: A concept analysis. *Journal of Advanced Nursing, 21*(1), 103–109.

Israel, B. A., Eng, E., Schulz, A. J., & Parker, E. A. (Eds.). (2005). *Methods for community-based participatory research for health.* San Francisco, CA: Jossey-Bass.

Kang, R. (1995). Building community capacity for health promotion: A challenge for public health nurses. *Public Health Nursing, 12*(5), 312–318.

Keller, L. O., Strohschein, S., Lia-Hoagberg, B., & Schaffer, M. A. (2004). Population-based public health interventions: Practice-based and evidence supported. Part 1. *Public Health Nursing, 21*(5), 453–468.

Kenny, G. (2002). Children's nursing and interprofessional collaboration: Challenges and opportunities. *Journal of Clinical Nursing, 11*(3), 306–313.

Kretzmann, J. P., & McKnight, J. (1993). *Building communities from the inside out: A path toward finding and mobilizing a community's assets.* Chicago, IL: ACTA Publications.

Lindsey, E., Sheilds, L., & Stajduhar, K. (1999). Creating effective nursing partnerships: Relating community development to participatory action research. *Journal of Advanced Nursing, 29*(1), 1238–1245.

Merrett, A., Thomas, P., Stephens, R. M., Moghabghab, R., & Gruneir, M. (2011). A collaborative approach to fall prevention. *Canadian Nurse, 107*(8), 24–29.

Miller, L. C., Jones, B. B., Graves, R. S., & Sievert, M. C. (2010). Merging silos: Collaborating for information literacy. *Journal of Continuing Education in Nursing, 41*(6), 267–272.

Morgan, A., & Ziglio, E. (2007). Revitalizing the evidence base for public health: Assets model. *Promotion & Education, Suppl. 2, 17*–22.

Pennington, K., Coast, M. J., & Kroh, M. (2010). Health care for the homeless: A partnership between a city and school of nursing. *Journal of Nursing Education, 49*(12), 700–703. doi:10.3928/01484834-20100930-02

Reilly, J. R., Hovarter, R., Mrochek, T., Mittelstadt-Lock, K., Schmitz, S., Nett, S., . . . Behm, L. (2011). Spread the word, not the germs: A toolkit for faith communities. *Journal of Christian Nursing, 28*(4), 205–211. doi:16.1097/CNJ.06013c31822afc7f

Savage, C. L., Xu, Y., Lee, R., Rose, B. L., Kappesser, M., & Anthony, J. S. (2006). A case study in the use of community-based participatory research in public health nursing. *Public Health Nursing, 23*(5), 472–478.

Schaffer, M. A. (2009). A virtue ethics guide to best practices for community-based participatory research. *Progress in Community Health Partnerships: Research, Education, and Action, 3*(1), 83–90. Retrieved from http://muse.jhu.edu/login?auth=0&type=summary&url=/journals/progress_in_community_health_partnerships_research_education_and_action/v003/3.1.schaffer.pdf

Seifer, S. D., & Connors, K. (Eds). (2007). Faculty toolkit for service-learning in higher education. Community-Campus Partnership for Health, Learn and Serve America's National Service-Learning Clearinghouse. Retrieved from http://www.servicelearning.org/filemanager/download/HE_toolkit_with_worksheets.pdf

Snow, L. K. (2004). *The power of asset mapping.* Herndon, VA: Alban Institute.

Thibault, G. E. (2012). Core competencies for inter-professional collaborative practice. Institute of Medicine Global Forum on Innovation in Health Professional Education. Retrieved from http://iom.edu/~/media/Files/Activity%20Files/Global/InnovationHealthProfEducation/2012-MAR-08/Thibault_Core-Competencies-for-Inter-Professional-Collaborative-Practice.pdf

Timmerman, G. M. (2007). Addressing barriers to health promotion in underserved women. *Family & Community Health, Supplement, 30*(15), S34–S42.

Tuckman, B. W. (1965). Development sequences in small groups. *Psychology Bulletin, 63*(6), 384–399.

Wang, C. C., Morrel-Samuels, S., Hutchison, P. M., Bell, L., & Pestronk, R. M. (2004). Flint PhotoVoice: Community building among youths, adults, and policymakers. *American Journal of Public Health, 94*(6), 911–913.

Wood, A., Middleton, S. G., Leonard, D. (2010). "When it's more than the blues": A collaborative response to postpartum depression. *Public Health Nursing, 27*(3), 248–254.

World Health Organization. (2010). Framework for action on interprofessional education and collaborative practice. Retrieved from http://whqlibdoc.who.int/hq/2010/WHO_HRH_HPN_10.3_eng.pdf

Chapter 6

2009 H1N1 Flu Pandemic: Dakota County's response. (2010, May). Dakota County Public Health Department.

American Lung Association. (2010). *About OAS.* Retrieved from http://www.lungusa.org/lung-disease/asthma/in-schools/open-airways/about-oas.html

American Nurses Association. (2013). *Public health nursing: Scope and standards of practice.* Silver Spring, MD: Author.

American Public Health Association. (2012). *Affordable Care Act Overview.* Retrieved from http://www.apha.org/advocacy/Health+Reform/ACAbasics/default.htm

Carter, K. F., Kaiser, K. L., O'Hare, P. A., & Callister, L. C. (2006). Use of PHN competencies and ACHNE essentials to develop teaching-learning strategies for generalist C/PHN curricula. *Public Health Nursing, 23*(2), 146–160.

Centers for Disease Control and Prevention. (2012). *Meaningful use introduction.* Retrieved from http://www.cdc.gov/EHRmeaningfuluse/introduction.html

Centers for Disease Control and Prevention. (2013a). *Electronic lab reporting.* Retrieved from http://www.cdc.gov/EHRmeaningfuluse/elr.html

Centers for Disease Control and Prevention. (2013b). *National Program of Cancer Registries: Meaningful use of electronic health records.* Retrieved from http://www.cdc.gov/cancer/npcr/meaningful_use.htm

Centers for Disease Control and Prevention (2013c). *National voluntary accreditation for public health departments.* Retrieved from: http://www.cdc.gov/stltpublichealth/hop/pdfs/NVAPH_Factsheet.pdf

Curtis, M. P. (2010). Community collaboration in a community H1N1 vaccination program. *Journal of Community Health Nursing, 27,* 121–125.

Encyclopedia of Everyday Law: Child Abuse/Child Safety/Child Discipline. (2010). Retrieved from http://www.enotes.com/everyday-law-encyclopedia/child-abuse-child-safety-discipline#history

Garwick, A. W., Seppelt, A., & Riesgraf, M. (2010). Addressing asthma management challenges in a multisite, urban Head Start Program. *Public Health Nursing, 27*(4), 329–336.

Georgia Department of Public Health. (n.d.). "Meaningful use" submissions of reportable laboratory results. Retrieved from http://www.health.state.ga.us/programs/meaningfuluse/labresults.asp

Health Resources and Services Administration. (2013). The business case for breastfeeding. Retrieved from http://mchb.hrsa.gov/pregnancyandbeyond/breastfeeding

HealthCare.gov. (2013a). *Glossary: Accountable care organizations.* Retrieved from http://www.healthcare.gov/glossary/a/accountable.html

HealthCare.gov. (2013b). *National Prevention Strategy: America's Plan for Better Health and Wellness.* Retrieved from http://www.healthcare.gov/news/factsheets/2011/06/prevention06162011a.html

Healthy People. (2013). *Preparedness.* Retrieved from http://www.healthypeople.gov/2020/topicsobjectives2020/overview.aspx?topicid=34

Horlich, G., Shaw, F. E., Gorji, M., & Fishbein, D. B. (2008). Delivering new vaccines to adolescents: The role of school-entry laws. *Pediatrics, 121,* S79–S84.

International Society for Disease Surveillance. (2012, November). *Electronic syndromic surveillance using hospital inpatient and ambulatory clinical care electronic health record data: Recommendations from the ISDS meaningful use workgroup.* Retrieved from http://www.syndromic.org/storage/ISDS_2012-MUse-Recommendations.pdf

Keller, L. O., & Litt, E. A. (2008). *Report on public health nurse to population ratio.* Association of State and Territorial Directors of Nursing (ASTDN).

Land, M., & Barclay, L. (2008). Nurses' contribution to child protection. *Neonatal, Paediatric and Child Health Nursing, 11*(10), 18–24.

Minnesota Department of Health. (2003a). *Communicable disease reporting and HIPAA. Immunization sharing and HIPAA.* Retrieved from http://www.health.state.mn.us/divs/idepc/dtopics/reportable/rule/hipaacomm.html.

Minnesota Department of Health. (2003b). *Immunization sharing and HIPAA.* Retrieved from http://www.health.state.mn.us/divs/idepc/immunize/hippadata.html

Minnesota Department of Health. (2005a). *Isolation and quarantine procedures.* Retrieved from http://www.health.state.mn.us/divs/opa/isolation05.pdf

Minnesota Department of Health. (2005b). *Communicable disease rule, Chapter 4605.* Retrieved from http://www.health.state.mn.us/divs/idepc/dtopics/reportable/rule/rule.html

Minnesota Department of Health. (2008). *Minnesota responds Medical Reserve Corps volunteer protections.* Minnesota Department of Health fact sheet. Retrieved from http://www.health.state.mn.us/divs/opa/mrcfs08.pdf

Minnesota Department of Health. (2009a). *Local Public Health Act Overview.* Retrieved from http://www.health.state.mn.us/divs/cfh/lph/docs/lphoverview_factsheet.pdf

Minnesota Department of Health. (2009b). *Ready to respond: MDH Preparedness Newsletter.* Retrieved from http://www.health.state.mn.us/oep/news/09july.pdf

Minnesota Department of Health. (2011). *Local public health act overview.* Retrieved from http://www.health.state.mn.us/divs/cfh/lph/docs/lphoverview_factsheet.pdf

Minnesota Department of Health. (2012). *Financing local public health services in Minnesota: Trends in local tax levy expenditures.* Retrieved from http://www.health.state.mn.us/divs/cfh/ophp/system/ran/docs/1210ran_lhdfinancing.pdf

Minnesota Department of Health. (2013). *Health care homes.* Retrieved from http://www.health.state.mn.us/healthreform/homes/index.html

Minnesota Department of Health State Community Health Services Advisory Committee. (1992). *Controlling public health nuisances: A guide for community health boards.* Retrieved from http://www.health.state.mn.us/divs/eh/local/chsboardguide.pdf

Minnesota Rulemaking Manual. (2009). *Chapter 3—Rule Development.* Retrieved from http://www.health.state.mn.us/rules/manual/chapters.html

Minnesota Statutes. (2005). *Section 144.419. Isolation and quarantine of persons.* Retrieved from http://www.revisor.leg.state.mn.us/data/revisor/statutes/2005/144/419.html

National Alliance on Mental Illness. (2006). *Understanding the civil commitment process.* Retrieved from http://www.namihelps.org/assets/PDFs/civilcommitmentSinglePg102108.pdf

National Association of County and City Health Officials (NACCHO). (2008a). *Fast facts: 2008 national profile of local health departments.* Retrieved from http://www.naccho.org/topics/infrastructure/profile/resources/2008report/upload/profilebrochure2009-10-17_COMBINED_post-to-web.pdf

National Association of County and City Health Officials (NACCHO). (2008b). *Medical Reserve Corps.* Retrieved from http://www.naccho.org/topics/emergency/MRC/index.cfm

National Association of County and City Health Officials (NACCHO). (2010). *Public health law.* Retrieved from http://www.naccho.org/topics/infrastructure/PHLaw/index.cfm

National Association of County and City Health Officials (NACCHO). (2011). *2010 national profile of local health departments.* Retrieved from http://www.naccho.org/topics/infrastructure/profile/resources/2010report/upload/2010_Profile_main_report-web.pdf

Office of the Reviser of Statutes. (2012). *2012 Minnesota Statutes. 626.556 Reporting of maltreatment of minors.* Retrieved from http://www.revisor.mn.gov/statutes/?id=626.556

Pozgar, G. D. (2005). *Legal and ethical issues for health professionals.* Sudbury, MA: Jones and Bartlett.

Rein, A. (2012, June 3). *Beacon policy brief 1.0: The Beacon Community Program: Three pillars of pursuit.* Academy Health and the Office of the National Coordinator for Health Information. Retrieved from http://www.healthit.gov/sites/default/files/beacon-brief-061912.pdf

Savage, R. (2011, September 15). *HL7 Version 2.5.1: Implementation guide for immunization messaging, release 1.3.* Centers for Disease Control and Prevention and American Immunization Registry Association. Retrieved from fhttp://www.cdc.gov/vaccines/programs/iis/technical-guidance/downloads/hl7guide-2011-08.pdf

Schwartz, M. B., & Brownell, K. D. (2007). Actions necessary to prevent childhood obesity: Creating the climate for change. *Journal of Law, Medicine & Ethics, 31*(1), 78–89.

Stanhope, M., & Lancaster, J. (2008). *Public health nursing: Population-centered health care in the community.* St. Louis, MO: Mosby Elsevier.

Chapter 7

Aiken, T. (2004). *Legal, ethical, and political issues in nursing.* Philadelphia, PA: Davis.

American Association of Colleges of Nursing. (2013). Nurse-managed health clinics: Increasing access to primary care and educating the healthcare workforce. Retrieved from http://www.aacn.nche.edu/government-affairs/FY13NMHCs.pdf

American Nurses Association. (2007). *Registered Nurses Utilization of Nursing Assistive Personnel in All Settings.* American Nurses Association Position Statement. Retrieved from http://ana.nursingworld.org/MainMenuCategories/HealthcareandPolicyIssues/ANAPositionStatements/uap.aspx

American Nurses Association. (2010). *Nursing scope and standards of practice* (2nd ed.). Silver Spring, MD: Nursebooks.org.

American Nurses Association. (2012) *Principles for delegation by registered nurses to unlicensed assistive personnel (UAP)*. Silver Spring, MD: Nursebooks.org.

American Nurses Association. (2013). *Public health nursing: Scope and standards of practice*. Silver Spring, MD: Nursebooks.org.

Association of Community Health Nurse Educators. (2009). *Essentials of baccalaureate nursing education for entry level community/public health nursing*. Wheat Ridge, CO: Author.

Barkauskas, V. H., Pohl, V. H., Tanner, C., Onifade, T., & Pilon, B. (2011). Quality of care in nurse-managed health centers. *Nursing Administration Quarterly, 35*(1), 34–43.

Beauchamp, T., & Childress, J. (1979). *Principles of biomedical ethics*. New York, NY: Oxford University Press.

Bredow, T. (2013). Personal communication. North Metro Pediatrics Clinic. http://www.northmetropeds.org/index.htm

California Board of Registered Nursing. (2006). *California nursing practice act with regulations and related statutes*. Charlottesville, VA: Matthew Bender & Company, Inc.

Clancy, A., & Svensson, T. (2007). "Faced" with responsibility: Levinasian ethics and the challenges of responsibility in Norwegian public health nursing. *Nursing Philosophy, 8*(3), 158–166.

Coddington, J. A., & Sands, L. P. (2008). Cost of health care and quality outcomes of patients at nurse-managed clinics. *Nursing Economics, 26*(2), 75–83.

Easley, C. E., & Allen, C. E. (2007). A critical intersection: Human rights, public health nursing, and nursing ethics. *Advances in Nursing Science, 30*(4), 367–382.

Evanson, T. A. (2006). Intimate partner violence and rural public health nursing practice: Challenges and opportunities. *Online Journal of Rural Nursing and Health Care, 6*(1), 7–20.

Gallop, R. (1998). Postdischarge social contact: A potential area for boundary violation. *Journal of the American Psychiatric Nurses Association, 4*(4), 105–110.

Griffith, R. (2007). Understanding confidentiality and disclosure of patient information. *British Journal of Community Nursing, 12*(11), 530–534.

Institute of Medicine. (2010). The future of nursing: Leading change, advancing change. Report Brief. Retrieved from http://www.iom.edu/~/media/Files/Report%20Files/2010/The-Future-of-Nursing/Future%20of%20Nursing%202010%20Report%20Brief.pdf

Jacobson, G. A. (2002). Maintaining professional boundaries: Preparing nursing students for the challenge. *Journal of Nursing Education, 41*(6), 279–281.

Jarrin, O. G. (2010). Core elements of U.S. nurse practice acts and incorporation of nursing diagnosis language. *International Journal of Nursing Terminologies and Classifications, 21*(4), 166–176. doi:10.1111/j.1744-618x.2010.01162.x

Keller, L. O., & Litt, E. A. (2008). Report on public health nurse to population ratio. Association of State and Territorial Directors of Nursing (ASTDN).

McGarry, J. (2003). The essence of "community" within community nursing: A district nursing perspective. *Health and Social Care in the Community, 11*(5), 423–430.

Minnesota Department of Health, Office of Public Health Practice. (2006). *A collection of "Getting Be-

hind the Wheel Stories" 2000–2006. Retrieved from http://www.health.state.mn.us/divs/opi/cd/phn/docs/0606wheel_stories.pdf

National Nursing Centers Consortium (2011). About nurse-managed care. Retrieved from http://www.nncc.us/site/index.php/about-nurse-managed-care

Oberle, K., & Tenove, S. (2000). Ethical issues in public health nursing. *Nursing Ethics, 7*(5), 425–438.

Przybilla, J., Johnson, A., Hooker, C. (2009). Perinatal hepatitis B prevention: Adapting public health services to meet the changing needs of a diverse community. *Public Health Reports, 124,* 454–457.

Purtilo, R. (2005). *Ethical dimensions in the health professions* (4th ed.). Philadelphia, PA: Elsevier Saunders.

Racher, F. E. (2007). The evolution of ethics for community practice. *Journal of Community Health Nursing, 24*(1), 65–76.

Robinson, K. M. (2010). Care coordination: A priority for health reform. *Policy, Politics, & Nursing Practice, 11,* 266–274. doi:10.1177/1527154410396572

Russell, K. A. (2012). Nurse practice acts guide and govern nursing practice. *Journal of Nursing Regulation, 3*(3), 36–40. Retrieved from www.journalofnursingregulation.com

Schneiderman, J. U. (2003). Exploration of the role of nurses in caring for children in foster care. (Doctoral Dissertation). University of Southern California. Los Angeles, CA.

Schneiderman, J. U. (2006). Innovative pediatric nursing role: Public health nurses in child welfare. *Pediatric Nursing, 32*(4), 321.

Scoville Walker, S. (2004). Ethical quandaries in community health nursing. In E. Anderson & J. McFarlane (Eds.) *Community as partner: Theory and practice in nursing,* 4th ed. (pp. 83–113). Philadelphia, PA: Lippincott, Williams & Wilkins.

Stanhope, M., & Lancaster, J. (2012). *Public health nursing: population-centered health care in the community.* Maryland Heights, MO: Elsevier.

Underwood, J. M., Mowat, D. L., Meagher-Stewart, D. M., Deber, R. B., Baumann, A. O., MacDonald, M. B., … Munroe, V. J. (2009). Building community and public health nursing capacity: A synthesis report of the national community health nursing study. *Canadian Journal of Public Health, 100*(5), 1–13.

Volbrecht, R. M. (2002). *Nursing ethics: Communities in dialogue.* Upper Saddle River, NJ: Prentice Hall.

Weydt, A. (2010). Developing Delegation Skills. *OJIN: The Online Journal of Issues in Nursing, 15*(2). Manuscript 1. (May 31). Retrieved from http://www.nursingworld.org/MainMenuCategories/ANAMarketplace/ANAPeriodicals/OJIN/TableofContents/Vol152010/No2May2010/Delegation-Skills.html

Williams, J. K., & Cooksey, M. M. (2004). Navigating the difficulties of delegation: Learn to improve teamwork in the unit by delegating duties appropriately. *Nursing, 34*(9), 32.

Chapter 8

Ahmed, O. H., Sullivan, S. J., Schneiders, A. G., Anderson, L., Paton, C, & Crory, P. R. (2013). Ethical considerations in using Facebook for health care support: A case study using concussion management. (2013). *Physical Medicine and Rehabilitation, 5,* 328-344. doi.org/10.1016.j.pmrj.2013.03.007

Bennett, G. G., & Glasgow, R. E. (2009). The delivery of public health interventions via the internet: Actualizing their potential. *Annual Review of Public Health, 30,* 273–293.

Black, A. (2008). Health literacy and cardiovascular disease: Fostering client skills. *American Journal of Health Education, 39*(1), 55–57.

Browne, A. J., Doane, G. h., Reimer, J., MacLeod, M., & McLellan, E. (2010). Public health nursing practice with 'high priority' families: The significance of contextualizing 'risk'. *Nursing Inquiry, 17*(1), 26-37.

Bull, S. S., Levine, D. K., Black, S. R., Schmiege, S. J., & Santelli, J. (2012). Social media-delivered sexual health intervention: A cluster randomized controlled trial. *American Journal of Prevention Medicine, 43*(5), pp. 467-474. http://dx.doi.org/10.1016/j.amepre.2012.07.022

Chaffee, M. (2000). Health communications: Nursing education for increased visibility and effectiveness. *Journal of Professional Nursing, 16*(1), 31–38.

Clark, M. J. (2008). *Community health nursing: Advocacy for population health.* Upper Saddle River, NJ: Pearson Education, Inc.

Centers for Disease Control and Prevention. (2011). The health communicator's guide to social media toolkit. Atlanta, GA: Author. Retrieved from http://www.cdc.gov/healthcommunication/ToolsTemplates/SocialMediaToolkit_BM.pdf

Currie, D. (2013, July). University of Maine nursing students spread health message via lessons in local schools. *The Nation's Health.* www.thenationshealth.org

DeBuono, B. A. (2002). *Pfizer health literacy initiative.* New York, NY: Pfizer Graphic.

Devereaux, L., & Schoon, P. M. (2013). Teaching plan. St. Catherine University.

Evans, D. E., & McCormack, L. (2008). Applying social marketing in health care: Communicating evidence to change consumer behavior. *Medical Decision Making, 28,* 781–792.

Goodrow, B., Scherzer, G., & Florence, J. (2004). An application of multidisclipinary education to a campus-community partnership to reduce motor vehicle accidents. *Education for Health, 17*(2), 152–162.

Green, A. (2006). A person-centered approach to palliative care nursing. *Journal of Hospice and Palliative Nursing, 8*(5), 294–301.

Harvard Medical School. (2011). Motivating Behavior Change. *Harvard Mental Health Letter, 27*(8). Retrieved from www.health.harvard.edu

Holmes, B. J. (2008). Communicating about emerging infectious disease: The importance of research. *Health, Risk & Society, 10*(4), 349–360.

Institute of Medicine. (2004). *Health literacy: A prescription to end confusion.* Washington, D. C.: National Academy Press.

Jakeway, C. C., Cantrell, E. E., Cason, J. B., & Talley, B. S. (2006). Developing population health competencies among public health nurses in Georgia. *Public Health Nursing, 23*(2), 161–167.

Jiménez-Muro, A., Nerín, I., Samper, P., Marqueta, A., Beamonte, A., Gargallo, P., … Rodríguez, G. (2013). A proactive smoking cessation intervention in postpartum women. *Midwifery, 29,* 240-245.

Karasz, J. N., Eiden, A., & Bogan, S. (2013). Text messaging to communicate with public health audiences: How the HIPAA Security Rule affects practice. *American Journal of Public Health, 103*(4), 617-622. doi:10.2105/AJPH.2012.300999

Katakura, N., Yamamot-Mitani, & Ishigaki, K. (2010). Home-visit nurses' attitudes for providing effective assistance to clients with schizophrenia. *International Journal of Mental Health Nursing, 19*, 102-109. doi: 10.1111/j.1447-0349.2009.00641.x

Keller, L. O., Strohschein, S., Lia-Hoagberg, B., & Schaffer, M. A. (2004). Population-based public health interventions: Practice-based and evidence-supported (Part I). *Public Health Nursing, 21*(5), 453–468.

Kolb, D. A. (1984) *Experiential learning experience as a source of learning and development.* Upper Saddle River, NJ: Prentice Hall.

Kolb, D. A. (2005). *The Kolb learning style inventory. Version 3.1.* David A. Kolb, Experience Based Learning Systems, Inc.

Kreps, G. L., & Sparks, L. (2008). Meeting the health literacy needs of immigrant populations. *Patient Education and Counseling, 71*(3), 328–332.

Levy-Storms, L. (2005). Strategies for diffusing public health innovations through older adults' health communication networks. *Generations, 29*(2), 70-75.

Miller, W. R. (2004). Motivational interviewing in service to health promotion. *American Journal of Health Promotion, 18*, A1–A10.

National Council of State Boards of Nursing. (2011, August). White Paper: A nurse's guide to the use of social media. Chicago, IL: Author. Retrieved from https://www.ncsbn.org/Social_Media.pdf

Onega, L. L., & Devers, E. (2008). Health education and group process. In M. Stanhope & J. Lancaster (Eds.), *Public health nursing: Population-centered health care in the community* (pp. 289–338). St. Louis, MO: Mosby Elsevier.

Osterman, R. (2011). Feasibility of using motivational interviewing to decrease alcohol consumption during pregnancy. *Journal of Addictions Nursing, 22*, 93-102. doi: 10.3109/10884602.2011.585723

Pfister-Minogue, K. A., & Salveson, C. (2010). Training and experience of public health nurses in using behavior change counseling. *Public Health Nursing, 27*(6), 544-551. doi: 10.1111/j.1525-1446.2010.00884.x

Public Health Nursing Section. (2001). *Public Health Interventions—Application for Public Health Nursing Practice.* St. Paul, MN: Minnesota Department of Health.

Richardson, L. (2012). Motivational interviewing: Helping patients move toward change. *Journal of Christian Nursing, 29*(1), 18-24. doi: 10.1097/CNJ:0b013.c381238c510

Russell, E. (2009). *Fundamentals of Marketing.* London, UK: Bloomsbury.

Shinitzky, H. E., & Kub, J. (2001). The art of motivating behavior change: The use of motivational interviewing to promote health. *Public Health Nursing, 18*(3), 178–185.

Sowan, N. A., Moffatt, S. G., & Canales, M. K. (2004). Creating a mentoring partnership model: A university-department of health experience. *Family & Community Health, 27*(4), 326-337.

Spector, N., & Kappel, D. M. (2102). Guidelines for using electronic and social media. *Online Journal of Issues in Nursing, 17*(3). doi: 10.3912/OJIN.Vol17No03Man01

Starkey, F., Audrey, S., Holliday, J., Moore, L., & Campbell, R. (2009). Identifying influential young people to undertake effective peer-led health promotion: The example of A Stop Smoking In Schools Trial (ASSIST). *Health Education Research, 24*(6), 977-988. http://dx.doi.org/10.1093/her/cyp045

Substance Abuse & Mental Health Service Administration Network. (1994). *You can prepare easy to read materials.* Technical Assistance Bulletin, National Clearinghouse for Alcohol and Drug Information. Retrieved from http://www.actforyouth.net/documents/YDM%20pdf6.4C%20handout.pdf

Thompson, D. R., Chair, S. Y., Chan, S. W., Astin, F., Davidson, P. M., & Ski, C. F. (2011). Motivational interviewing: A useful approach to improving cardiovascular health? *Journal of Clinical Nursing, 20,* 1236-1244. doi: 10.1111/j.1365-2702.2010.03558.x

Toofany, S. (2006). Patient empowerment: Myth or reality? *Nursing Management, 13*(6), 18–22.

Tveiten, S., & Severinsson, E. (2006). Communication—A core concept in client supervision by public health nurses. *Journal of Nursing Management, 14*(3), 235–243.

Weiss, B. D. (2007). *Health literacy and patient safety: Help patients understand.* Chicago, IL: American Medical Association Foundation and American Medical Association.

Westdahl, C., & Page-Goertz, S. (2006). Promotion of breastfeeding—Beyond the benefits. *International Journal of Childbirth Education, 22*(4), 8–16.

Whitman, N. I. (1998). Assessment of the learner. In M. D. Boyd, C. J. Gleit, B. A. Grahm, & N. I. Whitman (Eds.), *Health teaching in nursing practice: A professional model* (pp. 157–180). Stamford, CT: Appleton & Lange.

Wright, A. L, Naylor, A., Wester, R., Bauer, M., & Sutcliffe, E. (1997). Using cultural knowledge in health promotion: Breastfeeding among the Navajo. *Health Education & Behavior, 24*(5), 625–639.

Zahner, S. J., & Gredig, Q. B. (2005). Improving public health nursing education: Recommendations of local public health nurses. *Public Health Nursing, 22*(5), 445–450.

Chapter 9

Aronowitz, T. (2005). The role of "envisioning the future" in the development of resilience among at-risk youth. *Public Health Nursing, 22*(3), 200–208.

Austin, W., Bergum, V., & Dossitor, J. (2003). Relational ethics: An action ethic as a foundation for health care. In V. Tschudin (Ed.), *Approaches to ethics: Nursing beyond boundaries* (pp. 45–52). Woburn, MA: Buttersworth-Heinenmann.

Bender, A., Peter, E., Wynn, F., Andrews, G., & Pringle, D. (2011). Welcome intrusions: An interpretive phenomenological study of TB nurses' relational work. *International Journal of Nursing Studies, 48*(11), 1409–1419. doi:http://dx.doi.org/10.1016/j.ijnurstu.2011.04.012

Browne, A. J., Hartrick Doane, G., Reimer, J., MacLeod, M., & McLellan, E. (2010). Public health nursing practice with "high priority" families: The significance of contextualizing "risk." *Nursing Inquiry, 17*(1), 26–37.

Chafey, K. (1996). "Caring" is not enough: Ethical paradigms for community-based care. *Nursing and Health Care Perspectives on Community, 17*(1), 10–15.

Chismar, D. (1988). Empathy and sympathy: The important difference. *Journal of Value Inquiry, 22*(4), 257–266.

Crisp, B., & Lister, P. (2004). Child protection and public health: Nurses' responsibilities. *Journal of Advanced Nursing, 47*(6), 656–663.

Duiveman, T., & Bonner, A. (2012). Negotiating: Experiences of community nurses when contracting with clients. *Contemporary Nurse: A Journal for the Australian Nursing Profession, 41*(1), 120–125.

Fawcett, J. (2000). *Analysis and evaluation of contemporary nursing knowledge: Nursing models and theories.* Philadelphia, PA: F. A. Davis.

Fazzone, P. A., Barloon, L. F., McConnell, S. J., & Chitty, J. A. (2000). Personal safety, violence, and home health. *Public Health Nursing, 17*(1), 43–52.

Finfgeld-Connett, D. (2008). Qualitative convergence of three nursing concepts: Art of nursing, presence and caring. *Journal of Advanced Nursing, 63*(5), 527–534.

Fredriksson, L., & Eriksson, K. (2006). The ethics of the caring conversation. *Nursing Ethics, 13*(1), 138–148.

Gantert, T., McWilliam, C., Ward-Griffin, C., & Allen, N. (2009). Working it out together: Family caregivers' perceptions of relationship-building with in-home service providers. *Canadian Journal of Nursing Research, 41*(3), 44–63.

Gellner, P., Landers, S., O'Rourke, D., & Schlegel, M. (1994). Community health nursing in the 1990s—Risky business? *Holistic Nursing Practice, 8*(2), 15–21.

Heaman, M., Chalmers, K., Woodgate, R., & Brown, J. (2007). Relationship work in an early childhood home visiting program. *Journal of Pediatric Nursing, 22*(4), 319–330.

Jack, S. M., DiCenso, A., & Lohfeld, L. (2005). A theory of maternal engagement with public health nurses and family visitors. *Journal of Advanced Nursing, 49*(2), 182–190.

Jackson, C. (2010). Using loving relationships to transform health care: A practical approach. *Holistic Nursing Practice, 24*(4), 181–186.

Kendra, M. A., Weiker, A., Simon, S., Grant, A., & Shullick, D. (1996). Safety concerns affecting delivery of home health care. *Public Health Nursing, 13*(2), 83–89.

Ladd, R. E., Pasquerella, L., & Smith, S. (2000). What to do when the end is near: Ethical issues in home health care nursing. *Public Health Nursing, 17*(2), 103–110.

Marcellus, L. (2005). The ethics of relation: Public health nurses and child protection clients. *Journal of Advanced Nursing, 51*(4), 414–420.

Martins, D. C. (2008). Experiences of homeless people in the health care delivery system: A descriptive phenomenological study. *Public Health Nursing, 25*(5), 420–430.

McNaughton, D. B. (2005). A naturalistic test of Peplau's theory in home visiting. *Public Health Nursing, 22*(5), 429–438.

Morse, J. M., Bottorff, J., Neander, W., & Solberg, S. (1991). Comparative analysis of conceptualizations and theories of caring. *IMAGE: Journal of Nursing Scholarship, 23*(2), 119–126.

Morse, J. M., Solberg, S. M., Neander, W. L., Bottorff, J. L., & Johnson, J. L. (1990). Concepts of caring and caring as a concept. *Advances in Nursing Science, 13*(1), 1–14.

Nagano, H. (2000). Empathic understanding: Constructing an evaluation scale from the microcounseling approach. *Nursing and Health Sciences, 2*(1), 17–27.

Nurses Association of New Brunswick (2011). *Practice Standard: The Therapeutic Nurse-Client Relationship.* Retrieved from http://www.nanb.nb.ca/downloads/Practice%20Standard%20-%20 Nurse-Client%20Relationship%20-%20E.pdf

Olthuis, G., Dekkers, W., Leget, C., & Vogelaar, P. (2006). The caring relationship in hospice care: An analysis based on the ethics of the caring relationship. *Nursing Ethics, 13*(1), 29–40.

Porr, C., Drummond, J., & Olson, K. (2012). Establishing therapeutic relationships with vulnerable and potentially stigmatized clients. *Qualitative Health Research, 22*(3), 384–396.

Ridgeway, S. (2010). Lillian Wald founded public health nursing. *Working Nurse.* Retrieved from http://www.workingnurse.com/articles/Lillian-Wald-Founded-Public-Health-Nursing

Robert Wood Johnson Foundation [RWJF]. (2010). A new way to talk about the social determinants of health. Retrieved from http://www.rwjf.org/files/research/vpmessageguide20101029.pdf

Schaffer, M. A., Jost, R., Pederson, B. J., & Lair, M. (2008). Pregnancy-free club: A strategy to prevent repeat adolescent pregnancy. *Public Health Nursing, 25*(4), 304–311.

Schulte, J. (2000). Finding ways to create connections among communities: Partial results of an ethnography of urban public health nurses. *Public Health Nursing, 17*(1), 3–10.

Schulte, J. M., Nolt, B. J., Williams, R. L., Spinks, C. L., & Hellsten, J. J. (1998). Violence and threats of violence experienced by public health field workers. *Journal of the American Medical Association, 280*(5), 439–442.

Shores, C. I. (2012). Caring behaviors of faith community nurses. *International Journal for Human Caring, 16*(3), 74.

SmithBattle, L. (2003). Displacing the "rule book" in caring for teen mothers. *Public Health Nursing, 20*(5), 369–376.

SmithBattle, L., Diekemper, M., & Leander, S. (2004a). Getting your feet wet: Becoming a public health nurse, part 1. *Public Health Nursing, 21*(1), 3–11.

SmithBattle, L., Diekemper, M., & Leander, S. (2004b). Moving upstream: Becoming a public health nurse, part 2. *Public Health Nursing, 21*(2), 95–102.

SmithBattle, L., Drake, M. A., & Diekemper, M. (1997). The responsive use of self in community health nursing practice. *Advances in Nursing Science, 20*(2), 75–89.

Smith-Campbell, B. (1999). A case study on expanding the concept of caring from individuals to communities. *Public Health Nursing, 16*(6), 405–411.

Sundelof, A. E., Hansebo, G., & Ekman, S.-L. (2004). Friendship and caring communion: The meaning of caring relationship in district nursing. *International Journal for Human Caring, 8*(3), 13–20.

Warelow, P., Edward, K. L., & Vinek, J. (2008). Care: What nurses say and what nurses do. *Holistic Nursing Practice, 22*(3), 146–153.

Chapter 10

Alameda County Public Health Department (ACPHD). (2008). A framework for health equity. *Life and death from unnatural causes: Health and social inequity in Alameda County.* Oakland, CA: ACPHD, p. 4. Retrieved from http://www.acphd.org/media/53628/unnatcs2008.pdf

American Nurses Association (ANA). (2001). *Code of ethics for nurses with interpretive statements.* Washington, DC: Nursesbooks.org.

American Nurses Association (ANA). (2010a). *Guide to the code of ethics for nurses—Interpretation and application.* Silver Springs, MD: Nursebooks.org

American Nurses Association (ANA). (2010b). Nurses human rights. ANA position statements on ethics and human rights. Silver Springs, MD: Nursing World. Retrieved from http://www.nursingworld.org/MainMenuCategories/EthicsStandards/Ethics-Position-Statements.aspx

American Nurses Association (ANA). (2013). *Public health nursing: Scope & standards of practice.* Silver Springs, MD: Nursesbooks.org.

Baum, N., Gollust, S., Goold, S., & Jacobson, P. (2007). Looking ahead: Addressing ethical challenges in public health practice. *Journal of Law, Medicine, and Ethics, 35*(4), 657–667.

Bay Area Regional Health Inequities Initiative (BARHII). (2008). Health Inequities in the Bay Area. San Francisco, CA: BARHII. Retrieved from http://www.barhii.org/press/download/barhii_report08.pdf

Beauchamp, D. E. (2013). Public health as social justice. In M. T. Donohue (Ed.), *Public health and social justice* (pp. 11–19). San Francisco, CA: Jossey-Bass/John Wiley & Sons, Inc.

Brennen Ramirez, I. K., Baker, E. A., & Metzler, M. (2008). *Promoting Health Equity: A Resource to Help Communities Address Social Determinants of Health.* Atlanta, GA: U.S. Department of Health and Human Services: Centers for Disease Control and Prevention.

Broussard, B. B. (2011). The bucket list: A service-learning approach to community engagement to enhance community health nursing clinical learning. *Journal of Nursing Education, 50*(1), 40–43. doi:10.3928/01484834-20100930-07

Bu, X., & Jezewski, M. A., (2006). Developing a mid-range theory of patient advocacy through competency analysis. *Journal of Advanced Nursing, 57*(1), 101–110.

Budetti, P. (2008). Market justice and US healthcare. *Journal of the American Medical Association, 299*(1), 92–94.

California Newsreel. (2008). Backgrounders from the unnatural causes health equity data base. *Unnatural Causes.* Retrieved 2013, from http://www.unnaturalcauses.org/assets/uploads/file/primers.pdf

Cawley, T. & McNamara, P.M. (2011). Public health nurse perceptions of empowerment and advocacy in child health surveillance in West Ireland. *Public Health Nursing, 28*(2), 150–158. doi:10.1111/j.1525-1446.2010.00921.x

Center for Vulnerable Populations Research. (n.d.). Who are the vulnerable? Los Angeles, CA: University of California, Los Angeles, School of Nursing. Retrieved from http://nursing.ucla.edu/site.cfm?id=388

Centers for Disease Control and Prevention. (2011). CDC health disparities and inequality report – United States, 2011. *Morbidity and Mortality Weekly Report Supplement, 60.* Retrieved from http://www.cdc.gov/mmwr/pdf/other/su6001.pdf

Centers for Disease Control and Prevention. (2013). CDC Health Disparities & Inequalities Report (CHDIR), 2013. *Morbidity and Mortality Weekly Report Supplement, 62*(3), 1–187. Atlanta, GA: U.S. Department of Health and Human Services. Retrieved from http://www.cdc.gov/minorityhealth/CHDIReport.html

Congressional Budget Office. (2008). Growing disparities in life expectancy. *Economic and Budget Issue Brief*. Retrieved from http://www.cbo.gov/publication/41681

Curtin, L. (1979). The nurse as advocate: A philosophical foundation for nursing. *Advances in Nursing Science, 1*(3), 1–10.

Denehy, J. (2007). National Association of School Nurses: Speaking up for children. *Journal of School Nursing, 23*(3): 125–127.

Edmonson, C. (2010). Moral courage and the nurse leader. *Online Journal of Issues in Nursing, 15*(3). doi:10.3912/OJIN.Vol15No03Man05.

Ensign, J. (2001). The health of shelter-based foster youth. *Public Health Nursing, 18*(1), 19–23.

Falk-Rafael, A. (2005a). Speaking truth to power: Nursing's legacy and moral imperative. *Advances in Nursing Science, 28*(3), 212–223.

Falk-Rafael, A. (2005b). Advancing nursing theory through theory-guided practice—The emergence of a critical caring perspective. *Advances in Nursing Science, 28*(1), 38–49.

Falk-Rafael, A. (2006). Globalization and global health: Toward nursing praxis in the global community. *Advances in Nursing Science, 29*(1), 2–14.

Falk-Rafael, A., & Betker, C. (2012). Witnessing social injustice downstream and advocating for health equity upstream. *Advances in Nursing Science, 35*(2), 98–112. doi:10.1097/ANS.0b013e31824fe70f

Gadow, S. (1999). Relational narrative: The postmodern turn in nursing ethics. *Scholarly Inquiry for Nursing Practice: An International Journal, 13*(1), 57–70.

Galer-Unti, R. (2010). Advocacy 2.0: Advocating in the digital age. *Health Promotion Practice, 11*(6), 784–787.

Gallagher, A. (2011). Moral distress and moral courage in everyday nursing practice. *Online Journal of Issues in Nursing, 16*(2). doi:10.3912/OJIN.Vol16No02PPT03

Gebrke, P. M. (2008). Civic engagement and nursing education. *Advances in Nursing Science, 31*(1), 52–66.

Gruskin, S., Cottingham, J., Hilber, A. M., Kismodi, E., Lincetto, O., & Roseman, M. J. (2008). Using human rights to improve maternal and neonatal health: History, connections and a proposed practical solution. *Bulletin of the World Health Organization, 86*(8), 589–593.

Horton, S., & Johnson, R. J. (2010). Improving access to health care for uninsured elderly patients. *Public Health Nursing, 27*(4), 362–370.

Hughes, J. (2010). Putting the pieces together: How public health nurses in rural and remote Canadian communities respond to intimate partner violence. *Online Journal of Rural Nursing and Health Care, 10*(1), 34–47.

International Council of Nurses. (2006). The ICN position statement on nurses and human rights. Geneva, Switzerland: Author. Retrieved from http://www.icn.ch/images/stories/documents/publications/position_statements/E10_Nurses_Human_Rights.pdf

Iton, A. B. (2008). The ethics of the medical model in addressing the root causes of health disparities in local public health practice. *Journal of Public Health Management Practice, 14*(4), 335–339.

Keller, L. O. (2010). Table: Comparison of value structure. Unpublished, personal correspondence.

Kleinfehn-Wald, N. (2010). Social justice and human rights issues identified by practicing public health nurses. Unpublished research.

Lachman, V.D. (2010). Strategies necessary for moral courage. *Online Journal of Issues in Nursing, 15*(3). doi:10.3912/OJIN.Vol15No03Man03.

Lavery, S. H., Smith, M. L., Esparza, A. A., Hrushow, A., Moore, M., & Reed, D. F. (2005). The community action model: A community-driven model designed to address disparities in health. *American Journal of Public Health*, *95*(4), 611–616.

Ludwick, R., & Silva, M.C. (2000). Nursing around the world: Cultural values and ethical conflicts. *2000 Online Journal of Issues in Nursing, 5*(3). Retrieved from http://www.nursingworld.org/MainMenuCategories/ANAMarketplace/ANAPeriodicals/OJIN/Columns/Ethics

MacDonald, H. (2006). Relational ethics and advocacy in nursing: Literature review. *Journal of Advanced Nursing, 57*(2), 119–126.

Mallik, M. (1997). Advocacy in nursing—A review of the literature. *Journal of Advanced Nursing, 25*(1), 130–138.

Minnesota Department of Health (MDH). (2001). *Public health interventions—Application for public health nursing practice*. St. Paul, MN: MDH.

Murray, J.S. (2010). Moral courage in healthcare: Acting ethically even in presence of risk. *Online Journal of Issues in Nursing, 15*(3). doi: 10.3912/OJIN.Vol15No03Man02

National Research Council and Institute of Medicine. (2013). *U.S. health in international perspective: Shorter lives, poorer health.* Washington, D.C.: The National Academies Press, p. 32. Retrieved from http://www.nap.edu/catalog.php?record_id=13497

Office of the High Commissioner for Human Rights, United Nations Human Rights. (n.d.). Retrieved from http://www.ohchr.org/EN/Issues/Pages/WhatareHumanRights.aspx?Pages/WhatareHuman-Rights.aspx

Public Health Leadership Society. (2002). *Principles of the ethical practice of public health.* Version 2.2. Retrieved from http://phls.org/CMSuploads/Principles-of-the-Ethical-Practice-of-PH-Version-2.2-68496.pdf

Racher, F. E. (2007). The evolution of ethics for community practice. *Journal of Community Health Nursing, 24*(1), 65–76.

Redlener, I., & Grant, R. (2009). America's safety net and health care reform—What lies ahead? *New England Journal of Medicine, 361*(23), 2201–2204. doi:10.1056/NEJMp0910597

Reutter, L., & Kushner, K. E. (2010). "Health equity through action on the social determinants of health": Taking up the challenge in nursing. *Nursing Inquiry, 17*(3), 269–280.

Satcher, D., & Higginbotham, E. J. (2008). The public health approach to eliminating disparities in health. *American Journal of Public Health*, *98*, 400–403.

Schoon, P. M., Champlin, B., & Hunt, R. (2012). Developing a sustainable foot care clinic in a homeless shelter within an academic-community partnership through curricular integration and faculty engagement. *Journal of Nursing Education, 51*(12), 714–718. doi:10.3928/01484834-20121112-02

Schoon, P. M., Miller, T. W., Maloney, P., & Tasbir, J. (2012). Chapter 7: Power and politics. In P. Kelly & J. Tazbir (Eds.), *Essentials of leadership and management* (pp. 186–208). Clifton Park, NJ: Delmar/Centage.

Selanders, L. C., & Crane, P. C. (2012). The voice of Florence Nightingale on advocacy. *Online Journal of Issues in Nursing, 17*(1), 1–10. doi:10.3912/OJIN.Vol17No01Man01

Signal, L., Martin, J., Cram, F., & Robson, B. (2008). *The Health Equity Assessment Tool: A user's guide.* Wellington, New Zealand: Ministry of Health.

Singh, G. K., Siahpush, M., & Kogan, M. D. (2010). Rising social inequalities in US childhood obesity, 2003–2007. *Annals of Epidemiology, 20*(1), 40–52. http://dx.doi.org/10.1016/j.annepidem.2009.09.008. Retrieved from http://www.sciencedirect.com/science/article/pii/S104727970900324X

Strass, P., & Billay, E. (2008). A public health nursing initiative to promote antenatal health. *Canadian Nurse, 104*(2), 29–33.

United Nations. (1948). The universal declaration of human rights. Geneva, Switzerland: Author. Retrieved from http://www.un.org/en/documents/udhr/

United Nations. (2013). *The Millennium Development Goals report–2013.* Geneva, Switzerland: Author. Retrieved from http://www.un.org/millenniumgoals/pdf/report-2013/mdg-report-2013-english.pdf

U.S. Department of Health and Human Services. (2012). United States life tables, 2008. *National Vital Statistics Report, 61*(3), 3. Retrieved from http://www.cdc.gov/nchs/data/nvsr/nvsr61/nvsr61_03.pdf

U.S. Department of Health and Human Services. (2013). Infant mortality statistics from the 2009 period—Linked birth/infant death data set. *National Vital Statistics Report, 61*(8), 1.

Vanderburg, S., Wright, L., Boston, S., & Zimmerman, G. (2010). Maternal child home visiting program improves nursing practice for screening of woman abuse. *Public Health Nursing, 27*(4), 347–352.

Volbrecht, R. M. (2002). *Nursing ethics—Communities in dialogue.* Upper Saddle River, NJ: Pearson Prentice Hall.

Williams, D. R., Costa, M. V., Oduniami, A. O., & Mohammed, S. A. (2008). Moving upstream: How interventions that address social determinants of health can improve health and reduce disparities. *Journal of Public Health Management Practice. 14*(Suppl), S8–S17. doi:10.1097/01.PHH.0000338382.36695.42

World Health Organization. (n.d.). Social determinants of health—Key concepts. Retrieved from http://www.who.int/social_determinants/thecommission/finalreport/key_concepts/en/index.html

Chapter 11

Aston, M., Meagher-Stewart, D., Sheppard-Lemoine, D., Vukic, A., & Chircop, A. (2006). Family health nursing and empowering relationships. *Pediatric Nursing, 32*(1), 61–67.

Center for Spirituality and Healing [CSH]. (2013). *Deep Listening.* Retrieved from http://cityhill.org/media.php?pageID=96

Cioffi, J. (2003). Communicating with culturally and linguistically diverse patients in an acute care setting: Nurses' experiences. *International Journal of Nursing Studies, 40*(3), 299–306.

Dillon, R. (1992). Respect and care: Toward a moral integration. *Canadian Journal of Philosophy, 22*(1), 105–132.

Falk-Rafael, A., & Betker, C. (2012). The primacy of relationships: A study of public health nursing practice from a critical caring perspective. *Advances in Nursing Science, 35*(4), 315–332.

Flores, G. (2005). The impact of medical interpreter services on the quality of health care: A systematic review. *Medical Care Research Review, 62*(3), 255–299.

Garrett, P. (2009). Healthcare interpreter policy: Policy determinants and current issues in the Australian context. *Interpreting and Translation, 1*(2), 44–54.

Goldsborough, J. D. (1970). On becoming nonjudgmental. *American Journal of Nursing, 70*(11), 2340–2343.

Helleso, R., & Solveig Fagermoen, M. (2010). Cultural diversity between hospital and community nurses: Implications for continuity of care. *International Journal of Integrated Care, 10*, e036.

Kupperschmidt, B. R. (2006). Addressing multigenerational conflict: Mutual respect and carefronting as strategy. *Online Journal of Issues in Nursing, 11*(2).

Leininger, M. (1978). Transcultural nursing theories and research approaches. In M. Leininger (Ed.), *Transcultural Nursing* (pp. 31–51). New York, NY: Wiley.

Mack, M., Uken, R., & Powers, J. (2006). People improving the community's health: Community health workers as agents of change. *Journal of Health Care for the Poor and Underserved, 17*(1), 16–25.

Nagano, H. (2000). Empathic understanding: Constructing an evaluation scale from the microcounseling approach. *Nursing and Health Sciences, 2*(1), 17–27.

O'Brien, M. J., Squires, A. P., Bixby, R. A., & Larson, S. C. (2009). Role development of community health workers: An examination of selection and training processes in the intervention literature. *American Journal of Preventive Medicine, 37*(6), s262–s269.

Pasco, A. C. Y., Morse, J. M., & Olson, J. K. (2004). The cross-cultural relationships between nurses and Filipino Canadian patients. *Journal of Nursing Scholarship, 36*(3), 239–246.

Passel, J., & Cohn, D. (2008). U.S. Population Projections 2005–2050. Retrieved from http://www.pewhispanic.org/files/reports/85.pdf

Payne, R. K., DeVol, P. E., & Smith, T. D. (2001). *Bridges out of poverty: Strategies for professionals and communities.* Highlands, TX: aha! Process, Inc.

Pesznecker, B. L. (1984). The poor: A population at risk. *Public Health Nursing, 1*(4), 237–249.

Pirkey, J. M., Levey, J. A., Newberry, S. M., Guthman, P. L., & Hansen, J. M. (2012). Videoconferencing expands nursing students' cultural realm. *Journal of Nursing Education, 51*(10), 586–590.

Porr, C. (2005). Shifting from preconceptions to pure wonderment. *Nursing Philosophy, 6*(3), 189–195.

Porr, C., Drummond, J., & Olson, K. (2012). Establishing therapeutic relationships with vulnerable and potentially stigmatized clients. *Qualitative Health Research, 22*(3), 384–396.

Ramarajan, L., Barsade, S. G., & Burack, O. R. (2008). The influence of organizational respect on emotional exhaustion in the human services. *Journal of Positive Psychology, 3*(1), 3–18.

Segal, J., Smith, M. A., & Jaffe, J. (2013). *Nonverbal communication skills: The power of nonverbal communication and body language.* Retrieved from http://www.helpguide.org/mental/eq6_nonverbal_communication.htm

U.S. Census Bureau. (2013). U.S. Population Other Than White by State: 2000. Retrieved from http://www.census.gov/geo/maps-data/maps/pdfs/thematic/pct_otherthan_white_2000.pdf

Volbrecht, R. M. (2001). *Nursing ethics: Communities in dialogue.* Upper Saddle River, NJ: Prentice Hall.

Wright, L. M., & Leahey, M. (2005). *Nurses and families: A guide to family assessment and intervention*, 4th ed. Philadelphia, PA: F. A. Davis.

Chapter 12

Crisp, B. R., & Green Lister, P. (2004). Child protection and public health: Nurses' responsibilities. *Journal of Advanced Nursing, 47*(6), 656–663.

DeMay, D. A. (2003). The experience of being a client in an Alaska public health nursing home visitation program. *Public Health Nursing, 20*(3), 228–236.

Flynn, M. A., Hall, K., Noack, A., Clovechok, S., Enns, E., Pivnick, J., . . . Pryce, C. (2005). Promotion of healthy weights at preschool public health vaccination clinics in Calgary: An obesity surveillance program. *Canadian Journal of Public Health, 96*(6), 421–426.

Friedman, M. M., Bowden, V. R., & Jones, E. G. (2003). *Family nursing: Research, theory and practice*, 5th ed. Upper Saddle River, NJ: Prentice Hall.

Gerrity, P. (2010). And to think that it happened on 11th street: A nursing approach to community-based holistic care and health care reform. *Alternative Therapies in Health and Medicine, 16*(5), 62–67.

Hayden, D. (2011). Spirituality in end-of-life care: Attending the person on their journey. *British Journal of Community Nursing, 16*(11), 546–551.

Hayes, J. C., Davis, J. A., & Miranda, M. L. (2006). Incorporating a built environment module into an accelerated second-degree community health nursing course. *Public Health Nursing 23*(5), 442–452.

Hayter, M. (2005). Reaching marginalized young people through sexual health nursing outreach clinics: Evaluating service use and the views of service users. *Public Health Nursing, 22*(4), 339–346.

Kemp, L., Anderson, T., Travaglia, J., & Harris, E. (2005). Sustained nursing home visiting in early childhood: Exploring Australian nursing competencies. *Public Health Nursing, 22*(3), 254–259.

Kemper, A. R., Fant, K. E., & Clark, S. J. (2005). Informing parents about newborn screening. *Public Health Nursing, 22*(4), 332–338.

Labun, E. (1988). Spiritual care: An element in nursing care planning. *Journal of Advanced Nursing, 13*(3), 314–320.

McKeown, F. (2007). The experiences of older people on discharge from hospital following assessment by the public health nurse. *Journal of Clinical Nursing, 16*(3), 469–476.

McSherry, W., Cash, K., & Ross, L. (2004). Meaning of spirituality: Implications for nursing practice. *Journal of Clinical Nursing, 13*(8), 934–941.

Minnesota Department of Health (MDH). (2009). Early identification of young children with special health care needs. *Minnesota Department of Health Fact Sheet: Title V (MCH) Block Grant Children and Adolescents with Special Health Care Needs.* St. Paul, MN: Author.

Minnesota Department of Health (MDH). (2013a). *Adverse childhood experiences in Minnesota.* Retrieved from http://www.health.state.mn.us/divs/cfh/program/ace/content/document/pdf/acereport.pdf

Minnesota Department of Health (MDH). (2013b). *How-to: Community health assessment.* Retrieved from http://www.health.state.mn.us/divs/opi/pm/lphap/cha/howto.html

Mondy, C., Cardenas, D., & Avila, M. (2003). The role of an advanced practice public health nurse in bioterrorism preparedness. *Public Health Nursing, 20*(6), 422–431.

Olds, D. L., Kitzman, H., Hanks, C., Cole, R., Anson, E., Sidora-Arcoleo, K., . . . Bondy, J. (2007). Effects of nurse home visiting on maternal and child functioning: Age-9 follow-up of a randomized trial. *Pediatrics, 120*(4), 832–845.

Ricketts, S. A., Murray, E. K., & Schwalberg, R. (2005). Reducing low birthweight by resolving risks: Results from Colorado's Prenatal Plus Program. *American Journal of Public Health, 98*(11), 1952–1957.

Schim, S., Doorenbos, A., Benkert, R., & Miller, J. (2007). Culturally congruent care: Putting the puzzle together. *Journal of Transcultural Nursing, 18*(2), 103–110.

Schneiderman, J. U. (2006). Innovative pediatric nursing role: Public health nurses in child welfare. *Pediatric Nursing, 32*(4), 317–321.

Sittner, B., Hudson, D., & Defrain, J. (2007). Using the concept of family strengths to enhance nursing care. *MCN: American Journal of Maternal/Child Health Nursing, 32*(6), 353–357.

Somervell, A. M., Saylor, C., & Mao, C. L. (2005). Public health nurse interventions for women in a dependency drug court. *Public Health Nursing, 22*(1), 59–64.

Strass, P., & Billay, E. (2008). A public health nursing initiative to promote antenatal health. *Canadian Nurse, 104*(2), 29–33.

World Health Organization (WHO). (n.d.). *Environmental Health.* Retrieved from http://www.who.int/topics/environmental_health/en/

Chapter 13

American Nurses Association. (2013). *Public health nursing: Scope and standards of practice.* Silver Springs, MD: Nursesbooks.org.

American Public Health Association. (2010). *Top ten rules of advocacy.* Retrieved from http://www.apha.org

Avolio, B. J., Walumbwa, F. O., & Weber, T. J. (2009). Leadership: Current theories, research, and future directions. *Annual Review of Psychology, 60,* 421–449.

Blackburn, C. (1992). *Improving health and welfare work with families in poverty: A handbook.* Buckingham, UK: Open University Press.

Carnegie, E., & Kiger, A. (2009). Being and doing politics: An outdated model or 21st century reality? *Journal of Advanced Nursing, 65*(9), 1976–1984. doi:10.1111/j.1365-2648.2009.05084.x

Cohen, B. E., & Reutter, L. (2007). Development of the role of public health nurses in addressing child and family poverty: A framework for action. *Journal of Advanced Nursing, 60*(1), 96–107.

Dakota County Public Health (DCPH). (2004). *Dakota County Clinical Menu, modified from Henry Street Consortium Clinical Menu.* West St. Paul, MN: DCPH.

Deschaine, J., & Schaffer, M. (2003). Strengthening the role of public health nurse leaders in policy development. *Policy, Politics, and Nursing Practice, 4*(4), 266–274.

Des Jardin, K. (2001). Political involvement in nursing—Politics, ethics, and strategic action. *AORN Journal, 74*(5), 614–622.

Doody, O., & Doody, C. M. (2012). Transformational leadership in nursing practice. *British Journal of Nursing, (21)*20, 1212–1218.

Falk-Rafael, A. (2005). Speaking truth to power: Nursing's legacy and moral imperative. *Advances in Nursing Science, 28*(3), 212–223.

George, B., & Sims, P. (2007). *True north: Discover Your authentic leadership.* Hoboken, NJ: Jossey-Bass/Wiley.

Henry Street Consortium. (2003). *Population-based public health nursing competencies.* St. Paul, MN: Author. Retrieved from http://www.health.state.mn.us/divs/opi/cd/phn/henrystreet/docs/0303henryst_corecomp.pdf

Henry Street Consortium. (2004). *The Henry Street Consortium Clinical Menu.* St. Paul, MN: HSC. Retrieved from http://www.health.state.mn.us/divs/opi/cd/phn/henrystreet/

Hill, K. S. (2008). Leading change: The creativity of a public health nurse leader. *Journal of Nursing Administration, 38*(11), 459–460.

Kalb, K. B., Cherry, N. M., Kauzloric, J., Brender, A., Green, K., Miyagawa, L. . . . & Shinoda-Mettler, A. (2006). *A competency-based approach to public health nursing performance appraisal.* Public Health Nursing, 29(3), 115–138.

Mason, D. J., Backer, B. A., & Georges, C. A. (1991). Toward a feminist model for the political empowerment of nurses. *Image Journal of Nursing Scholarship, 23*(2), 72–77.

Meagher-Stewart, D., Underwood, J., MacDonald, M., Schoenfeld, B., Blythe, J., Knibbs, K., . . . Crea, M. (2010). Organizational attributes that assure optimal utilization of public health nurses. *Public Health Nursing, 27*(5), 433–441.

Minnesota Department of Health. (2001). *Public health interventions—Applications for public health nursing practice.* St. Paul, MN: Author. Retrieved from http://www.health.state.mn.us/divs/opi/cd/phn/wheel.html

Morrison, R. S., Jones, L., & Fuller, B. (1997). The relation between leadership style and empowerment on job satisfaction of nurses. *Journal of Nursing Administration, 27*(5), 27–34.

Murphy, L. G. (2012). Authentic leadership—Becoming and remaining an authentic nurse leader. *Journal of Nursing Administration, 42*(11), 507–512.

Nissen, L. B., Merrigan, D. M., & Kraft, M. K. (2005). Moving mountains together: Strategic community leadership and systems change. *Child Welfare, 84*(2), 123–140.

O'Neill, J. A. (2013). Advancing the nursing profession begins with leadership. *Journal of Nursing Administration,43*(4), 179–181.

Quad Council of Public Health Nursing Organizations. (2011). *Quad Council Competencies for Public Health Nurses.* Retrieved from http://www.achne.org/files/Quad%20Council/QuadCouncilCompetenciesforPublicHealthNurses.pdf

Racher, F. (2007). The evolution of ethics for community practice. *Journal of Community Health Nursing, 24*(1), 65–76.

Schoon, P. (2013). *Shared leadership enhances nursing care in homeless shelter.* Unpublished manuscript.

Underwood, J. M., Mowat, D. L., Meagher-Stewart, D. M., Deber, R. B., Baumann, A. O., MacDonald, M. B., . . . Munroe, V. J. (2009). Building community and public health nursing capacity: A synthesis report of the national community health nursing study. *Canadian Journal of Public Health, 100*(5), I-1–I-11.

U.S. Department of Health and Human Services. (n.d.). *Healthy People 2020—About Healthy People.* Retrieved from http://www.healthypeople.gov/hp2020

Volbrecht, R. M. (2002). *Nursing ethics: Communities in dialogue.* Upper Saddle River, NJ: Pearson Prentice Hall.

Wolf, G. A. (2012). Transformational leadership: The art of advocacy and influence. *Journal of Nursing Administration, 42*(6), 309–310.

Wong, C. A, Spence Laschinger, H. K., & Cummings, G. G. (2010). Authentic leadership and nurses' voice behavior and perceptions of care equity. *Journal of Nursing Management, 18*, 889–900.

Chapter 14

Keller, L. O., Schaffer, M. A., & Reckinger, D. (2013). Visibility for public health nursing. Unpublished paper.

Minnesota Department of Health. (2006). Wheel of public health interventions: A collection of "Getting Behind the Wheel" stories, 2000–2006. Office of Public Health Practice. Retrieved from http://www.health.state.mn.us/divs/opi/cd/phn/docs/0606wheel_stories.pdf

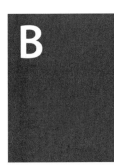

Chapter 1

Professional Associations

American Public Health Association—Professional organization for public health professionals, including a public health nursing section. http://www.apha.org

Association of Public Health Nurses (formally the Association of State and Territorial Directors of Nursing)—PHNs promoting health and safety of populations across 50 states. http://www.astdn.org

Association of State and Territorial Health Officials. http://www.astho.org

Online Public Health Certificate Program

Foundations of Public Health Certificate Program—Free online courses with foundational knowledge for public health workers with limited formal education or training in public health. http://www.foundationsofph.org

Public Health Nurse Ready—Free online certificate program for nurses to enhance their skills in public health nursing. www.empirestatephtc.org

Healthy People 2020

Determinants of Health: A Framework for Reaching Healthy People 2020 Goals. http://www.youtube.com/watch?v=5Lul6KNIw_8

Healthy People 2020 LHI Infographic Gallery. http://www.healthypeople.gov/2020/LHI/infographicGallery.aspx

Public Health Online Videos

The Deadly History of Public Health. http://www.youtube.com/watch?v=KS76_gfmlNk

This Is Public Health. http://www.youtube.com/watch?v=Bpu42LmLo4U&list=PL2927BB296090A6A6

WHO—Health Profession's Role in Primary Health Care—Nurses and Midwives. http://www.who.int/hrh/nursing_midwifery/films/en/

Public Health and Public Health Nursing Online Videos

David Reyes—A Public Health Nursing Story. http://www.youtube.com/watch?v=tVkO4dpPIwE

History of Nursing and Public Health—Student-Created Video. http://www.youtube.com/watch?v=joGYymjkGzk

Is a Career in Public Health Right for Me? http://www.youtube.com/watch?v=XwgTfCRYD3s

Just the Job Video—Public Health Nurse—Ireland. http://www.youtube.com/watch?v=hb4dZ7MusnI

Public Health Nurse—Interview With PHN Who Works in TB Control. http://www.youtube.com/watch?v=UIBhTb11qOo

Public Health Nurses—Profile. http://www.youtube.com/watch?v=g-79UCQ-7bY

Roles of Public Health Nurse—School Nursing (Student-Created Video). http://www.youtube.com/watch?v=96ZLPtUwizw

The Frontier Nursing Service. http://www.youtube.com/watch?v=OWu5IuzOt9c

The Many Faces of Public Health Nursing. http://www.youtube.com/watch?v=cA2zIvaMmVw

What Is a Public Health Nurse? (Salary and Job Description). http://www.youtube.com/watch?v=umWzRu-tD0E

Why Choose Public Health Nursing? http://www.youtube.com/watch?v=9PEOYW69Z5c

Journal Articles

Abrams, S. E. (2010). Hints for the aspiring public health nurse. *Public Health Nursing, 27*(2), 196–199. doi:10.1111/j.1525-1446.2010.00844.x

Kelly, K. K. (2011). Practice development in community nursing: Opportunities and challenges. *Nursing Standard, 10*(52), 38–44.

Markham, T., & Carney, M. (2007). Public health nurses and the delivery of quality nursing care in the community. *Journal of Clinical Nursing 17*(10), 1342–1350. doi:10.1111/j.1365-2702.2006.01894.x

Riner, M. E. (2013). Globally engaged nursing education with local immigrant populations. *Public Health Nursing, 30*(3), 246–253. doi:10.1111/phn.12026

Chapter 2

Agency for Healthcare Research and Quality. Database of evidence reports. http://www.ahrq.gov/legacy/clinic/epcindex.htm#prep

Centers for Disease Control and Prevention (CDC). Stacks—Repository of public health research and recommendations. http://stacks.cdc.gov

The Cochrane Library. (n.d.). International database of systematic reviews owned by the Cochrane Collaboration. http://www.thecochranelibrary.com/view/0/index.html

College of Community Health Sciences, the University of Alabama. (n.d.). Evidence-Based Public Health Internet Resources. http://cchs.ua.edu/library/public-health-resources/evidence-based-public-health-internet-resources

Evidence-Based Project for Public Health Practice. (n.d.). Evidence-based resources for public health practice (annotated listing of 13 database resources). Lamar Soutter Library, UMass Medical School. http://library.umassmed.edu/ebpph/ebresources.pdf

Home Visiting Evidence of Effectiveness (HOMVEE). (n.d.). Discussion of models and programs, whether they meet Department of Health and Human Services (DHHS) criteria, the target population, and whether research shows positive effectiveness. http://homvee.acf.hhs.gov/programs.aspx

National Institutes of Health. Guidelines for evaluating web-based health resources. http://nccam.nih.gov/health/webresources

New York Department of Health. (n.d.). Prevention agenda toward the healthiest state—Evidence-based public health. http://www.health.ny.gov/prevention/prevention_agenda/evidence_based_public_health.htm

Southern Cross University Library Guides. (n.d.). Public health—Guides for EBP databases and Cochrane Library tutorials. http://libguides.scu.edu.au/content.php?pid=90595&sid=674679

Evidence-Based Practice Videos and Tutorials

Cousineau, R. (n.d.). Why we need evidence-based health care. U.S. Department of Veterans Affairs. http://www.youtube.com/watch?v=OeA_OKqqBJ4

Melnyk, B. (n.d.). Healthcare needs to be evidence-based. Ohio State University. http://www.youtube.com/watch?v=MXEiRBJJKlk

Duke Medical Library. (n.d.). Introduction to evidence-based practice. http://guides.mclibrary.duke.edu/content.php?pid=431451&sid=3529499

My Source for Public Health, University of South Carolina. (n.d.). Framework for evidence-based public health. http://www.youtube.com/watch?v=_etctHCE1To

San Jose State University. (n.d.). Evidence-based practice—Nursing. http://www.youtube.com/watch?v=h7-b9Z6eNms

University of Minnesota, Health Sciences Library. (n.d.). Evidence-based practice. http://hsl.lib.umn.edu/learn/ebp/mod01/index.html

Journal Articles

Bigbee, J. L., & Issel, M. (2012). Conceptual models for population-focused public health nursing interventions and outcomes: The state of the art. *Public Health Nursing, 29*(4), 370–379. doi:10.1111/j.1525-1446.2011.01006.x

Chan, R. J., & Wong, A. (2012). Guest editorial—Two decades of exceptional achievements: Does the evidence support nurses to favour Cochrane systematic reviews over other systematic reviews? *International Journal of Nursing Studies, 49*, 773–774.

Mays, G. P., & Hogg, R. A. (2012). Expanding delivery system research in public health settings: Lessons learned from practice-based research networks. *Journal of Public Health Management Practice, 18*(6), 485–498. doi:10.1097/PHH.0b013e31825f75c9

McDonald, L. (2001). Florence Nightingale and the early origins of evidence-based nursing. *Evidence-Based Nursing, 4*(3). http://ebn.bmj.com/content/4/3/68.full

Chapter 3

Community Assessment Online

Community Assessment Windshield Survey—Windshield Survey of Marinette, 2011, University of Wisconsin, Student Survey. http://www.youtube.com/watch?v=TGXMoQjXbUk

The Community Toolbox. (n.d.). Windshield and Walking Surveys. http://ctb.ku.edu/en/tablecontents/chapter3-section21-main.aspx

Windshield Survey—Saukville, 2010, University of Wisconsin, Student Survey. http://www.youtube.com/watch?v=FGFA3_gdTpY

Family Assessment: Genograms and Ecomaps

Genogram Tutorial. http://www.youtube.com/watch?v=m0u9Nqoca-Y

GenoPro. (n.d.). Introduction to the Genogram. http://www.genopro.com/genogram

Green, C. D. (n.d.). Tracing family traits using a genogram. http://broadcast.lds.org/elearning/FHD/Community/en/Community/Cynthia%20Doxey%20Green/Tracing_Family_Traits_Using_a_Genogram/Genograms.pdf

Naidoo, M. (n.d.). Family Systems: Genograms and Ecomaps. http://www.kznhealth.gov.za/family/pres13.pdf

Strong Bonds Fact Sheet—Simple Guide to Ecomaps. http://www.strongbonds.jss.org.au/workers/cultures/ecomaps.pdf

Public Health Nursing Practice and Process

Public Health Nursing Process and Documentation—County of Los Angeles, California. http://www. publichealth.lacounty.gov/phn/docs/Documentation12_02_08.pdf

Wisconsin's Public Health Nursing Practice Model—Linking Education and Practice for Excellence in Public Health Nursing Project (LEAP Project). http://videos.med.wisc.edu/videoInfo.php?videoid=3385

Public Health Nursing Stories

Case Study on Indoor Air Quality in Family With Young Children. http://www.medscape.com/viewarticle/718616_5

National Association of School Nurses Radio. http://www.nasn.org/Default.aspx?tabid=597

Nurse-Family Partnership Stories. http://www.nursefamilypartnership.org/nurses/stories-from-nurses

Public Health Nursing Stories. http://www.health.state.mn.us/divs/cfh/connect/index.cfm?article=phstories. categorysearch&qCategoryId=200029

Public Health Planning, Community Assessment, and Intervention Strategies

Community Preventive Services Task Force. (n.d.). The Guide to Community Preventive Services. http://www.thecommunityguide.org/index.html

Healthy People 2020. (n.d.). MAP-IT. Implementing Healthy People 2020. http://www.healthypeople. gov/2020/implement/MapIt.aspx

National Association of City and County Health Officials (NACCHO). (n.d.). A Strategic Approach to Community Health Improvement: Mobilizing for Action Through Planning and Partnership (MAPP)—Field Guide. http://www.naccho.org/topics/infrastructure/mapp/upload/mapp_field_guide2.pdf

National Prevention, National Promotion, and Public Health Council. (2013). National Prevention Strategy—Annual Status Report 2013. http://www.surgeongeneral.gov/initiatives/prevention/2013-npc-status-report.pdf

Work Group for Community Health and Development. (n.d.). The Community Tool Box. University of Kansas. http://ctb.ku.edu/en/tablecontents/chapter_1002.aspx

Publications

Berger, K. S. (2014). *Invitation to the life span,* 2nd ed. New York, NY: Worth Publishers.

Langan, J. C., & James, D. C. (2005). *Preparing Nurses for Disaster Management.* Upper Saddle River, NJ: Pearson/Prentice Hall.

Lewenson, S. B., & Truglio-Londrigan, M. (2013). Public health nursing assessment tool. In M. Truglio-Londrigan, & S. B. Lewenson, *Public health nursing—Practicing population-based care,* pp. 67–101. Burlington, MA: Jones and Bartlett Learning.

Maxwell, M. I. (2014). *Understanding environmental health,* 2nd ed. Burlington, MA: Jones and Bartlett Learning.

Chapter 4

About John Snow: http://www.ph.ucla.edu/epi/snow.html

Agency for Healthcare Research and Quality Home Page (AHRQ): http://www.ahrq.gov

Balshem, M. (1993). *Cancer in the community: Class and medical authority.* Washington, DC: Smithsonian Institution Press.

Brooks, G. (2001). *Year of wonders: A novel of the plague.* London, UK: Penguin Books.

California Department of Public Health Network for a Healthy California GIS Map Viewer: http://www.cnngis.org

CDC Wonder: http://wonder.cdc.gov

Census Bureau Home Page: http://www.census.gov

Centers for Disease Control and Prevention (CDC): http://www.cdc.gov

Epidemiology and Disease Control Program—Maryland Department of Health: http://edcp.org

Epidemiology Data Center: http://www.edc.gsph.pitt.edu

Fed Stats: http://www.fedstats.gov

Indian Health Service (HIS): http://www.ihs.gov

Maternal and Child Health Bureau. Life course resources: http://mchb.hrsa.gov/lifecourseresources.htm

National Center for Health Statistics: http://www.cdc.gov/nchs

National Institute of Nursing Research (NINR): http://www.ninr.nih.gov

Pan American Health Organization (PAHO): http://new.paho.org

Population Reference Bureau: http://www.prb.org

Resources for Creating Public Health Maps: http://www.cdc.gov/epiinfo/maps.htm

U.S. Environmental Protection Agency (EPA): http://www.epa.gov

U.S. Health Resources and Services Administration (HRSA): http://www.hrsa.gov/index.html

Chapter 5

Community-Campus Partnerships for Health (CCPH). *A nonprofit organization that promotes health (broadly defined) through partnerships between communities and higher educational institutions. CCPH has many resources for partnership development.* http://www.ccph.info

Community Tool Box. Identifying community assets and resources. (2009). University of Kansas: Work Group for Community Health and Development. http://ctb.ku.edu/en/tablecontents/sub_section_main_1043.htm

Core Competencies for Interprofessional Collaborative Practice. (2011). Interprofessional Education Collaborative. http://www.aacn.nche.edu/education-resources/ipecreport.pdf

Grant R. W., Finnocchio, L. J, & the California Primary Care Consortium Subcommittee on Interdisciplinary Collaboration (1995). Common barriers to interprofessional team work. In *Interdisciplinary Collaborative Teams in Primary Care: A Model Curriculum and Resource Guide.* San Francisco, CA: Pew Health Professions Commission. Retrieved from http://www.med.mun.ca/getdoc/5662c96a-7a26-4fcf-b19c-ccb806a5df44/Common-barriers-to-interprofessional-healthcare-te.aspx

Lasker, R. D., & Guidry, J. A. (2009). Engaging the community in decision making: Case studies in tracking participation, voice and influence. Jefferson, NC: McFarland and Company, Inc. http://www.mcfarlandpub.com

Narsavage, G., & Lindell, D. (2001). Community engagement through service learning manual. Fort Collins, CO: Case Western Reserve University & Frances Payne Bolton School of Nursing. http://depts.washington.edu/ccph/pdf_files/CETSLmanual4.pdf

Public Health Interventions—Applications for Public Health Nursing Practice. St. Paul: Minnesota Department of Health. (2001). (Collaboration is located on pp. 177–210.) http://www.health.state.mn.us/divs/cfh/ophp/resources/docs/phinterventions_manual2001.pdf

Reilly, J. R. (2011). Spread the word, not the germs: A toolkit for faith communities. *Journal of Christian Nursing, 28*(4), 205–211. A voluntary workgroup of public health personnel and parish nurses in Wisconsin collaborated to develop the Infection Control and Emergency Preparedness Toolkit for the Faith Community.

World Health Organization. (2010). Framework for action on interprofessional education and collaborative practice. http://whqlibdoc.who.int/hq/2010/WHO_HRH_HPN_10.3_eng.pdf

Chapter 6

Affordable Care Act

Health Care Reform Hits Main Street (video): http://kff.org/health-reform/video/health-reform-hits-main-street

Centers for Disease Control (CDC)

Government website with health statistics and evidence for public health interventions: http://www.cdc.gov

Confidentiality

The Health Insurance Portability and Accountability Act of 1996 (HIPAA) Privacy and Security Rules: http://www.hhs.gov/ocr/privacy

Emergency Preparedness

http://emergency.cdc.gov/planning/

International Nursing Coalition for Mass Casualty Education—*Nursing Curriculum for Emergency Preparedness*. The five Learning Modules are at http://webapps.nursing.vanderbilt.edu/incmcemodules2/main.html#progress

Module 1: Tipping Point

Module 2: Incident Management System

Module 3: Biological

Module 4: Radiological

Module 5: Nuclear

Natural Disasters and Severe Weather

http://emergency.cdc.gov/disasters/

Nurses on the Front Line: Preparing for Emergencies and Disasters. The National Nurse Emergency Preparedness Initiative (NNEPI). http://nnepi.gwnursing.org. Emergency preparedness is a required outcome for BSN graduates. This online course offered free through George Washington University and sponsored by the Department of Homeland Security will help you to meet this BSN outcome. It takes about 6 hours to complete.

Floods

Katrina "Nature at its worst. Nursing at its best" (YouTube video). http://www.youtube.com/watch?v=JPSbDq2NjDg&feature=channel

Minnesota Department of Health. (2010). Floods: Caring for yourself. Retrieved http://www.health.state.mn.us/divs/eh/emergency/natural/floods/selfcare.html

Minnesota Department of Health. (2010). Floods: Protecting your health. http://www.health.state.mn.us/divs/eh/emergency/natural/floods/index.html

Minnesota Department of Health. (2010). Information and guidelines for healthcare facilities and providers in the event of spring flooding or other natural disasters. http://www.health.state.mn.us/divs/fpc/profinfo/ib10_2.html

Influenza Information

Information and resources for individuals, families, and professionals about influenza. www.flu.gov

Resources about immunization for nurses. American Nurses Association. ANA immunize. www.anaimmunize.org

Nutrition Policy for School Children

Centers for Disease Control and Prevention. (2008). Make a difference at your school: Key strategies to prevent obesity. http://www.cdc.gov/HealthyYouth/KeyStrategies

Centers for Disease Control and Prevention. (2013). Competitive Foods in School. http://www.cdc.gov/healthyyouth/nutrition/standards.htm

Robert Wood Johnson Foundation. (2009). Improving child nutrition policy: Insights from national USDA study of school food environments. http://www.rwjf.org/content/dam/web-assets/2009/02/improving-child-nutrition-policy

U.S. Department of Agriculture, Food and Nutrition Service. (2013). Nutrition Standards for School Meals. http://www.fns.usda.gov/cnd/governance/legislation/nutritionstandards.htm

U.S. Department of Agriculture, Food and Nutrition Service. (2013). Nutrition education. http://www.fns.usda.gov/fns/nutrition.htm

U.S. Department of Health and Human Services. (2013). Dietary guidelines for Americans. http://www.health.gov/dietaryguidelines

Public Health Law

The Network for Public Health Law: http://www.networkforphl.org

Reducing Youth Access to Tobacco

Centers for Disease Control. (2013). Youth tobacco prevention. http://www.cdc.gov/tobacco/youth

Minnesota Department of Health. (2013). Youth Tobacco Prevention. http://www.health.state.mn.us/divs/hpcd/tpc/youth

Minnesota Department of Health. (2013). Youth Tobacco Reports. http://www.health.state.mn.us/divs/chs/tobacco/youth.html

Chapter 7

Confidentiality

The Health Insurance Portability and Accountability Act of 1996 (HIPAA) Privacy and Security Rules. Retrieved from http://www.hhs.gov/ocr/privacy

Delegation

American Nurses Association. (2012). *Principles for Delegation by Registered Nurses to Unlicensed Assistive Personnel (UAP)*. Silver Spring, MD: Author.

National Council of State Boards of Nursing and American Nurses Association. Joint Statement on Delegation. (2006). Retrieved from https://www.ncsbn.org/Delegation_joint_statement_NCSBN-ANA.pdf

Ethics Resources

American Nurses Association. The Center for Ethics and Human Rights. Code of Ethics, Genetics and Genomics, ANA Positions on Ethics and Human Rights. Retrieved from http://nursingworld.org/MainMenuCategories/EthicsStandards/Ethics-Position-Statements.aspx

American Nurses Association. Code of Ethics for Nurses. Retrieved from http://www.nursingworld.org/MainMenuCategories/EthicsStandards/CodeofEthicsforNurses.aspx

Fowler, M. D. M. (Ed.). (2008). *Guide to the code of ethics for nurses: Interpretation and application*. Silver Springs, MD: American Nurses Association.

North Carolina Institute for Public Health. Offers a short course on ethics—offers questions about ethics in public health. Retrieved from http://oce.sph.unc.edu/phethics

Nursing Ethics (journal). Retrieved from http://nej.sagepub.com

Professional Boundaries

Professional Boundaries: A Nurse's Guide to the Importance of Professional Boundaries. National Council of State Boards of Nursing. Retrieved from https://www.ncsbn.org/Professional_Boundaries_2007_Web.pdf

Chapter 8

Email Communication

Effective email communication. University of North Carolina at Chapel Hill Writing Center. http://writingcenter.unc.edu/files/2012/09/Effective-E-mail-Communication-The-Writing-Center.pdf

Netiquette guidelines for ethical and respectful online communication. http://www.albion.com/netiquette

Health Communication and Social Marketing

Gateway to Health Communication & Social Marketing Practice. Access resources to help build health communication or social marketing campaigns and programs. http://www.cdc.gov/healthcommunication

Using Social Media

Centers for Disease Control and Prevention. (2011). The health communicator's guide to social media toolkit. Atlanta, GA: Author. Retrieved from http://www.cdc.gov/healthcommunication/ToolsTemplates/SocialMediaToolkit_BM.pdf

National Council of State Boards of Nursing. (2011, August). *White Paper: A nurse's guide to the use of social media.* Chicago, IL: Author. Retrieved from https://www.ncsbn.org/Social_Media.pdf

Social Media: A Guide for Researchers: Links and Resources. Research Information Network. http://www.rin.ac.uk/system/files/attachments/links_and_resources_0.pdf

Social Media Guidelines for Nurses (video). National Council of State Boards of Nursing website. https://www.ncsbn.org/3493.htm

General Health Information

Online Source for Health Information. Centers for Disease Control and Prevention. (2010). Health and safety topics. http://www.cdc.gov

Health Literacy

Health Literacy: Accurate, Accessible and Actionable Health Information for All. Centers for Disease Control website – access health literacy activities by state. http://www.cdc.gov/healthliteracy/

Improving Communication from the Federal Government to the Public. www.plainlanguage.gov

Simply Put: A Guide for Creating Easy-To-Understand Materials (2009). Centers for Disease Control and Prevention. http://www.cdc.gov/healthcommunication/toolstemplates/simply_put_082010.pdf

What We Know About Health Literacy. (2009). Centers for Disease Control. http://www.cdc.gov/health-communication/toolstemplates/healthliteracy.pdf

Motivational Interviewing

Behavior Change Counseling Index (BECCI)—Tool for evaluating practitioner competence in use of behavior change counseling skills. You can find the tool here: Pfister-Minogue, K. A., & Salveson, C. (2010). Training and experience of public health nurses in using behavior change counseling. *Public Health Nursing, 27*(6), 544–551. doi:10.1111/j.1525-1446.2010.00884.x

Health Promotion Topics

(These are only some examples. You will find many more topics on the CDC's website.)

Adolescent and School Health

Centers for Disease Control and Prevention—tools, curriculum, statistics. http://www.cdc.gov/HealthyYouth/index.htm

Flu Vaccine

Centers for Disease Control and Preventiuon. Public and Prevention Service Message

YouTube Video: Why Flu Matters: Personal Stories From Families Affected by Influenza (for parents). http://www.youtube.com/user/cdcflu

Handwashing

Hand hygiene print materials, signs, posters, brochures, manuals, curricula, and other hand hygiene materials that you can print and use. http://www.health.state.mn.us/handhygiene/materials.html

Oral Health

Guidelines, assessment tools, anticipatory guidance, posters, and public education materials. http://www.mchoralhealth.org/Toolbox/professionals.html

Minnesota Department of Health Child and Teen Checkups—Five modules. http://www.health.state.mn.us/divs/fh/mch/webcourse/dental/index.cfm

Physical Activity

Blue Cross Blue Shield of Minnesota "Do" Campaign. **Do** is based on a simple idea: By moving your body each day, you can improve your overall health and reduce your risk of heart disease, stroke, diabetes, and other illnesses. The *do* physical activity campaign was developed by Blue Cross and Blue Shield of Minnesota, based on guidelines set by the Centers for Disease Control and Prevention and the American Heart Association. http://www.do-groove.com

Tobacco Prevention and Control

North Carolina Division of Public Health. Provides information on preventing the initiation of smoking and other tobacco use, eliminating exposure to secondhand smoke, helping tobacco users quit, and addressing tobacco-related health disparities. http://www.tobaccopreventionandcontrol.ncdhhs.gov/

Chapter 9

Relationship Building

Henry Street Settlement: http://www.henrystreet.org/site/PageServer?pagename=abt_lwald

Jewish Women's Archives: http://jwa.org/historymakers/wald

Visiting Nurse Service of New York: http://www.vnsny.org/community/our-history/lillian-wald

Working Nurse: http://www.workingnurse.com/articles/Lillian-Wald-Founded-Public-Health-Nursing

Caring Relationships

Anderson, M., & Braun. J. (1995). *Caring for the elderly client*. Philadelphia, PA: F. A. Davis Company.

MacKay, R., Hughes, J., & Carver, E. (Eds.). (1989). *Empathy in the helping relationship*. New York, NY: Springer.

Chapter 10

Online Resources

Advocacy and Initiatives

American Nurses Association—Practice standards, position papers, and publications. http://www.nursingworld.org

American Public Health Association—Position papers. http://www.apha.org

Health in Mind: Improving Education Through Wellness. http://bit.ly/13DpNBv

Human Rights Watch. http://www.hrw.org

International Council of Nurses—Practice standards and position papers. http://www.icn.ch/

Kaiser Foundation—Health policy explained. http://www.KaiserEDU.org

National Association of Free and Charitable Clinics. http://www.nafcclinics.org

National Center for Cultural Competence—Cultural assessment and intervention tools. http://nccc.georgetown.edu/resources/assessments.html

National Partnership for Action to End Health Disparities. http://minorityhealth.hhs.gov/npa/templates/browse.aspx?lvl=1&lvlid=13

National Association of County and City Health Officials: Public Health Advocacy. http://www.naccho.org/advocacy

Nursing in America: A History of Social Reform. http://www.youtube.com/watch?v=dI4IFqHx1zA

The Provider's Guide to Quality and Culture. http://erc.msh.org/mainpage.cfm?file=1.0.htm&module=provider&language=english

Think Cultural Health: Advancing Health Equity at Every Point of Contact. https://www.thinkculturalhealth.hhs.gov

Unnatural Causes: Is Inequality Making Us Sick?—Social determinants of health. http://www.unnaturalcauses.org

Global Health

Gapminder. http://www.gapminder.org

Global Health Equity. http://www.youtube.com/watch?v=pzW7lQ9asRQ

Global Health: Health as a Human Right. http://www.youtube.com/watch?v=0hkhJxXMiDo

Global Health Watch. http://www.ghwatch.org

United Nations Foundation. http://unfoundation.org

United Nations: Millennium Development Goals and Beyond 2015. http://www.un.org/millenniumgoals

World Health Organization. http://www.who.int/en

Health Disparities

Centers for Disease Control and Prevention

  Morbidity and Mortality Weekly Report: Health Disparities and Inequalities Report: United States, 2011. http://www.cdc.gov/mmwr/pdf/other/su6001.pdf

  Minority Health. http://www.cdc.gov/minorityhealth

Fair Society, Healthy Lives—Yale University presentation   http://www.youtube.com/watch?v=FF2SV-VfaC0

Health Disparities. http://www.youtube.com/watch?v=FGeRg8_5TYo

Healthy People 2020. http://www.healthypeople.gov/2020

Institute of Medicine Reports—Search term "health disparities." http://www.iom.edu/Reports.aspx

Kids Count—State-by-state infant mortality data. http://datacenter.kidscount.org/data/tables/6051-infant-mortality?loc=1&loct=2#ranking/2/any/true/133/any/12719

Office of Minority Health's Knowledge Center Library Catalog. http://www.Minorityhealth.hhs.gov/templates/opac.aspx

Robert Wood Johnson Foundation

  Finding Answers: Disparities Research for Change. http://www.solvingdisparities.org/about

    Health Disparities. http://www.rwjf.org/en/search-results.html?u=&k=health+disparities

  The Health Equity Assessment Tool: A User's Guide. http://www.pha.org.nz/documents/health-equity-assessment-tool-guide1.pdf

Surgeon General's Reports—Search term "health disparities." http://www.surgeongeneral.gov/library

Social Determinants of Health

Framing Social Determinants of Health in Kent County. http://www.youtube.com/watch?v=xSPyjzJbqRw

Robert Wood Johnson Foundation

  Social Determinants of Health. http://www.rwjf.org/en/topics/search-topics/S/social-determinants-of-health.html

Social Determinants of Health—Three videos. http://www.youtube.com/watch?v=XgZyB3rwMRs&list=PLF3C4B4D0BE1708C0

The Social Determinants of Health. http://www.youtube.com/watch?v=IZZA4SSHm1k

Social Determinants of Health HKR 3400—Student-created video. http://www.youtube.com/watch?v=2yU_62aWU9A

Unnatural Causes 2. http://www.youtube.com/watch?v=RVMyunin5H8

What's Your Health Code? http://www.youtube.com/watch?v=DtLGXrxA8wk

Publications

American Nurses Association (ANA). (2010). Position statement: The nurse's role in ethics and human rights: Protecting and promoting individual worth, dignity, and human rights in the practice setting. Retrieved from ANA website: http://www.nursingworld.org/MainMenuCategories/EthicsStandards/Ethics-Position-Statements/-Nursess-Role-in-Ethics-and-Human-Rights.pdf

Benatar, S. R., Gill, S., & Bakker, I. (2011). Global health and the global economic crisis. *American Journal of Public Health, 101*(4), 646–653. doi:10.2105/AJPH.2009.188458

Donahoe, M. T. (2013). *Public health and social justice.* San Francisco, CA: John Wiley & Sons, Inc.

Fahrenwald, N. L. (2003). Teaching social justice. *Nurse Educator, 28*(5), 222–226.

Falk-Rafael, A. (2006). Globalization and global health: Toward nursing praxis in the global community. Advances in

Nursing Science, 29(1), 2–14.Hilfinger Messias, D. K. (2001). Globalization, nursing, and health for all. *Journal of Nursing Scholarship, 33*(1), 9–11.

Ivanov, L. L., & Oden, T. L. (2013). Public health nursing, ethics and human rights. *Public Health Nursing, 30*(3), 231–238. doi:10.1111/phn.12022

Lashley, M. (2007). Nurses on a mission: A professional service learning experience with inner-city homeless. *Nursing Education Perspectives, 28*(1), 24–26.

Ramal, E. (2008). Integrating caring, scholarship, and community engagement in Mexico. *Nurse Educator, 34*(1), 34–37.

Chapter 11

Bridges out of Poverty (Note that this presents examples at the individual level primarily.) A curriculum and a DVD series provide communities with strategies to address poverty. YouTube link for the DVD series: http://www.youtube.com/watch?v=G_8F7XQSX4Y

Lipson, J. G., & Dibble, S. L. (Eds.). (2005). *Culture and clinical care.* San Francisco, CA: UCSF Nursing Press.

O'Connor, A. (2001). *Poverty knowledge: Social science, social policy, and the poor in twentieth-century u.s. history* (Politics and Society in Twentieth-Century America). Princeton, NJ: Princeton University Press.

Pipher, M. (2002). *The middle of everywhere.* San Diego, CA: Harcourt, Inc. (Helping refugees enter the American community)

Rosenberg, M. (2003). *Nonviolent communication.* Encinitas, CA: Puddledancer Press.

Strachan, D. (2006). *Making questions work.* San Francisco, CA: Jossey-Bass.

Unnatural Causes DVD series: http://www.unnaturalcauses.org

Whitney, D. (2010). *The power of appreciative inquiry.* San Francisco, CA: Berrett-Koehler Publishers.

Chapter 12

American Association of Poison Control Centers. http://www.aapcc.org/dnn/default.aspx

Centers for Disease Control and Prevention (CDC). http://www.cdc.gov

Child Development Screening Instruments. Ages and Stages and the ESI-R: http://www.health.state.mn.us/divs/fh/mch/devscrn/glance.html

Environmental Pollution Agency (EPA)—Indoor Air Quality for Schools. http://www.epa.gov/iaq/schools/toolkit.html

EPA—Healthy School Environments. http://www.epa.gov/schools/

Health Care Without Harm. http://www.noharm.org

Home Safety Council. http://www.homesafetycouncil.org

Immunization Action Coalition. http://www.immunize.org

Kids Health. http://kidshealth.org

NCAST programs include screening tools used in public health nursing practice to assess the relationship and bonding between mother/parent and infant/child. http://www.ncast.org/index.cfm?category=2

Pediatric Home Assessment Tool for asthma. http://www.healthyhomestraining.org/Nurse/PEHA.htm

Solchany, J. E. (2001). *Promoting maternal mental health during pregnancy.* Seattle, WA: University of Washington, NCAST Programs.

Chapter 13

Online Resources

Alliance of Young Nurse Leaders and Advocates. http://www.aynla.org

American Nurses Association, Leadership and Leadership Institute. http://www.nursingworld.org/MainMenuCategories/ThePracticeofProfessionalNursing/Leadership

Robert Wood Johnson Foundation—Leadership resources—Webinars: http://www.rwjfleaders.org/resources

United Nations Millennium Development Goals. http://mdgs.un.org/unsd/mdg/Default.aspx

Online Videos and Tutorials

25 Most Famous Nurses in History. http://onlinebsn.org/2009/25-most-famous-nurses-in-history/

Colin Powell's 13 Rules of Leadership. http://www.youtube.com/watch?v=C-vve55FDaU&feature=related

Katrina—Nature at its worst. Nursing at its best. http://www.youtube.com/watch?v=JPSbDq2NjDg&feature=channel

Nursing Empowerment. http://www.youtube.com/watch?v=lzjbe7ZOCKk&feature=related

Regina Clark—7 Cs of Leadership on YouTube. http://www.youtube.com/watch?v=dACu_ucghuA

The Ten Most Influential Nurses in History. http://health.howstuffworks.com/medicine/healthcare/10-most-famous-nurses-in-history.htm

Publications

Dickenson-Hazard, N. (2008). *Ready, set, go lead!* Indianapolis, IN: Sigma Theta Tau International.

Gebbie, K. M., Wakefield, M., & Kerfoot, K. (2000). Nursing and health policy. *Journal of Nursing Scholarship, 32*(3), 307–315.

George, B. (2003). *Authentic leadership: Rediscovering the secrets to creating lasting value.* San Francisco: Jossey-Bass/Wiley.

Hansen-Turton, T., Sherman, S., & Ferguson, V. (2009). *Conversations with leaders: Frank Talk from nurses (and others) on the frontlines of leadership.* Indianapolis, IN: Nursing Knowledge International.

Houser, B. P., & Player, K. (2007). *Pivotal Moments in Nursing: Leaders who changed the path of a profession,* Vol. 1. Indianapolis, IN: Sigma Theta Tau International, Center for Nursing Press.

Houser, B. P., & Player, K. (2010). *Pivotal moments in nursing: Leaders who changed the path of a profession,* Vol. 2. Indianapolis, IN: Sigma Theta Tau International.

Maxwell, J. C. (2005). *The 21 irrefutable laws of leadership: Follow them and people will follow you.* Nashville, TN: Thomas Nelson Books.

Robert Wood Johnson Foundation. (n.d.). Strengthening public health nursing—Part II: How nurse leaders in policy making positions are transforming public health nursing. *Charting Nursing's Future,* 1–8. Retrieved from http://www.rwjf.org/content/dam/farm/reports/issue_briefs/2008/rwjf32669

Comparison of Henry Street Entry-Level PHN Competencies to Other Public Health Practice Frameworks

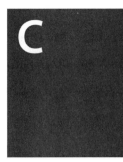

Entry-Level Population-Based PHN Competencies Henry Street Consortium, 2003 *11 Competencies*	Core Competencies for Public Health Professionals Council on Linkages, 2001; QUAD Council [ANA, APHA, ACHNE, ASTDN] Competencies, 2003 *18 Domains*	Scope and Standards of Public Health Nursing American Nurses Association, 2007 *6 Standards of Care; 8 Standards of Professional Performance*	Essential Public Health Services Core Public Health Functions Steering Committee, 1994 *10 Core Functions*
#1 Applies the public health nursing process to communities, systems, individuals, and families	• Analytic/Assessment Skills • Policy Development and Program Planning Skills • Cultural Competency Skills • Community Dimensions of Practice Skills	*Standards of Care* Assessment; Diagnosis; Outcome Identification; Planning; Assurance; Evaluation	• Monitor Health • Diagnose and Investigate • Inform, Educate, and Empower • Link to/Provide Care • Evaluate • System Management and Research
#2 Utilizes basic epidemiological principles (the incidence, distribution, and control of disease in a population) in public health nursing practice	• Analytic/Assessment Skills • Community Dimensions of Practice Skills • Basic Public Health Sciences Skills	*Standards of Care* Assessment; Diagnosis; Outcome Identification; Planning; Assurance; Evaluation	• Diagnose and Investigate

Entry-Level Population-Based PHN Competencies Henry Street Consortium, 2003 *11 Competencies*	Core Competencies for Public Health Professionals Council on Linkages, 2001; QUAD Council [ANA, APHA, ACHNE, ASTDN] Competencies, 2003 *18 Domains*	Scope and Standards of Public Health Nursing American Nurses Association, 2007 *6 Standards of Care; 8 Standards of Professional Performance*	Essential Public Health Services Core Public Health Functions Steering Committee, 1994 *10 Core Functions*
#3 Utilizes collaboration to achieve public health goals	• Communication Skills • Leadership and Systems Thinking Skills	Collaboration Collegiality	• Mobilize Community Partnerships • Link to/Provide Care
#4 Works within the responsibility and authority of the governmental public health system	• Policy Development and Program Planning Skills • Cultural Competency Skills • Community Dimensions of Practice Skills • Financial Planning and Management Skills • Leadership and Systems Thinking Skills	Quality of Care Performance Appraisal Resource Utilization	• Develop Policies • Enforce Laws
#5 Practices public health nursing within the auspices of the Nurse Practice Act	• Analytic/Assessment Skills • Policy Development and Program Planning Skills • Community Dimensions of Practice Skills	*Standards of Care* Assessment; Diagnosis; Outcome Identification; Planning; Assurance; Evaluation	• Assure Competent Workforce
#6 Effectively communicates with communities, systems, individuals, families and colleagues	• Communication Skills • Cultural Competency Skills • Financial Planning and Management Skills	Education	• Link to/Provide Care

Entry-Level Population-Based PHN Competencies Henry Street Consortium, 2003 *11 Competencies*	Core Competencies for Public Health Professionals Council on Linkages, 2001; QUAD Council [ANA, APHA, ACHNE, ASTDN] Competencies, 2003 *18 Domains*	Scope and Standards of Public Health Nursing American Nurses Association, 2007 *6 Standards of Care; 8 Standards of Professional Performance*	Essential Public Health Services Core Public Health Functions Steering Committee, 1994 *10 Core Functions*
#7 Establishes and maintains caring relationships with communities, systems, individuals, and families	• Communication Skills • Cultural Competency Skill • Leadership and Systems Thinking Skills	Quality of care Education Ethics	• Inform, Educate, and Empower • Mobilize Community Partnerships • Link to/Provide Care
#8 Shows evidence of commitment to social justice, the greater good, and the public health principles	• Analytic/Assessment Skills • Communication Skills • Leadership and Systems Thinking Skills	Quality of Care Ethics	• Inform, Educate, and Empower • Mobilize Community Partnerships • Develop Policies
#9 Demonstrates nonjudgmental and unconditional acceptance of people different from self	• Communication Skills • Cultural Competency Skills • Leadership and Systems Thinking Skills	Ethics	• Inform, Educate, and Empower • Mobilize Community Partnerships
#10 Incorporates mental, physical, emotional, social, spiritual, and environmental aspects of health into assessment, planning, implementation, and evaluation	• Analytic/Assessment Skills • Cultural Competency Skills	*Standards of Care* Assessment; Diagnosis; Outcome Identification; Planning; Assurance; Evaluation	• Inform, Educate, and Empower • Link to/Provide Care

Entry-Level Population-Based PHN Competencies Henry Street Consortium, 2003 *11 Competencies*	Core Competencies for Public Health Professionals Council on Linkages, 2001; QUAD Council [ANA, APHA, ACHNE, ASTDN] Competencies, 2003 *18 Domains*	Scope and Standards of Public Health Nursing American Nurses Association, 2007 *6 Standards of Care; 8 Standards of Professional Performance*	Essential Public Health Services Core Public Health Functions Steering Committee, 1994 *10 Core Functions*
#11 Demonstrates leadership	• Policy Development and Program Planning Skills • Communication Skills • Community Dimensions of Practice Skills • Financial Planning and Management Skills • Leadership and Systems Thinking Skills	Quality of Care Performance Appraisal Education Collegiality Ethics Collaboration Resource Utilization	• Mobilize Community Partnerships • Develop Policies • Assure Competent Workforce

Index

acceptance of others
   community, 317–318, 322
   definition of, 308
   individual/family, 316–317, 322
   intra-agency, 320–321, 323
   promoting increase of, 325–326
   systems, 319–320, 322
Accountable Care Organization (ACO), 180
accreditation programs, 168
ACHNE (Association of Community Health Nurse
   Educators)
   curriculum core competencies, 10–11
   education requirements, 212
ACIP (Advisory Committee on Immunization Practice),
   98
ACO (Accountable Care Organization), 180
action stage, behavior change, 225
*Adapting Your Practice:General Recommendations for the
   Care of Homeless Patients,* 155
Advisory Committee on Immunization Practice (ACIP),
   98
advocacy
   community level, 292
   definition of, 274
   empowerment of clients about healthcare needs, 69
   in digital age, 299
   framework for empowerment of clients and self, 278
   individual/family level, 289–290
   systems level, 292
advocacy-based leadership, 358–360
   definition of, 354
   political process, 373–376
Affordable Care Act
   Accountable Care Organization (ACO), 180
   Cancer Registry, 181
   Electronic Laboratory Reporting (ELR), 180
   healthcare or Medical Home, 180
   Health Information Technology for Economic and
      Clinical Health (HITECH), 180–181

health insurance exchange, 180
Immunization Information Systems (IIS), 180
interoperable electronic health records (EHRs),
   180–181
key provisions
   health system reform, 179–180
   insurance reform, 179
National Prevention Strategy, 179–180
Syndromic Surveillance (SS), 180
age groups in U.S. population, 310
agents
   definition of, 112
   epidemiological triangle, 130–131
American Nurses Association (ANA)
   Code of Ethics, 275
   Cornerstones of Public Health Nursing, 9
   delegation of duties, 210
   leadership standards, 364
   Principles of Public Health Nursing Practice, 9
   public health nursing, threats to future of, 6
   Public Health Nursing: Scope and Standards of Practice
      credentials requirement, 212
      ethical accountability, 207–209
      nursing process, levels of practice, 34–35
      standards of performance, 175–176
      standards of practice (list), 12–13
American Public Health Association (APHA),
   375–376
America's Plan for Better Health and Wellness,
   179–180
ANA (American Nurses Association)
   Code of Ethics, 275
   Cornerstones of Public Health Nursing, 9
   delegation of duties, 210
   leadership standards, 364
   Principles of Public Health Nursing Practice, 9
   public health nursing, threats to future of, 6
   Public Health Nursing: Scope and Standards of Practice
      credentials requirement, 212
      ethical accountability, 207–209
      nursing process, levels of practice, 34–35

standards of performance, 175–176
standards of practice (list), 12–13
APHA (American Public Health Association),
    375–376
assessment, 21–22, 35, 331–333
    all levels of practice
        for intervention strategies, 338–339
        mental, physical, emotional, social, spiritual, and
            environmental health, 331–332
    community level of practice, 68, 81–90
        health determinants, 83–87
        health status analysis, 21–22, 87–89
        needs assessments *versus* asset mapping, 152
        relationship with health department programs, 117
        subpopulations, 91–92
        vital signs of population, 81
        windshield surveys, 89–90
    definition of, 330
    environmental health, 77
    ethical actions, 103, 347
    government agencies' core functions, 14–15
    individual/family level, 74–78
        basic family functions, 75
        definition of, 68
        environment, 77
        family characteristics, 74–77
        focused or problem-specific assessments, 78
    overview, 73–74, 331–333, 336–337
    safety checklists, elderly person, 333–335
    systems level, 338–339
        health priorities, identifying and setting, 93–95
        overview, 93
        population risk diagnosis, 95
asset mapping
    examples, 153–154
    versus needs assessments, 152
Association of Community Health Nurse Educators
    (ACHNE)
    curriculum core competencies, 10–11
    education requirements, 212
authentic leadership, 358
    definition of, 354
    ongoing challenges, 356

B

Bachelor of Science in Nursing (BSN) degrees, 10–11, 212
Behavior Change Counseling Index, 226
behavior health changes
    health determinants model, 22
    motivational interviewing, 225–226
    stages of, 224–225

best practices
    collaboration, 145
    definition of, 49–50
    evidence-based practice, 50–51
        PICOT approach to clinical problem solving,
            53–54, 56
    experimental research, 50
    interventions, 97–100
    in public health nursing, 50–51, 53–54
    RCT reviews, 50
biology, health determinants model, 22
bioterrorism planning, 348–349
BSN (Bachelor of Science in Nursing) degrees, 10–11, 212

C

Cancer Registry, 181
caring relationships
    with all levels of clients, 252–258
    characteristics of
        embodiment, 265
        empathy, 255–256
        empathy *versus* sympathy, 255–257
        engaged interactions, 265
        environment, 266
        follow-up with commitments, 259
        interactions and interventions, 252
        respect, 255, 265
        tact and diplomacy, 239–242, 263
        trust, 252–254
    definition of, 250–251
    maintenance of, 263–264
    Smith-Campbell Caring Community Model, 257–258
case management for interventions, 38
    all levels of clients, 42–43
    in other non-public health settings, 391
    scope of, 197–198
case studies
    delegation, 211
    fall prevention programs for the elderly, 43
    health determinants analysis, 23
    MVNA evidence-based practice in maternal/cihild
        health home visiting, 57–58
    Scope of Public Health Nursing Practice, 215
CDC (Centers for Disease Control and Prevention)
    CDC Stacks, 53
    Health Communicator's Social Media Toolkit, 227–228
    health disparities, 283
    immunization guidelines, 51
    increase in pertussis cases, 119–120
    Lyme disease data, 125
    online research, 53

child abuse
    example cases of, 378
    mandated reporting of, 172
CINAHL database, 52
civil commitment, public health law example, 172
civil engagement
    definition of, 274
    as social justice intervention, 293
clients, definition of, 4
clinical appraisals of literature, definition of, 34
Cochrane Database of Systematic Reviews, 50
Cochrane Library, 53
collaboration
    all levels of practice, 145
    among individuals and organizations, 142–143, 146,
        150
    best practices, 145
    definition of, 142
    ethical issues, 156–157
collective social responsibility, 275
Commission on the Social Determinants of Health, 280
communicable diseases/surveillance of
    communicability, definition of, 112
    local public health departments, 178
    mandated reporting of, 172
communication skills
    Behavior Change Counseling Index, 226
    behavior changes, stages of, 224–225
    ethical issues, 236–237
    Health Communicator's Social Media Toolkit, 227–228
    importance of, 222–224
    information
        free content creation tools, 234
        Internet distribution, 233–234
        interpretation of, 226–227
        text messaging, 235
        writing tips, 229–230
    listening in unbiased manner, 311–312
    motivational interviewing, strategies, 225–226
    real-time communications, advocacy for justice, 299
    social marketing, 230–232
        definition of, 222
        guidelines for effectiveness, 230–232
    social networking sites, 233
        interpersonal skills, 235–236
        Netiquette, 235
    teaching-learning principles, 228–229
        Teaching Plan template, 239–242
    verbal/nonverbal listening, 312
community assets
    asset mapping
        examples, 153–154
        versus needs assessments, 152

community-based participatory research (CBPR),
        154–155
    definition of, 142
    planning interventions, 151
    promotions with questions, 153
    strengths-based interventions, 151
community engagement
    as advocacy, 293–295
        community and systems levels, 295
    definition of, 274
community level of practice, 17–19, 68
    3 Es of PHNs, 69
    acceptance of others, 317–318, 322
    advocacy, 292
    assessment, 21–22, 68, 81–90
        determinants of health, 83–87
        health status analysis, 87–89
        for intervention strategies, 338–339
        mental, physical, emotional, social, spiritual, and
            environmental health, 331–332
        relationship with health department programs, 117
        subpopulations, 91–92
        vital signs of population, 81
        windshield surveys, 89–90
    definition of, 4, 17, 68
    epidemiological triangle, 130–133
    health determinants model, 21–22
    intervention levels, 43, 340
        best practices, 97–99
        effective interventions, 46
        goals, 99–100
        planning using community assets, 151
    nursing process, 25
    partnering with PHNs, 69, 149–150
    populations served
        population at risk, 17
        population of interest, 17
    prevention levels, 43
    protective and risk factors for childhood
        communicable diseases, 20–21
    relationships with individuals/families and systems,
        18–19
confidentiality
    definition of, 194
    establishing and maintaining, 206–207
    Health Insurance Portability and Accountability Act
        (HIPAA), 206
contemplation stage, behavior change, 225
Cornerstones of Public Health Nursing, public health
    nursing practice
    ANA principles of, 9
    key component of, 14
County Health Rankings & Roadmaps, 128–129

D

data collection and management
  electronic health records (EHRs), 70–71
    definition of, 68
    federal mandate concerning, 73
    importance of, 101
  ethical issues, 103
  graphs, showing trends, 121–123
  health and disease mysteries solutions, 113–115
  health information systems (HIS), 70–71, 101
  health statistical data, 71
  importance before interventions, 100–102
  information sources
    Healthy People 2020 website, 121
    national *versus* global sources, 125–126
    obtaining/interpreting, 121
    state *versus* national sources, 124–125
  innovative methods, 128–129
  Omaha System
    components, 70
    quality improvement strategy, 101
  population trends, 126–127
  risk ratios and odds ratios, 127–128
daycare center inspections, 178
delegation, definition of, 194
determinants of health. *See* health determinants
DHHS (Department of Health and Human Services). *See also* CDC; Healthy People program; HIPAA
  federal level of public health, 167
  Geographic Information System (GIS), promotion of quality of life and health, 129
  Medicare and Medicaid Services, 167
diagnosis in nursing process, 35
  components of, 78–79
  NANDA classification system, 78
  population risks, 95
Dietary Guidelines for Americans, 48
Directly Observed Therapy (DOT), 289
diversities in patients, 309
  unconditional acceptance of, 313–315
  of U.S. population, 310
DOT (Directly Observed Therapy), 289
downstream approach, reduction of health disparities, 287–288

E

EBSCO, CINAHL database, 52
egalitarian relationships with clients, 69

EHRs (electronic health records)
  local health departments, 178
  provisions of Affordable Care Act, 180–181
ELR (Electronic Laboratory Reporting), 180
emotional health interventions, 339–340
empathy, 255–256
  versus sympathy, 255–257
  unconditional acceptance of others, 314
empowerment of clients
  to advocate for and manage own healthcare needs, 69
  framework for, 278
environmental health
  assessment of, 77, 331–332
  caring relationships, 266
  definition of, 112, 330
  Environmental Quality LHIs, 80
  epidemiological triangle, 130–133
  interventions considering all types of health, 339–340, 348
  physical and social, 84–86
  surveillance by local public health departments, 178
epidemiological triangle. *See also* epidemiology/epidemiologists
  application for all clients, 130–133
  definition of, 112
  environment, 130–133
  hosts, 130–131
    definition of, 112
  life course epidemiology, 133
epidemiology/epidemiologists. *See also* epidemiological triangle
  definition of, 112
  epidemics, definition of, 112
  and public health nursing process
    activities and interventions, 115–117
    ethical actions, 134–135
  questions asked regularly, 113
  solving mysteries, 114–117
ethical issues
  acceptance of others, 323–324
  assessment activities, 103, 347
  bioethics perspective, 208
  caring relationships, 265–267
  collaboration, 156–157
  communication skills, 236–237
  data collection and management, 103
  epidemiological principles, 134–135
  evaluation, 347
  government health agencies, 183–184
  health disparities, 277
  immunizations for children, 183–184
  implementation, 347

interventions, 347
planning, 347
professional boundaries, 212–213
for social justice and advocacy, 296–298
types of ethics, 207–208
ethnic/racial groups in U.S. population, 310–311
evidence-based examples
    acceptance of others
        Interpreter Services and Healthcare Quality, 319
        Nurse-Mother Relationship—What Moms Want
            and Nurses Can Offer, 316
        Quantitatively Assessing Empathy, 317
    Advocating for All, 99
    assessment
        Elementary School Health Assessment, 91–92
        Holistic Public Health Nursing for the Family, 332
        Minnesota Department of Health Adverse
            Childhood Experiences (ACE) Project, 335
    asset mapping
        Partnership to Decrease Childhood Obesity., 154
        Promoting Healthy Eating Behaviors, 153–154
    Best Practice Evidence Leads to Pediculosis
        Management Guidelines, 55
    caring relationships
        Caring PHN-Family Relationships, 260
        Phases of Relationship Building, 253
        Public Health Nursing Practice With "High-
            Priority" Families: The Significance of
            Contextualizing "Risk," 254
        Theory of Maternal Engagement With PHNs, 253
        Welcome Intrusions: An Interpretive
            Phenomenological Study of TB Nurses'
            Relational Work, 259
    case management
        Case Management of Children in Foster Care, 197
        Hepatitis B Prevention in Case Management for
            Pregnant Women, 197
        PHN Prenatal Care Case Management, 342
    communication skills
        Delivering Public Health Interventions Through the
            Internet, 233
        Effectiveness of Motivational Interviewing, 226
        Presenting Data on Improving Walking Path Safety,
            227
    community-based participatory research (CBPR)
        Improving maternal and infant health in an
            African-American community, 154
        PhotoVoice as a CBPR method for influencing
            social change, 154–155
    confidentiality, Maintaining Boundaries and
        Confidentiality in Working With Families with
        Intimate Partner Violence, 206–207
    Ecosocial Framework Applied to Childhood Lead
        Poisoning, 132

effective communication skills, Developing
    Relationships, 223–224
Elementary School Health Assessment, 91–92
ethical issues, Ethical Problems in Public Health
    Nursing, 209
government health service delivery
    Action Plan for Asthma Management, 176
    Business Case for Breastfeeding, 176
    Mock Vaccination Exercise, 176
health disparities, Immunization Rates in Shelter-
    Based Foster Youth, 282
health priorities, Population Needs in a Rural/
    Suburban County, 94–95
Healthy People 2020 Goals, 97
interpersonal collaboration (IPC)
    Collaborating for Information Literacy, 147
    Collaborative Approach to Fall Prevention, 147
    Collaborative Response to Postpartum Depression,
        147
interventions
    Community-Based Holistic Care, 343
    Evidence for Home Visits With Mothers and
        Children, 345
    Health Department Partnerships to Prevent Obesity
        Among Cognitively Challenged Persons, 341–
        342
    Independent Practice of Public Health Nurses, 198
    In-Home Influenza Immunizations, 98
    PHN Home Visits to Elderly Clients, 345–346
    PHN Prenatal Care Case Management, 342
    Teen Parent Program, 102
    Use of Epidemiological Tuberculosis Data to Inform
        a New York State Corrections Intervention, 123
leadership
    Bringing About Social Change to Reduce Child
        Poverty, 369
    Organizational Attributes That Support Public
        Health Nursing Practice, 368
    PHN Student Initiative Demonstrates Leadership
        and Improves Population Health, 359–360
    Shared Leadership Enhances Nursing Care in a
        Homeless Center, 366
nonprofit organization resources, American Lung
    Association Open Airways for Schools, 181
Nurse Practice Act, Core Elements of U.S. Nurse
    Practice Acts, 195
nursing evaluations, Comparing Maternal Child
    Health Problems and Outcomes Across PHN
    Agencies, 101
nursing within child welfare systems, Independent
    Practice of Public Health Nurses, 198
Origins of Epidemiology and Nursing, 114
planning and implementation, Healthy People 2020
    Goals, 97

Population Needs in a Rural/Suburban County, 94–95
professional boundaries
    Caring PHN-Family Relationships, 260
    Defining Boundaries in Public Health Nursing, 205
    Maintaining Boundaries and Confidentiality in Working With Families with Intimate Partner Violence, 206–207
public health nursing practice, Nurse-Managed Health Clinics (NMHCs), 198
Screening for Neurodevelopmental Delays in Four Communities in Mexico and Cuba, 130
social determinants of health, Safe Motherhood Initiative, 281
social justice
    National Association of School Nurses: Speaking Up for Children, 293
    Social Justice and Human Rights Issues Identified by Practicing PHNs, 279
social marketing
    Breastfeeding on a Navajo Reservation, 232
    Stop Smoking in Schools Trial (ASSIST), 232
evidence-based practice
    acceptance of others
        community, 317–318, 322
        individual/family, 316–317, 322
        intra-agency, 320–321, 323
        systems, 319–320, 322
    best practices, 50–51
    database and Internet searches, 52–53
    definition of, 34
    education, 47–48
    interventions, 45–47
    Johns Hopkins Nursing Evidence-Based Practice Model, 47–48
    PICOT approach to clinical problem solving, 53–54, 56
    practice, 47–48
    problem-solving process, 44–45
    questions for articles/other publications, 55
        research- and non-research-based literature, 55
    research, 47–48, 51–52
    translating evidence into practice, 56
experimental research, best practices, 50

Facebook, 233
    advocacy for justice, 299
    public health interventions, 233
federal health departments. *See also* government health agencies
    definition of responsibilities, 167
    H1N1 flu clinic, example
        coordination with state and federal, 168
        essential services, 170–171

feminist ethics in nursing process
    acceptance of others, 324
    assessment activities, 103, 347
    caring relationships, 267
    collaboration, 157
    communication skills, 237
    epidemiological principles, 134
    immunizations for children, 184
    leadership, 377
    professional accountability, 207–208
    professional boundaries, 213
    for social justice and advocacy, 298
food-safety education, 178
food service establishment inspections, 178
foreign-born in U.S. population, 310
funding streams, definition of, 166

GIS (Geographic Information System)
    County Health Rankings & Roadmaps, 128–129
    Lyme disease data, 124
global public health
    cross-border health risks, attention to, 6
    versus public health, 6
    status measures, 81
government health agencies. *See also* federal, state, and local health departments; public health departments
    accreditation programs, 168
    coordination between agencies, example, 168
    core functions, 14–15
    delivery of services, examples, 176
    ethical issues, 183–184
    funding streams, 177
    human rights responsibilities, 275
    legal issues
        data privacy, 182–183
        mandated reporting, 183
        school-entry laws, 183

H

Healthcare or Medical Home, 180
Health Communicator's Social Media Toolkit, 227–228
health determinants
    childhood communicable diseases, protective and risk factors, 20–21
    community level assessment
        behaviors, 83
        biology, 83–87
        environment, physical, 84
        environment, social, 84–86
        policy and interventions, 86–87

definition of, 4
health determinants model, 21–22
individual/family level, 290
key component of public health nursing, 14
health disparities
children and poor health, 283
definition of, 274
ethical principles confronting, 277
Health Equity Assessment Tool (HEAT), 285
health inequities and inequalities, 282
life expectancy, 283–284
mortality rates, 284–286
reduction by downstream or upstream approach, 287–288
health equity, 275
advocacy for, 292
definition of, 274
health inequities and inequalities, 282
Health Equity Assessment Tool (HEAT), 285
health information systems (HIS), 70
Health Information Technology for Economic and Clinical Health (HITECH), 180–181
health insurance exchange, 180
Health Insurance Portability and Accountability Act (HIPAA)
confidentiality, 206
data privacy, 182–183
mandated reporting, 183
school-entry laws, 183
health literacy, definition of, 222
health status
community assessment process, 21
analysis of, 87–89
definition of, 4
health determinants model, 21–22
indicators
definition of, 68
measurable outcomes, 97
health system reform, 179–180
Healthy People program
activities emphasizing nonjudgmental acceptance of others, 315
collaborations and partnership building, 150
data on multiple topics, 121
Health Communication and Information Technology, 232
immunizations for children, 366
Interventions and Resources, 204, 232
Leading Health Indicators (LHIs), 26–27
Environmental Quality, 80
Maternal, Infant, and Child Health, 204
mission and goals, 26
2010 *versus* 2020, 96–97

national health priorities, 26
Preparedness, 182
promotion strategies, 250
Social Determinants of Health, 204, 280
HEAT (Health Equity Assessment Tool), 285
herd immunity, definition of, 112
HIPAA (Health Insurance Portability and Accountability Act)
confidentiality, 206
data privacy, 182–183
mandated reporting, 183
school-entry laws, 183
HIS (health information systems), 70
HITECH (Health Information Technology for Economic and Clinical Health), 180–181
holistic treatment
definition of, 330
ethical actions, 347
family care, 332
home care nursing
versus public health nursing, 5
safety precautions, 261–262
homeless patients, 155
HOMVEE (Home Visiting Evidence of Effectiveness), 52
hospice care nursing *versus* public health nursing, 5
hosts
definition of, 112
epidemiological triangle, 130–131
human rights
definition of, 274
government responsibilities, 275
guiding principles, 275
priorities, 279
vulnerable populations, 279–280

I

IIS (Immunization Information Systems), 180
immunization programs
ethical issues, children, 183–184
immunity, definition of, 112
local public health departments, 178
incidence/incidents, definition of, 113
independent practice
coordination with physicians, 196
definition of, 194
individual/family level of practice, 16–17
3 Es of PHNs, 69
acceptance of others, 316–317, 322
advocacy, 289–290
assessment, 74–78
basic family functions, 75

definition of, 68
environment, 77
family characteristics, 74–77
focused or problem-specific assessments, 78
for intervention strategies, 338–339
mental, physical, emotional, social, spiritual, and
environmental health, 331–332
collaboration, 145
effective communication skills, 222–224
epidemiological triangle, 130–133
health determinants model, 21–22
intervention levels, 42, 340
best practices, 97–99
effective interventions, analysis of, 46
effective interventions, examples of, 45
goals, 99–100
planning using community assets, 151
nursing process, 25
partnering with PHNs, 69, 149–150
prevention levels, 42
protective and risk factors for childhood
communicable diseases, 20–21
relationships with systems and communities, 18–19
information interpretation strategies, 226–227
Instagram, 233
insurance reform, 179
International Council of Nurses, 275
Internet
advocacy for justice, 299
CDC as source, 53
content creation tools, 234
database and information searches, 52–53
information distribution, 233–234
social networking sites, 233
avoiding problems, 235–236
interoperable electronic health records (EHRs), 180–181
interpersonal collaboration (IPC)
common barriers/strategies for overcoming, 144
definition of, 142
different perspectives and ideas, 147–148
evidence-based examples, 147
four domains of, 143
understanding, of group development and dynamics,
148
interventions, 36–41
advocacy, 40
at community and systems levels, 295
in other practice settings, 391
best practices, 97–100
caring relationships, 259
case finding, 38, 42
case management, 38
all levels of clients, 42–43

in other non-public health settings, 391
scope of, 197–198
coalition building, 40, 46
in other practice settings, 391
collaboration, 39
all levels of clients, 42–43, 391
community assets, 151
community organizing, 40, 340, 391
consultation, 39, 391
counseling, 39, 45, 391
definition of, 23, 330
delegated functions, 39
in other practice settings, 391
disease and health event investigation, 37, 390
effectiveness of, 45–46
ethical actions, 347
evidence-based practice, 45
health teaching, 39, 42–46, 198, 391
home visiting, 45
impact of, 344–346
individual/family level, 340
Johns Hopkins Nursing Evidence-Based Practice Model,
47–48
key interventions, 23–24
nonjudgmental attitude for patients' differences, 313
outreach, 38, 43
in other practice settings, 390
policy development and enforcement, 41, 391
practice levels, 42–43
primary prevention levels, 42–43, 338
Public Health Intervention Wheel, 36–41
referral and follow-up, 38, 42–43, 198
in caring relationships, 259
in other practice settings, 391
from research and non-research, 47–48
screening, 38, 42–43, 198, 343–344, 391
secondary prevention levels, 42–43, 338
social marketing, 40, 43
in other practice settings, 391
strategies for all levels of practice, 338–339
surveillance, 37, 46, 198
systems level, 340
tertiary prevention levels, 42–43, 339
intervention scheme, Omaha System, 70
interviewing
examples of, 223–224
motivational
definition of, 222
teaching-learning principles, 228–229
IPC (interpersonal collaboration)
common barriers/strategies for overcoming, 144
definition of, 142
different perspectives and ideas, 147–148

evidence-based examples, 147
four domains of, 143
understanding, of group development and dynamics, 148

Joanna Briggs Institute, 50
Johns Hopkins Nursing Evidence-Based Practice Model (JHNEBP), 47

leadership. *See also* leadership journey
advocacy-based, 358–360
    definition of, 354
    political process, 373–376
ANA standards, 364
authentic, 358
    definition of, 354
    ongoing challenges, 356
community level, 369–370
competency expectations, 363–365
definition of, 354
ethical considerations, 376–377
leadership, 354, 359
organizational culture, 368–369
responsibilities, 6
role of, 355
shared, 359
    definition of, 354
    example, 366–367
skill requirements, 360–363
leadership journey
challenges, 355
definition of, 354
entry-level
    competencies developed, 371–372
    expectations, 372–373
personal experiences, 357–358
Leading Health Indicators (LHIs), 26–27, 48
learning examples
acceptance of others, 324–326
assessment, 348–349
caring relationships, 268
collaboration
    Infection Control and Emergency Preparedness Toolkit for the Faith Community, 158
    Project Hope: A Partnership Between a City and a School of Nursing, 159
    Worksite Health Promotion, 159
communication skills, 238
government agencies, working with
    Emergency Preparedness, 185

Implementing Nutrition Policy for School Children, 185–186
Reducing Youth Access to Tobacco, 186
Updating Immunization Records, 185
leadership
    Action in Response to Suspicion of Child Abuse, 378
    Groundwater Contamination in a Rural Community, 379
    Infection Control Interventions With a Day Care, 379
    Nurses Day on the Hill, 379
professional boundaries and ethical actions, 214–215
public health nursing process, 348–349
    Combining Community Assessment and Change Projects to Make a difference, 105
    Effective Use of Epidemiologic Principles, 135–137
    Establishing a Foot Care Clinic in a Homeless Shelter, 105
    Partnering With Faith Communities, 105
    PHN Clinical in Nicaragua, 104
    Population-Focused Analysis Project (PFAP), 105
legal issues, Health Insurance Portability and Accountability Act (HIPAA)
data privacy, 182–183
mandated reporting, 183
school-entry laws, 183
LHIs (Leading Health Indicators), 26–27, 48
life course epidemiology, definition of, 113
LinkedIn, 233
listening, verbal/nonverbal, 312
local health departments. *See also* government health agencies
definition of responsibilities, 167
H1N1 flu clinic, example
    coordination with state and federal, 168
    essential services, 170–171
IT (information technology) use, 178
National Association of County and City Health Officials (NACCHO), 178
nonprofit organization contributions, 181
programs offered, 178

maintenance stage, behavior change, 225
market justice
definition of, 274
versus social justice, 286–287
medical models, definition of, 166
mental health interventions, 339–340
Millennium Development Goals (MDG), 280–281

motivational interviewing
  behavior changes, stages of, 224–225
  definition of, 222
  strategies, 225–226
mutuality, 314

NACCHO (National Association of County and City
  Health Officials), 178
NANDA (North American Nursing Diagnosis
  Association), classification system for diagnosis, 78
National Academy of Sciences, 285
National Association of School Nurses, Speaking Up for
  Children program, 293
National Institutes of Health (NIH), credible search
  sources, 52
National Prevention Strategy, 179–180
NCAST (Nursing Child Assessment Satellite Training),
  211
Netiquette, 235
Network for Public Health Law, 172
Nightingale, Florence, 114–115
NIH (National Institutes of Health), credible search
  sources, 52
NMHCs (Nurse-Managed Health Clinics), 198
nonjudgmental of patients' differences
  definition of, 308
  diversity types, 309
  ethical actions, 323–324
  implementation of, 308–310
  in interventions, 313
  promotion of diverse opinions/perspectives, 313
  respect
    caring relationships, 255, 265
    of others' points of view, 312, 313–314
nonverbal listening, 312
North American Nursing Diagnosis Association
  (NANDA), classification system for diagnosis, 78
Nurse-Managed Health Clinics (NMHCs), 198
Nurse Practice Act
  components o, 195
  core elements in all states, 195
  credentials requirement, 212
  definition of, 194
  delegation, 209–210
    accountability, 209
    authority, 209
    care provisions, 210
    responsibility, 209
  supervision, 209
Nurses Association of New Brunswick, 255

Nursing Child Assessment Satellite Training (NCAST),
  211
nursing diagnosis components, 78–79
nutrition services, 178

Omaha System, data collection and management
  components, 70
  quality improvement strategy, 101

partnerships
  building with clients, 149–150
  definition of, 142
  guidelines for effective partnerships, 150
PCAs (Personal Care Attendants), 320
PHAB (Public Health Accreditation Board), 168
PHN (public health nurses/nursing)
  best practices, 50–51
  components of, 14
  Cornerstones of Public Health Nursing, 10
  credentials required, 212
  impact if no services are available, 392–393
  personal reflections, 397
  registration, definition of, 194
  requirements
    knowledge areas, 385–386
    personal characteristics, 386–387
  students
    learning from their stories, 393–395
    transitioning to practice, 396
  threats to future of, 6
Physical Activity Guidelines, 48
physical environment, health determinants model, 22
PICOT approach to clinical problem solving, 53–54, 56
Pinterest, 233
planning in nursing process, 35
population-based practices, 7
  criteria for, 7
  definition of, 4
population(s)
  definition of, 4, 68
  served by public health, 17
pre-contemplation stage, behavior change, 224
preparation stage, behavior change, 225
prevalence, definition of, 113
prevention levels
  Affordable Care Act, 179
  definition of, 4
  key interventions, 23–24
  primary level, 23–24
    community, 43

individual/family, 42
   systems, 43
and public health nursing
   key component of, 14
   prevention continuum, 24
secondary level, 23–24
   community, 43
   individual/family, 42
   systems, 43
stages of health, 23–24
tertiary level, 23–24
   community, 43
   individual/family, 42
   systems, 43
Principles of Public Health Nursing Practice, ANA, 9
Pringle, Dorothy, 259
priority settings, definition of, 68
problem classification scheme, Omaha System, 70
problem rating scale for outcomes, Omaha System, 70
professional boundaries
   versus caring relationships, 259–261
   definition of, 194
   establishment of, 204–205
   with ethical actions, 212–215
   management of relationships, 263–264
   relationships, definition of, 250
   safety precautions, 261–262
   situations for possible violations, 205, 260
   tact and diplomacy, 239–242, 263
protective factors
   definition of, 113
   and risk factors and health issues, 118–120
   vaccinations as, 120
public health
   core functions of professional of government agencies
      assessment, 14–15
      assurance, 14–15
      policy development, 14
   definition of, 4
   versus global public health, 6
   importance to nursing, 6
   informatics, definition of, 68
   models
      definition of, 166
      versus medical models, 172–174
      childhood obesity prevention example, 174
   nuisances, 171
   nursing leadership responsibilities, 6
   Ten Essential Services of Public Health, 14–16
   threats to, 6
Public Health Accreditation Board (PHAB), 168

public health departments. *See also* government health
   agencies
   definition of, 166
   essential services
      in H1N1 flu clinic, example, 168, 170–171
      time dedicated to, 169
   Public Health Accreditation Board (PHAB), 168
Public Health Intervention Wheel. *See also* interventions
   elements of, 36–41
   interdisciplinary nature of, 98
   leadership examples, 371–372
   public health nursing
      applications in other practice settings, 390–391
      key component of, 14
      scope of, 196
public health nurses/nursing (PHN)
   best practices, 50–51
   components of, 14
   Cornerstones of Public Health Nursing, 10
   credentials required, 212
   impact if no services are available, 392–393
   personal reflections, 397
   registration, definition of, 194
   requirements
      knowledge areas, 385–386
      personal characteristics, 386–387
   students
      learning from their stories, 393–395
      transitioning to practice, 396
   threats to future of, 6
public health nursing practice
   Affordable Care Act's influence on, 179–181
   ANA principles, 9
   applications in other practice settings, 387–390
   concepts shaping, 8
   criteria for population-based, 7
   definition of, 4, 8
   versus home care nursing, 5
   scope of, 196–198
   standards, 11–14
public health nursing process, 21–22
   3 Es, 69
   definition of, 34, 68
   home visiting, 71–72
      components, 72–73
      federal mandate, EHRs, 73
      and nursing process, 72–73
   overview, 34–35
   planning and implementation process, 96–97
Public Health Nursing: Scope and Standards of Practice,
   ANA
   credentials requirement, 212
   ethical accountability, 207–209

healthcare for poor, 318
nursing process, levels of practice, 34–35
standards of performance, 175–176
standards of practice (list), 12–13
PubMed database, 52

quality improvement *versus* evidence-based practice, 51–52
quarantines, 171

racial/ethnic groups in U.S. population, 310–311
RCTs (randomized controlled trials), 48
experimental research, 50
systematic reviews of, 50
research *versus* evidence-based practice, 51–52
risk factors
definition of, 113
and diseases, 127–128
health determinants analysis, 290
obtaining/interpreting information, 121
and odds factors, 127–128
and protective factors and health issues, 118–120
rule ethics in nursing process
acceptance of others, 323
assessment activities, 103, 347
caring relationships, 267
collaboration, 156
communication skills, 236
epidemiological principles, 134
immunizations for children, 184
leadership, 377
professional accountability, 207–208
professional boundaries, 213
for social justice and advocacy, 297

safety checklists, 333–335
school inspections, 178
screening for interventions, 38, 42–43, 198, 343–344, 391
shared leadership, 359
definition of, 354
example, 366–367
Sigma Theta Tau International, *Worldviews on Evidence-Based Nursing,* 50
Smith-Campbell Caring Community Model, 257–258

social determinants of health
Commission on the Social Determinants of Health, 280
community level, 290
definition of, 4, 21, 274
interventions considering all types of health, 339–340
Millennium Development Goals (MDG), 280–281
reduction of disparities by downstream or upstream approach, 287–288
systems level, 290
targets and progress, 281
vulnerable populations, 280
social environment
health determinants model, 22
interventions considering all types of health, 339–340
social justice
civil engagement as, 293
definition of, 274
guiding principles, 275
versus market justice, 286–287
priorities, 279
vulnerable populations, 279–280
social marketing, 230–232
definition of, 222
guidelines for effectiveness, 230–232
social networking sites, 233
advocacy for justice, 299
interpersonal skills, 235–236
Netiquette, 235
spiritual health
definition of, 330
interventions considering all types of health, 339–340
SS (Syndromic Surveillance), 180
state health departments. *See also* government health agencies
definition of responsibilities, 167
H1N1 flu clinic, example
coordination with state and federal, 168
essential services, 170–171
statutory authorities
definition of, 166
implementation of laws, 171–172
Network for Public Health Law, 172
strengths-based interventions, 151
supervision, definition of, 194
surveillance in interventions, 37, 46, 113, 198, 390
Syndromic Surveillance (SS), 180
systematic reviews of RCTs, best practices, 50
systems level of practice, 17
acceptance of others, 319–320, 322

advocacy, 292
assessment
    health priorities, identifying and setting, 93–95
    for intervention strategies, 338–339
    mental, physical, emotional, social, spiritual, and
        environmental health, 331–332
    overview, 93
    population risk diagnosis, 95
collaboration, 145
definition of, 4
health determinants model, 21–22
intervention levels, 43, 340
    best practices, 97–99
    effective interventions, analysis of, 46
    examples of effective interventions, 46
    goals, 99–100
    planning using community assets, 151
nursing process, 25
partnering with PHNs, 149–150
prevention levels, 43
protective and risk factors for childhood
    communicable diseases, 20–21
relationships with individuals/families and
    communities, 18–19

TB (tuberculosis) cases
    data trends
        in graphs, 122–123
        and prevention measures, 123
    screening/treatment, 178
    WHO as data source, 125–126
teaching-learning principles and template, 228–229,
    239–242
Ten Essential Services of Public Health, 14–16
text messaging, 235
transformational leadership, 354, 359
Tumblr, 299
Twitter, 233

unconditional acceptance of others
    definition of, 308
    ethical actions, 323–324
    implementation of, 310
    interactions with respect, 252, 255, 265, 312–315
    promotion of diverse opinions/perspectives, 313
United Nations
    Millennium Development Goals (MDG), 280–281
    Universal Declaration of Human Rights, 275–276

unlicensed assistive personnel (UAP), 209
upstream approach, reduction of health disparities,
    287–288
U.S. Surgeon General, source for online research, 53

verbal/nonverbal listening, 312
virtue ethics in nursing process
    acceptance of others, 324
    assessment activities, 103, 347
    caring relationships, 267
    collaboration, 156
    communication skills, 237
    epidemiological principles, 134
    immunizations for children, 184
    leadership, 377
    professional accountability, 207–208
    professional boundaries, 213
    for social justice and advocacy, 298
vital signs of population health status, 81

Wald, Lillian, 114–116, 251
WHO (World Health Organization)
    Commission on the Social Determinants of Health,
        280
    data sources, 125–126
    public health, definition of, 5
    vulnerable populations, 280
WIC (Women, Infants, and Children) services, 178, 201
windshield surveys, 89–90
Women, Infants, and Children (WIC) services, 178, 201
World Health Association, 6
World Health Organization (WHO)
    Commission on the Social Determinants of Health,
        280
    data sources, 125–126
    public health, definition of, 5
    vulnerable populations, 280
Worldviews on Evidence-Based Nursing, 50

YouTube, 233